The Diet Detective's
COUNT DOWN

7,500 of Your Favorite Food Counts with
Their Exercise Equivalents for Walking, Running,
Biking, Swimming, Yoga, and Dance

Charles Stuart Platkin

A FIRESIDE BOOK
Published by Simon & Schuster
New York   London   Toronto   Sydney

FIRESIDE
Rockefeller Center
1230 Avenue of the Americas
New York, NY 10020

FIRESIDE and colophon are registered trademarks
of Simon & Schuster, Inc.

For information regarding special discounts for bulk purchases,
please contact Simon & Schuster Special Sales at 1-800-456-6798 or
business@simonandschuster.com.

Manufactured in the United States of America

10   9   8   7   6   5   4   3   2   1

Library of Congress Cataloging-in-Publication Data

ISBN-13: 978-0-7432-9800-1
ISBN-10:   0-7432-9800-4

This book is dedicated to my daughter,
Parker South, a constant inspiration; to my parents,
Linda and Norton, who have always been and continue to
be a driving force in my life; and to my wife, a patient,
considerate, and caring friend, Shannon.

Contents

Introduction: What Are Exercise Equivalents?

Have you ever found yourself debating whether or not to buy "just one" bag of chips? Or grab a little candy bar for the road? Consider this: what if the nutritional labels on your favorite foods spelled out exactly the amount of activity you would have to engage in to burn those calories? It might change your shopping and snacking habits.

We all know we're supposed to reduce our calorie intake and increase our physical activity to lose weight—so why is it that, as a country, we're still getting fatter? Maybe it's because we have no idea what a calorie really represents. Despite the ubiquitous promotion of weight-loss campaigns and diets, the concept of a calorie remains somewhat nebulous. What if the Food and Drug Administration required restaurants and food manufacturers to put an "exercise equivalent" on menus and food labels? Instead of calories, the labels would tell us how long we'd have to exercise to burn off what we were about to eat.

Just think about the implications. Knowing that we have to walk for fourteen hours, roughly forty-three miles, in order to burn off one pound of fat would certainly increase the likelihood of our skipping dessert. After all, it's much easier to imagine passing up a day of overeating ice cream, chips, and fried chicken than it is to see oneself walking forty-three miles.

That's why I decided to write this book. The idea is to learn the costs of what you're eating. My goal is not to sit here and tell you which foods you should or shouldn't be eating. Of course some carbohydrates (such as whole grains, fruits, and vegetables) and some fats (such as unsaturated as opposed to saturated) are better than others. And yes, eating protein can help you control cravings and keep you feeling full. But in the end, long-term weight control is about energy regulation or how many calories you consume as opposed to how many you burn.

Sometimes I'm asked what my diet philosophy is—low carb, low fat, diet or no diet, glycemic index, or calorie counting. The answer is that my philosophy doesn't matter much, because it's really about what works for each individual behaviorally. What are *you* willing to do for the rest of your life? This book can help you make better choices. So whether you're on a low- or a high-carb diet, this book can help you recognize the better calorie deals—or Calorie Bargains. It will also help you see those that are worse—or Calorie Rip-Offs. But again, these are a matter of individual preference. You might look at a big, fat, juicy steak and say, "Wow, this is really worth the ten hours of walking it will take to burn it off," while someone else might say, "Forget it. The chicken breast will fill me up just as well."

Read on and use this book as a fun and entertaining reference that can make you much more aware of the costs and benefits of the foods you eat. And the next time you're faced with a box of Double Stuf Oreos, you'll have a real-life, quantifiable basis for deciding whether or not to stuff one more cookie down your throat. You may think that this kind of information will "ruin" the pleasure you take in eating, but it's quite the contrary. Although knowing the "true value" of your food choices may be uncomfortable at first, choosing your personal Calorie Bargains will actually change the way you feel about food and make what you do eat more, not less, enjoyable.

Think of it this way: what if you went to a foreign country and walked into a furniture store. You love what you see, but everything is priced in a foreign currency—"dowleys." The price tag on the couch you adore reads 5 million dowleys—what does that mean? What is the price of the couch? You really don't have any idea, do you? It could be $500, or could be $5,000,

Even Lettuce Has Calories to Burn

Knowing the exercise equivalents of lettuce and the 7,500 other foods in this book serves a dual purpose. First, it gives you a chance to see that eating any food provides energy—energy to help you live. For instance, knowing that one apple provides enough energy to keep walking for about nineteen minutes—well, that tells you something. Secondly, including many different foods, both high- and low-calorie options, helps you make choices. If you see that it takes three hours to walk off an ice cream cone and only thirty minutes for a piece of fruit, don't you think that would influence your decision? Is the ice cream worth that much more? Maybe to you it is, but at the very least you're making an informed decision, which will lead you to make better decisions in the long run.

or even $15,000. Now you might be able to guess that based on the quality it is within a certain range, but that would be a pretty wide range. If you found out the couch was only $500, you'd be excited and you'd definitely buy it. But if, on the other hand, it was $15,000 and out of your budget, you would probably pass it up because it just wasn't affordable.

To a certain degree, that's what it's like when you're trying to understand what a calorie means. And once you can relate to a calorie on your own terms, you'll acquire a certain level

Don't Worry: You Don't Have to Swim for Fifteen Hours to Burn Off What You Ate Today

Remember, you don't start out with zero calories; you get a daily allowance of calories to use at your discretion based on your metabolic rate and *your current level of activity*. Find out how many calories you use each day by turning to page 60. Once you know how many calories you burn through your normal daily activities, you can then look at the exercise equivalents for those extra foods to help you make better choices.

of clarity about your own eating and activity habits. That's not to say that all of a sudden you're going to magically lose weight, but you will develop a certain level of consciousness and intuitiveness that will help you control your weight.

The COUNT DOWN method is effective because the information is simple and accessible. You can start by looking for a few specific foods, and I guarantee that you will immediately want to know more. Just how much yoga does it take to burn fifteen potato chips (about an ounce)? And how long do you need to swim if you drink a can of Coke? The statistics are not only tools that will help you to improve your health; they're also fun, surprising, and interesting in their presentation.

COUNT DOWN provides the fast, accessible, simple information that I know you're hungry for. It cuts through the jargon of rigid diet prescriptions and pedantic health instructions and lets you see for yourself just how much damage nibbling and snacking can do when you choose calorie-packed foods. It will also alert you to the benefits of activity. You will quickly be able to see the differences in energy needed to do yoga versus walking or running. And it vividly illustrates the fact that you need calories to keep moving.

How COUNT DOWN Works

The *last thing* I want you to do is sit there and start counting every calorie you've eaten for the day and then calculate how many hours of walking, biking, running, or swimming you would have to do to burn them off. Wow!

Using COUNT DOWN

1. Figure out your daily calorie needs.

2. Hunt for Calorie Bargains.

3. Take the three-day food challenge.

4. Stay on the lookout for Calorie Bargains and Calorie Rip-Offs by comparing the amount of exercise necessary to burn the foods you currently eat with others you might substitute.

5. Think before you eat by using the Exercise Equivalents, and keep COUNT DOWN handy so you can check to see the "splurgeworthyness" of the food you're about to eat.

That would be a huge mistake, because I'll show you how to figure out your basic calorie budget—the number of calories you can eat each day without gaining weight. The problem begins when you go over your budget and begin to stockpile energy, which then turns into fat.

Once you've calculated your daily calorie budget, I will teach you how to use exercise equivalents to help you lose weight—forever. How can I make such a claim? The idea behind COUNT DOWN is to first get you thinking about what you are eating, because being a conscious eater is half the battle. Then, once you become more aware of the costs and benefits of eating, you will learn about making substitutions—the right ones. You will notice that things start to click—you will have an "aha" moment when you realize, finally, what weight control is all about. But don't be too hard on yourself for not getting it sooner. More than likely, you were never really taught the value of a calorie in the first place.

Calorie Overview

Calories have been getting a bad rap. When you hear the word, it conjures up images of eating cakes, candies, and other sin foods. COUNT DOWN can help you appreciate calories rather than seeing them as something evil that ends up ruining your day. A calorie should be viewed as energy that keeps you going. The only problem is that if you eat more of them than you need to keep going, you end up stockpiling them, and that's what turns into fat.

Okay, what exactly *is* a calorie? It's a measure of energy, the capacity to do work. Science defines a calorie as the amount of energy required to raise the temperature of 1 gram of water by 1 degree Celsius. But in our everyday struggle to eat well and exercise, it is easy to forget that the simple functional purpose of calories is to fuel our body's day-to-day activities.

Calories at Rest: If you want to start keeping track of your calories in order to lose weight, the first thing you need to know is how many calories you should eat each day. Sounds simple, right? Well, maybe not.

There are a variety of methods for estimating caloric needs, including a complex equation called Harris-Benedict, considered the "gold standard," which takes into account your height, weight, gender, and age and determines your basal metabolic rate (BMR, sometimes referred to as resting metabolic rate). Your BMR is the number of calories you need to support the ongoing, unconscious work of your body (your heart beating, breathing, body temperature). It accounts for the largest component of your daily energy needs, usually around 60 to 70 percent. But two people of the same height, weight, gender, and age can have very different BMRs. "In fact, one of the biggest determinants of BMR is body composition, specifically the ratio of muscle to fat," says Linda Bandini, Ph.D., R.D., a professor of nutrition at Boston University. Basically the more muscle you have, the more calories you'll burn during your resting state.

Once you've determined your BMR, you probably think all you have to do to lose weight is cut down on the number of calories you consume. But that's not the whole story. Knowing your metabolic rate basically tells you how many calories you need to operate your body if you do nothing—that's all. If you simply cut calories from your BMR, you will lose weight, but the wrong kind of weight—mostly lean muscle tissue.

BMR Calculations Are Not 100 Percent Accurate

The BMR you calculate should be used as a guideline, sort of a starting point. That's why it's acceptable that these measurements are not 100 percent accurate. Ideally, you should also weigh yourself at least every thirty days, because the scale doesn't lie. Then adjust your eating accordingly. If you see you're gaining weight, you may need to cut calories; if you are losing weight too rapidly, you may need to bump up your calories.

What About Activity? Your resting metabolic rate is only a part of the equation for determining your caloric needs. After you figure that out, you need to factor in your activity level—and this is where the problems begin. To determine how many calories you're burning from activity, you would typically choose from a predetermined scale ranging from "sedentary" (you sit, drive, lie down, or stand in one place for most of the day and don't do any type of exercise), which would mean tacking on about 20 percent more calories to your BMR, all the way to "extreme activity" (heavy manual labor, army and marine recruit training, or competitive athletes), which would allow you to eat more than double the calories required simply to maintain your body weight.

Trying to estimate someone's activity level is no easy task, and standards can easily be misapplied. What is moderate activity for an elite athlete is quite different from what's moderate for the average Joe. For instance, according to the guidelines, a competitive athlete might burn 2,400 calories per day at rest. Double that, according to the guidelines, and the same person's caloric needs should be 4,800 per day. But someone training for the Tour de France, for example, might actually burn 10,000 calories per day—so the formula can be significantly inaccurate.

There are many Web sites (e.g., kidsnutrition.org/caloriesneed.htm) that let you plug in personal information and give you a relatively accurate BMR. Or you can use a simple formula such as figuring 10 to 11 calories per pound of body weight for your basal metabolic rate and factoring in the proper percentage for your physical activity level.

However, the following (Harris-Benedict equation) is the most widely accepted method of determining your calorie needs:

Step 1: Calculate your resting or basal metabolic rate (BMR)

Female: $655.1 + (4.35 \times \text{weight in pounds}) + (4.699 \times \text{height in inches}) - (4.676 \times \text{age})$

Male: $66.5 + (6.25 \times \text{weight in pounds}) + (12.71 \times \text{height in inches}) - (6.775 \times \text{age})$

Step 2: Calculate Your Caloric Needs

Now that you've determined your BMR, multiply it by your activity factor:

- Sedentary: 1.2 (You sit, drive, lie down, or stand in one place for most of the day and don't do any type of exercise.)
- Light activity: 1.3 to 1.4 (You're sedentary for most of the day and do light activity, such as walking, for no more than two hours daily.)
- Moderate activity: 1.5 (You're on your feet most of the workday, with light lifting only, and do no structured exercise.)
- Very active: 1.6 to 1.7 (Your typical workday includes several hours of physical labor, such as light industry and construction-type jobs.)
- Extreme activity: 2 to 2.4 (You do heavy manual labor, do army and marine recruit training, or are a competitive athlete.)

Your BMR multiplied by your activity factor is your total daily calorie allowance for weight maintenance.

To lose weight, you will need to increase your level of activity and/or decrease your caloric intake until you are burning more calories than you consume.

Bargain Hunting

With prices on the rise and the health of the economy questionable, bargain hunting is back in vogue. We look for bargains in clothing, electronics, food, and travel—just to name a few. We go to discount price clubs and wait until things go on sale so that we can get more for less. We want to spend wisely so we know we're getting the most for our money.

What if we were as cost-conscious about our calorie consumption as we are about our spending?

Unfortunately, we have a finite number of calories in our bodies' budgets, just as we have limited funds in our pocketbooks. So how can we be sure we're making good use of the calories we consume? The answer: look for Calorie Bargains. Calorie Bargains are foods that are relatively low in calories but still taste great and satisfy your strongest temptations. You use these "cheaper" foods to replace others you eat regularly that are more calorically "expensive." But remember, if it doesn't satiate you, a Calorie Bargain can easily turn into a Calorie Rip-Off, which means you'll end up eating more food, consuming more calories, and gaining more weight.

Here's one of mine. I used to eat chips, cookies, and ice cream, averaging about 600 calories in an evening. Now I substitute pan popcorn. I don't love air-popped corn, so I started experimenting and found a way to use regular kernels, a skillet, and cooking spray. Put the kernels in a deep pot lightly coated with vegetable cooking spray, cover, and turn on the heat. Make sure to open the lid slightly from time to time to release the steam. Shake the pot during cooking. After a number of burned batches I was finally able to get it right: 5 cups (popped) equals 150 calories. Calorie savings: About 450.

Having Trouble Finding Your Calorie Bargains? Take the Three-Day Food Challenge

If you've never kept a food diary and you want to see what works best for you, try our Three-Day Food Challenge. It's a real challenge to take a good, hard look at what you eat for three straight days, but if you're honest and diligent about it, you can learn a lot about your eating habits in this short period of time and discover clues that will help you develop a diet plan.

Celebrity Calorie Bargains

I've spent years finding Calorie Bargains for myself and getting tips on others from readers, so I began to wonder what health "celebrities" do to create the Calorie Bargains that help them stay fit. Here are a few notables:

Mike Huckabee, governor of the state of Arkansas, who lost more than one hundred pounds and made healthy living a priority for his administration. Used to eat: Premium ice cream: 2 cups, 550 calories.

Calorie Bargain: Yarnell's "Carb Aware" guilt-free ice cream made with Splenda. "You can't tell the difference between this and regular premium ice cream, which it has replaced in my diet. Yarnell's is amazingly good, and it's what we serve at the governor's mansion. Guests are shocked to find out it's a sugar-free, low-fat, low-carb product." Breakdown: 2 cups, 250 calories.

Calorie savings: 300.

Bobby Flay, chef/restaurateur, cookbook author, and television personality. Used to eat: "When I was younger, I loved eating breakfast sandwiches consisting of fried eggs, bacon, and cheese every morning on my way to work." Breakdown: 440 calories.

Calorie Bargain: "Now I prepare healthy smoothies for breakfast or yogurt with fresh fruit." Breakdown: 16-ounce low-calorie smoothie (no sugar), about 150 calories; low-fat yogurt with fruit, 220 calories.

Calorie savings: About 250.

Denise Austin, fitness expert, author, fitness DVD personality (star of more than forty exercise videos and DVDs). Used to eat: Baked potato (100 calories) with 2 tablespoons of sour cream (about 120 calories) and 1 tablespoon butter (60 calories) for a total of 280 calories. Frappuccino and whipped cream at Starbucks, 390 calories.

Calorie Bargain: "I've replaced the sour cream and butter with 2 tablespoons of salsa for 30 calories. And you can make your own coffee treat with a lot less calories. Use ice cubes, ½ cup skim milk (about 50 calories), and ½ cup decaf coffee. Froth it up and blend it."

Calorie savings: 150 for the potato extras; 340 for the coffee drink.

Step 1: Keep a Food Diary

- Keep it real: Record everything that goes into your mouth, including beverages, bites off someone else's plate, or samples at the grocery store.

The Advantages of Keeping a Three-Day Food Diary

- It creates a tangible, in-your-face record of your everyday eating habits.
- You'll be able to see what you're eating at all times, which can help you realize what you shouldn't be eating.
- You can pinpoint "unconscious eating times" as well as times of day when you overeat most of your calories.

- Portion distortion: Learn to be honest about portion size. As a general rule, assume you're eating 30 to 40 percent more than you think.
- No excuses: Use this guide to track your food! Keep blank journals in your office, car, purse, and/or briefcase!

Step 2: Evaluate Your Food Diary

At the end of three days, your diary should provide you with a clear picture of what, how, when, and why you eat what you eat. Here's what you should look for:

- Triggers: A trigger is anything—a mood, an event, even a certain food—that makes it difficult for you to stick to your goal of losing weight. Look for patterns of emotions, foods, or times of day that contribute to excess calorie consumption.

- Meal patterns: Skipping meals or waiting too long to eat can lead to overeating later in the day. If your meals are more than four hours apart, try scheduling a snack in between.

- Unconscious eating: It's easy to consume massive amounts of high-calorie and high-fat foods while sitting in front of the TV or at the computer. Keeping a food diary helps you keep this unconscious eating in check.

- Failure to plan: If high-calorie and high-fat fast foods or vending-machine snacks appear frequently on your food diary, it may be a sign of poor planning. A food diary allows you to see your weak spots and plan for them.

- Unbalanced meals: Are some of your meals heavy on the carbs? Or maybe a protein overdose? Not choosing balanced meals can lead to excessive hunger, which in turn can result in overeating.

- Fruits and veggies: These are your weight-loss allies. Your ultimate goal is to eat at least five servings a day. If you're not having any now, work your way up slowly.

Create Your Own Food Diary

Here's a rundown of exactly what you should be recording:

Meal, Time, and Place

Record the approximate time you sit down to eat. This will help you find the eating schedule that works best for you. Also, record which meal it was (e.g., breakfast, midmorning, etc.) and where you ate it—whether is it on the run, sitting at your desk, at a restaurant, etc.

Hunger Level

Record your level of hunger on a scale of 1 to 5, 1 being the least hungry and 5 being the most hungry. Aim to be between 3 and 4 when you're eating. You never want to let yourself get too hungry, and you certainly don't want to eat when you're not hungry at all.

Dining Companions

Write down who you ate with and what you talked about. This information could offer clues to unconscious eating or stress eating.

Feelings and Mood

Record how you feel before, during, and after you eat. Before is probably the most important because it can have the greatest effect on how and what you eat. Try to keep track of whether you have general feelings, such as being happy or sad, or specific ones, such as "stressed at work," "angry at spouse," or "having a great day." You will see that this really helps you pinpoint which emotions affect your eating habits the most.

Food and Drink

Record all the individual foods you eat and beverages you drink, including accurate portion sizes and even brand names (food nutrients vary by brand). Anything that goes in your mouth should be in your food diary—including drinks, little nibbles from the refrigerator, and bites from other people's plates!

Nutrient Information and Exercise Equivalents

Use the information in COUNT DOWN to record the calories (and/or carbs), and the Exercise Equivalents for each food/meal you eat. Total your calories at the end of the day to make sure you are staying within your goal. You can do this at home while relaxing.

At the end of three days, your diary should provide you with a clear picture of what, how, when, and why you eat what you eat.

Step 3: Review Your Diary

Your diary will show you which foods you eat most often—which is where COUNT DOWN comes in. Look for other foods that are lower in calories to use as substitutes or replacements—these are your Calorie Bargains. For example, if you typically use Breakstone's All Natural Salted Butter (3 tablespoons, 300 calories), switching to I Can't Believe It's Not Butter! Fat Free (3 tablespoons, 15 calories) would save you 285 calories.

Increase Your Physical Activity

Another benefit of COUNT DOWN is that it will help you understand how and why increasing your activity level matters when it comes to long-term weight control.

This may seem obvious, but it's an important concept considering that the scientific journal *Health Education & Behavior* has found that even though people might not identify themselves as "exercisers," they claim to get enough physical activity just from "caregiving, housekeeping, and workday activities." The problem is that you need to *increase* these activities if they are to have an effect on your weight.

Staying Motivated

Okay, so you now have a bit of incentive to increase your activity. The question is, how do you stay motivated and excited?

Calorie Burning Per Minute of Exercise

	Easy	*Moderate*	*Brisk/Fast*
Walking	4 cal/min	4.5 cal/min	5 cal/min
Biking	7 cal/min	11 cal/min	13.5 cal/min
Running	9 cal/min	13 cal/min	15 cal/min

If you're already doing these things, that's wonderful, but remember, they don't count as an increase in physical activity. You have to *add new activities* to increase your caloric expenditure.

Most experts say the key is to make exercise "intrinsic"—or internally motivating. To really stay active, you need to be doing something because you value the actual experience—you appreciate the activity for what it is, not just what it's doing for you. Here are a few tips to increase the pleasure you get from the experience and keep you motivated.

Enjoy It: Focus on the feelings of competence and social interaction you get from the experience. A study in the *International Journal of Sport Psychology* showed that a group who participated in aerobic exercise to improve their physical appearance didn't stick with it nearly as long as a group who did martial arts because they enjoyed it. And a study in *Health Education Research* reported that the activity you decide to increase should be chosen carefully, with an emphasis on moderation in intensity and integration into your lifestyle—don't just start to increase your physical activity doing something you don't like. So if you can't find something that you love right away, at the very least find something you don't hate. It's important to find as many redeeming qualities as possible for any of the exercises that you choose.

Experiment and Match: Try a variety of activities. If you don't like to walk, how about biking, dancing, hiking, or golfing? To spice things up, try listening to music or watching TV while you're working out. There is an exercise for everyone; you just have to find the one that you love.

Go Slow: People who tell me they want to start exercising often have grandiose ideas of getting up every morning, going to the gym, and then running five miles. If you've never been physically active before, it's best to start slowly— even two or three times a week is better than nothing. In the initial stages, you really need to cut yourself a bit of slack, meaning that if you miss a day or two, you don't have to give up completely. As you can tell by looking at the exercise equivalents in this book, you don't need to push so hard; it's more important just to do something.

Excuses, Excuses, Excuses: We have many great excuses why we *can't* increase our physical activity levels, ranging from time constraints to lack of money to lack of energy to no place to "do it" to bad weather to physical discomfort. Do you have excuses? Brainstorm and write down all the reasons you can think of for *not* working toward your fitness goals. Remember to include your self-doubts, fears, and insecurities—these are excuses too! Be honest.

Next, punch holes in your excuses until they are no longer airtight. Do this by coming up with counterarguments for every single excuse you may have for not exercising—this is called Excuse Busting.

Make It Social: There is a plethora of research demonstrating that working out with a group on a regular basis increases your likelihood of sticking with your routine. One study found that married couples who worked out together had a significantly higher attendance and a lower dropout rate than married people who worked out alone. Find a regular fitness class you know you'll enjoy. Organize a group of friends, coworkers, or neighbors to participate in some regular fitness activity. Get yourself a workout buddy. Not only will you increase your fitness level and improve your appearance, but you'll also reduce stress and increase the effectiveness of your immune system (social groups do that). And you will probably have a good time as well!

Have a Plan and Set Goals: Don't just decide that "starting next week" you're going to walk every day—especially if you don't like walking. Investigate your options, write them down, and make the decision as if it's something that's important to you. Come up with a plan for exercise that will keep you excited for longer than twenty-four hours. Keep in mind that one of the most important things is to remain flexible about everything—including your exercise, your time, and yourself.

Visualize Your Future: Being able to see yourself in a positive situation in the future will keep you focused on your exercise path. Create a "Life Preserver"—that is, an imagined future event in which you have achieved your fitness goal. For example, think of how excited you'll be when you've completed your first two-hour hike or finished a scenic bike tour.

After the Fat

With all the talk about getting extra weight off your body, there's a lot less being said about how to *keep it off*—an elusive concept that is still poorly understood by the average dieter. Yet if you really think about it, weight maintenance is significantly more important and more difficult than losing weight. I can hear all of you saying, "That's ridiculous. In order to keep weight off, you have to lose it first." That is certainly true, but think about how many times you've actually lost weight. Five, ten, maybe twenty times?

It's ironic that we focus on weight loss when the real challenge is keeping weight off. Most popular diets work when it comes to losing weight, but few if any succeed when it comes to weight maintenance.

Why don't we pay more attention to the most important aspect of weight control? Probably because weight maintenance is just not as sexy. No downward movement of the scales, no dramatic before-and-after experiences; it's a routine and, as a result, it can be boring.

Weight Loss versus Weight Maintenance: They're different processes. There are many ways to lose weight but not many ways to keep it off. In fact, the truth is that almost anyone can lose weight in the short run using almost any method. However, when it comes to weight maintenance, fewer strategies work. The reason is that most of us use temporary, prescriptive, and restrictive programs to lose the weight, which don't teach methods of incorporating and adjusting your unique dieting pattern. So when it's time to switch from weight loss to weight maintenance, we're typically tired of the "diet" and want to go back to a "normal" life.

You Can Do It: One of the most popular myths about losing weight is that everyone who loses will eventually gain it back. However, the concept that no more than 2 percent of dieters can actually maintain their weight loss is based on only one or two studies that are now decades old.

So what do you do after the fat is gone? You need to learn the techniques that other successful weight-loss maintainers follow and develop strategies that will last a lifetime.

Keep Your Pants On: The National Weight Control Registry has determined that almost all successful weight-loss maintainers have some kind of "five-pound warning system"—a way of measuring and/or monitoring their weight before it gets out of control. It could be something as simple as keeping a "thin" pair of pants or a skirt they try on periodically instead of getting on the scale, but they all have some way of knowing when they are slipping and have a backup plan ready to put into action as soon as they receive their warning.

Walk: It seems that walking is an important key to long-term weight maintenance. The theory is that as you lose weight you need something

Where to Walk

Look for parks, paths, and trails in your area. Even your neighborhood sidewalks can be perfect, and on rainy or cold days, consider your local mall to be your indoor track. The level flooring (fewer injuries) and climate control are excellent motivators. Also, make arrangements to walk with friends, family, or coworkers—socializing helps get you there and keeps you busy with gossip, so you actually have fun.

to compensate for the lower metabolism—that's right, you burn fewer calories as you lose weight. Physical activity keeps your calorie-burning capacity high. Walking is easy to do and easy to maintain no matter where you are or what you're doing. In fact, according to the National Weight Control Registry, 77 percent of successful losers use walking as their primary means of physical activity. How long do weight maintainers engage in physical activity each day?

At least an hour more than they did before they lost the weight. Notice I used the phrase physical activity, not "exercise," because it's not about exercise. The goal is to increase your physical activity each day, and it doesn't even have to be all at once. For instance, you might take a twenty-to-thirty minute walk in the morning, increase your walking during the day (by parking a bit further than necessary, taking the stairs, or making other similar adjustments), and dedicate ten to fifteen minutes when you first get home to cleaning the house, doing yoga, going for a bike ride, walking the dog, or doing anything else that will keep your body moving—and consequently burning calories. As long as these little activities are additional—that is, an increase from the amount of activity you used to get—they will help you get and stay in shape.

Make It Automatic: Successful maintainers have figured out ways to make their behaviors and choices second nature. It's based on the concept of automaticity—the subconscious ways we perform daily behaviors. Activities like setting your alarm clock at night, putting on your shoes before leaving the house, and remembering how to drive to work do not require much thought. The idea is to apply the same principle to your diet. Arrange your personal environment to maximize your chances of losing and maintaining your weight loss and minimize your chances of slipping up. Avoid cues that tempt you. If you drive by Dunkin' Donuts on the way to work and can't resist stopping for a box of doughnuts, change your route. Don't leave foods in the house that are going to "set you off"—or at least put them out of reach.

No Days Off Necessary: There is no calorie vacation on this plan, no days off for you to just "let yourself go." Save that for when you're "on a diet." According to research at Brown University Medical School, a major predictor of successful weight maintenance is dietary consistency. This means that those who maintain the same diet regimen across the week and year are more likely to maintain their weight loss over the following year than those who diet more strictly on weekdays and/or during nonholiday periods.

This is not about dieting—it's about making changes that will last, making better food decisions, and finding Calorie Bargains that you can actually see yourself eating for the rest of your life. That's how you need to think about your food choices to start out, then periodically you should reevaluate those choices to make sure they're still working for you. So focus on making the adjustments that will keep you happy—and make sure you don't feel like you're making huge sacrifices; if you do, chances are they won't last long.

The "Fast-Metabolism-I-Can-Eat-Whatever-I-Want" Club: Does this sound familiar? After losing those pounds you suddenly feel that, magically, your body has changed, making you a charter member of the exclusive "fast-metabolism-I-can-eat-whatever-I want" club. For the first few weeks in your new, fit body, you are confident that the weight is off for good. You indulge, and the diet you had been on is now ancient history because all along you knew you could never live on that diet for the rest of your life. Weight control is a forever process, so you need to create practices you can live with forever.

Be Diet Savvy—Watch Out for Diet Traps

Unconscious Eating: Eating without paying attention.

Zap this trap: No matter what else you're doing, always stop to think about what you're about to eat and whether you really want it—or whether it's just a big waste. If snacking makes the experience sweeter or the studying easier, you don't have to give it up—just go for the option that's healthiest and lowest in calories: baby carrots, grape tomatoes, an orange, an apple, a small bowl filled with a measured amount of pretzels or chips. (Put the rest of the bag back in the kitchen!) If you decide ahead of time to eat only a healthy amount, you'll be able to enjoy every bite, knowing you're treating yourself—and your body—right.

Eating Alarm Times: Specific times of day you're most likely to overeat.

Zap this trap: Since you know you're going to be tempted to overeat at certain times, have Calorie Bargain snacks at the ready. And be careful—carrots and celery might not always cut it as a replacement for ice cream, doughnuts, or Doritos. So if you normally eat chips while sitting in front of prime-time TV, make sure to come up with a variety of alternatives that'll keep you satisfied, even on your most "splurgeworthy" days.

Diet Busters: Foods or events that can throw a wrench in your diet routine.

Zap this trap: The key here is preparation. Identify your top Diet-Buster moments—those circumstances, situations, or events that are, and probably always have been, most difficult for you. Once you know what they are, you'll be able to figure out how to control them. Decide beforehand what you're going to eat and how much you're going to have—that way you won't be caught off guard.

A Final Word About Using COUNT DOWN

Again, COUNT DOWN is meant to be a guide you can keep in your desk at work, in your briefcase or purse, or in the kitchen—anywhere you'll have easy and quick access to it when you're around food and making food decisions. It's divided into categories to make it easier to find the foods you're looking for. Browse through the Deli Section if you're looking for Calorie Bargain meats, or check out the Dessert Section to see which kind of ice cream will have you swimming the fewest laps. Or if you absolutely *must* have those chocolate chip cookies, well, at least take a look at how long you'll need to be sitting in that yoga pose after you eat them.

Whatever diet you're on, whether it's Weight Watchers, Jenny Craig, Atkins, South Beach, or another weight-loss eating plan, COUNT DOWN can help you realize your weight-loss goals. This book is designed to help you develop a new way of thinking about food.

The Diet Detective's

COUNT DOWN

*All exercise equivalents
are in minutes.

Dairy (Including Eggs)

FOOD	AMOUNT	CAL	CARBS	FAT	WALK	RUN	BIKE	SWIM	YOGA	DANCE
Butter										
Salted butter	1 tbsp	102	0	12	26	11	14	12	35	17
Whipped butter with salt	1 tbsp	67	0	8	17	7	10	8	23	11
Breakstone's Lightly Salted Butter	1 tbsp	100	0	11	26	11	14	12	34	17
Breakstone's Whipped Butter	1 tbsp	70	0	7	18	7	10	9	24	12
Land O' Lakes Butter	1 tbsp	100	0	11	26	11	14	12	34	17
Land O' Lakes Whipped Butter	1 tbsp	50	0	6	13	5	7	6	17	9
Margarine										
Margarine (stick)	1 tsp	33	0	4	9	4	5	4	11	6
Margarine (iquid)	1 tsp	34	0	4	9	4	5	4	12	6
Blue Bonnet Margarine (stick)	1 tbsp	100	0	11	26	11	14	12	34	17
Fleischmann's Light Margarine	1 tbsp	50	0	6	13	5	7	6	17	9
Fleischmann's Margarine (stick)	1 tbsp	100	0	11	26	11	14	12	34	17
Fleischmann's Soft Margarine	1 tbsp	100	0	11	26	11	14	12	34	17
I Can't Believe It's Not Butter! (soft)	1 tbsp	80	0	9	21	9	11	10	27	14
I Can't Believe It's Not Butter! (stick)	1 tbsp	90	0	10	23	10	13	11	31	15
I Can't Believe It's Not Butter! Fat Free	1 tbsp	5	0	0	1	1	1	1	2	1
I Can't Believe It's Not Butter! Light (soft)	1 tbsp	50	0	5	13	5	7	6	17	9
I Can't Believe It's Not Butter! Light (stick)	1 tbsp	50	0	6	13	5	7	6	17	9
I Can't Believe It's Not Butter! Spray	1.25 sprays	0	0	0	0	0	0	0	0	0
I Can't Believe It's Not Butter! Squeeze	1 tbsp	60	0	7	15	6	9	7	20	10
Land O' Lakes Margarine (stick)	1 tbsp	100	0	11	26	11	14	12	34	17
Land O' Lakes Soft Margarine	1 tbsp	100	0	11	26	11	14	12	34	17
Mazola Margarine	1 tbsp	100	0	11	26	11	14	12	34	17
Move Over Butter	1 tbsp	90	0	10	23	10	13	11	31	15

FOOD	AMOUNT	CAL	CARBS	FAT	WALK	RUN	BIKE	SWIM	YOGA	DANCE
Parkay Margarine	1 tbsp	100	0	11	26	11	14	12	34	17
Parkay Soft Margarine	1 tbsp	100	0	11	26	11	14	12	34	17
Parkay Squeezable Margarine	1 tbsp	90	0	10	23	10	13	11	31	15
Promise Buttery Spread	1 tbsp	80	0	8	21	9	11	10	27	14
Promise Light Buttery Spread	1 tbsp	45	0	5	12	5	6	5	15	8
Smart Balance Buttery Spread	1 tbsp	80	0	9	21	9	11	10	27	14
Smart Balance Light Buttery Spread	1 tbsp	45	0	5	12	5	6	5	15	8
Smart Balance Omega Plus Buttery Spread	1 tbsp	80	0	9	21	9	11	10	27	14
Smart Beat Smart Squeeze	1 tbsp	7	1	0	2	1	1	1	2	1
Smart Beat Super Light (no saturated fat)	1 tbsp	22	0	2	6	2	3	3	8	4
Weight Watchers Light Margarine	1 tbsp	45	2	4	12	5	6	5	15	8
Weight Watchers Margarine (stick)	1 tbsp	60	0	7	15	6	9	7	20	10
Weight Watchers Tub Margarine	1 tbsp	50	0	6	13	5	7	6	17	9
Cheese										
■ American										
American cheese	1 oz	106	0	9	27	11	15	13	36	18
American cheese food	1 oz	93	2	7	24	10	13	11	32	16
American cheese spread	1 oz	82	2	6	21	9	12	10	28	14
Fat-free American cheese	1 slice (.75 oz)	31	3	0	8	3	4	4	11	5
Boar's Head American	1 oz	100	1	9	26	11	14	12	34	17
Borden American	1 oz	110	1	9	28	12	16	13	37	19
Borden Light American	1 oz	70	1	4	18	7	10	9	24	12
Borden Nonfat American	1 oz	40	4	0	10	4	6	5	14	7
Healthy Choice Low Fat American	1 slice	40	2	1	10	4	6	5	14	7
Kraft Fat-Free Singles, American	1 slice	31	2	0	8	3	4	4	11	5
Kraft Singles, American	1.2 oz	110	3	8	28	12	16	13	37	19
Kraft Reduced Fat Singles, American	.75 oz	50	2	3	13	5	7	6	17	9
Smart Beat Nonfat American	1 slice	25	3	0	6	3	4	3	9	4

FOOD	AMOUNT	CAL	CARBS	FAT	WALK	RUN	BIKE	SWIM	YOGA	DANCE
■ Cheddar										
Cheddar	1 cup, diced	532	2	44	137	57	75	65	181	91
Low-fat Cheddar	1 cup, diced	228	3	9	59	24	32	28	78	39
Kraft Off the Block Natural Cheddar, Extra Sharp	1 oz	120	0	10	31	13	17	15	41	20
Cracker Barrel Reduced Fat Vermont Sharp Cheddar	1 oz	90	0	6	23	10	13	11	31	15
Laughing Cow Cheddar	1 oz	110	0	9	28	12	16	13	37	19
■ Cottage Cheese										
Cottage cheese, small or large curd	4 oz	116	3	5	30	12	17	14	40	20
Cottage cheese, with fruit	1 cup	219	10	9	57	23	31	27	75	37
Cottage cheese, with vegetables	1 cup	215	7	9	55	23	30	26	73	37
Fat-free cottage cheese	1 cup	123	3	1	32	13	17	15	42	21
1% cottage cheese	1 cup	163	6	2	42	17	23	20	55	28
1% cottage cheese, with vegetables	1 cup	151	7	2	39	16	21	18	51	26
2% cottage cheese	1 cup	203	8	4	52	22	29	25	69	35
Breakstone's 4% Cottage Cheese, Large Curd	.5 cup	120	5	5	31	13	17	15	41	20
Breakstone's 4% Cottage Cheese, Small Curd	.5 cup	120	5	5	31	13	17	15	41	20
Breakstone's Fat Free Cottage Cheese	.5 cup	80	6	0	21	9	11	10	27	14
Light n' Lively 1% Cottage Cheese	.5 cup	80	5	1	21	9	11	10	27	14
■ Cream Cheese										
Cream cheese	2 tbsp	101	1	10	26	11	14	12	34	17
Low-fat cream cheese	2 tbsp	69	2	5	18	7	10	8	23	12
Philadelphia Cream Cheese	2 tbsp	100	1	10	26	11	14	12	34	17
Philadelphia Fat Free Cream Cheese	2 tbsp	30	2	0	8	3	4	4	10	5
Philadelphia Whipped Cream Cheese	2 tbsp	70	0	7	18	7	10	9	24	12
Philadelphia Chive & Onion Cream Cheese	2 tbsp	110	2	10	28	12	16	13	37	19
Temptee Cream Cheese	2 tbsp	80	<1	8	21	9	11	10	27	14

FOOD	AMOUNT	CAL	CARBS	FAT	WALK	RUN	BIKE	SWIM	YOGA	DANCE
Temptee Whipped Cream Cheese	1 oz	100	1	10	26	11	14	12	34	17
Tofutti Better Than Cream Cheese	1 tbsp	40	1	4	10	4	6	5	14	7
■ **Mozzarella**										
Mozzarella, whole milk	1 cup, shredded	336	2	25	87	36	48	41	114	57
Mozzarella, whole milk, low moisture	1 oz	90	1	7	23	10	13	11	31	15
Mozzarella, part skim	1 oz	72	1	5	19	8	10	9	24	12
Mozzarella, part skim, low moisture	1 cup, diced	399	5	26	103	42	57	48	136	68
Fat-free mozzarella	1 cup, shredded	168	4	0	43	18	24	20	57	29
Mozzarella, cheese substitute	1 cup, shredded	280	27	14	72	30	40	34	95	48
Healthy Choice String Cheese	1 oz	50	1	2	13	5	7	6	17	9
Kraft Pizza Cheese	.33 cup	120	1	9	31	13	17	15	41	20
Kraft Reduced Fat Pizza Cheese	.33 cup	90	1	6	23	10	13	11	31	15
Kraft Part Skim Shredded Mozzarella	.33 cup	90	0	6	23	10	13	11	31	15
Kraft Reduced Fat Shredded Mozzarella	.33 cup	80	0	5	21	9	11	10	27	14
Kraft Deli Thin Part Skim Mozzarella	1 slice	80	0	5	21	9	11	10	27	14
Kraft Fat Free Shredded Mozzarella	.25 cup	45	2	0	12	5	6	5	15	8
Kraft Part Skim String Cheese	1 piece	80	0	6	21	9	11	10	27	14
Polly-O Lite Mozzarella	1 oz	70	1	4	18	7	10	9	24	12
Polly-O String Cheese	1 slice (1 oz)	90	2	6	23	10	13	11	31	15
Weight Watchers Mozzarella	1 oz	70	1	4	18	7	10	9	24	12
■ **Muenster**										
Muenster	1 cup, diced	486	1	40	125	52	69	59	165	83
Low-fat Muenster	1 cup, shredded	310	4	20	80	33	44	38	105	53
Alpine Lace Muenster	1 oz	100	1	8	26	11	14	12	34	17
Boar's Head Muenster	1 oz	100	0	8	26	11	14	12	34	17
Dorman's Muenster	1 oz	110	0	9	28	12	16	13	37	19

FOOD	AMOUNT	CAL	CARBS	FAT	WALK	RUN	BIKE	SWIM	YOGA	DANCE
Hickory Farms Muenster	1 oz	100	0	9	26	11	14	12	34	17
■ Parmesan										
Grated parmesan	1 cup	431	4	29	111	46	61	52	147	73
Parmesan, hard	1 oz	111	1	7	29	12	16	14	38	19
Shredded parmesan	1 tbsp	21	0	1	5	2	3	3	7	4
Kraft Parm Plus Parmesan, with seasoning	2 tsp	15	2	0	4	2	2	2	5	3
Kraft 100% Grated Parmesan	2 tsp	20	0	2	5	2	3	2	7	3
■ Swiss										
Swiss cheese	1 oz	95	1	7	24	10	13	12	32	16
Low-fat Swiss	1 slice (1 oz)	50	1	1	13	5	7	6	17	9
Borden's Nonfat Swiss	1 oz	40	4	0	10	4	6	5	14	7
Health Favorites Lowfat Swiss	1 oz	80	1	4	21	9	11	10	27	14
Kraft Natural Swiss	1 slice	90	0	7	23	10	13	11	31	15
Kraft Reduced Fat Natural Swiss	1 slice	130	0	9	34	14	18	16	44	22
Kraft Singles, Swiss	1 oz	90	0	7	23	10	13	11	31	15
Kraft Nonfat Singles, Swiss	.75 oz	30	3	0	8	3	4	4	10	5
Weight Watchers Natural Swiss	1 oz	90	1	5	23	10	13	11	31	15
Weight Watchers Nonfat Swiss	1 slice	30	2	0	8	3	4	4	10	5
■ Other Cheeses										
Laughing Cow Babybel	1 oz	91	0	7	23	10	13	11	31	16
Laughing Cow Mini Babybel	.75 oz	74	0	6	19	8	10	9	25	13
Laughing Cow Bonbel	1 oz	100	0	8	26	11	14	12	34	17
Laughing Cow Mini Bonbel	.75 oz	74	0	6	19	8	10	9	25	13
Blue	1 cubic inch	61	0	5	16	7	9	7	21	10
Brick	1 cup, diced	490	4	39	126	52	69	60	167	83
Brie	1 cup, melted	802	1	66	207	85	114	98	273	137
Camembert	1 cup	738	1	60	190	79	105	90	251	126
Dorman's 50% Camembert	1 oz	89	0	7	23	9	13	11	30	15
Sargento Camembert	1 oz	90	0	7	23	10	13	11	31	15
Caraway	1 oz	107	1	8	27	11	15	13	36	18

FOOD	AMOUNT	CAL	CARBS	FAT	WALK	RUN	BIKE	SWIM	YOGA	DANCE
Cheshire	1 oz	110	1	9	28	12	16	13	37	19
Colby	1 cup, diced	520	3	42	134	55	74	63	177	89
Low-fat Colby	1 cup, diced	228	3	9	59	24	32	28	78	39
Sargento Colby	1 oz	110	1	9	28	12	16	13	37	19
Weight Watchers Colby	1 oz	80	1	5	21	9	11	10	27	14
Edam	1 oz	101	0	8	26	11	14	12	34	17
Dorman's 45% Edam	1 oz	91	0	7	23	10	13	11	31	16
Land O' Lakes Edam	1 oz	100	1	8	26	11	14	12	34	17
Sargento Edam	1 oz	100	0	8	26	11	14	12	34	17
Hickory Farms Light Farmer Cheese	1 oz	90	1	7	23	10	13	11	31	15
Hickory Farms Farmer Cheese	1 oz	90	1	7	23	10	13	11	31	15
Feta	1 cup, crumbled	396	6	32	102	42	56	48	135	67
Dorman's 45% Feta	1 oz	91	0	7	23	10	13	11	31	16
Sargento Feta	1 oz	80	1	6	21	9	11	10	27	14
Fontina	1 cup, diced	513	2	41	132	55	73	62	175	87
Gjetost	1 oz	132	12	8	34	14	19	16	45	23
Goat cheese, hard	1 oz	128	1	10	33	14	18	16	44	22
Goat cheese, semi-soft	1 oz	103	1	8	27	11	15	13	35	18
Goat cheese, soft	1 oz	76	0	6	20	8	11	9	26	13
Gouda	1 oz	101	1	8	26	11	14	12	34	17
Dorman's Gouda	1 oz	100	1	8	26	11	14	12	34	17
Sargento Gouda	1 oz	100	1	8	26	11	14	12	34	17
Gruyere	1 cup, diced	545	0	43	141	58	77	66	185	93
Boar's Head Havarti	1 oz	110	0	10	28	12	16	13	37	19
Dorman's 45% Havarti	1 oz	91	0	7	23	10	13	11	31	16
Sargento Havarti	1 oz	120	0	11	31	13	17	15	41	20
Limburger	1 cup	438	1	37	113	47	62	53	149	75
Sargento Limburger	1 oz	90	0	8	23	10	13	11	31	15
Monterey	1 cup, diced	492	1	40	127	52	70	60	167	84
Low-fat Monterey	1 cup, diced	413	1	29	106	44	59	50	141	70

FOOD	AMOUNT	CAL	CARBS	FAT	WALK	RUN	BIKE	SWIM	YOGA	DANCE
Kraft Monterey Jack	1 oz	110	0	9	28	12	16	13	37	19
Weight Watchers Monterey Jack	1 oz	80	1	5	21	9	11	10	27	14
Neufchâtel	1 oz	74	1	7	19	8	10	9	25	13
Pimento cheese	1 cup, diced	525	2	44	135	56	74	64	179	89
Port du Salut	1 cup, diced	465	1	37	120	49	66	57	158	79
Provolone	1 cup, diced	463	3	35	119	49	66	56	158	79
Kraft Smoked Provolone	1 slice	150	0	11	39	16	21	18	51	26
Ricotta, whole milk	1 cup	428	7	32	110	46	61	52	146	73
Ricotta, part skim	1 cup	339	13	19	87	36	48	41	115	58
Breakstone's Ricotta	.25 cup	110	3	8	28	12	16	13	37	19
Polly-O Part Skim Ricotta	2 oz	90	2	6	23	10	13	11	31	15
Polly-O Whole Milk Ricotta	2 oz	100	2	7	26	11	14	12	34	17
Romano	1 oz	110	1	8	28	12	16	13	37	19
Kraft 100% Grated Romano	2 tsp	20	0	2	5	2	3	2	7	3
Roquefort	1 oz	105	1	9	27	11	15	13	36	18
Queso Anejo	1 cup, crumbled	492	6	40	127	52	70	60	167	84
Queso Asadero	1 cup, diced	470	4	37	121	50	67	57	160	80
Queso Chihuahua	1 cup, diced	494	7	39	127	53	70	60	168	84
■ **Cheese Spreads and Sauces**										
Cheese fondue	1 cup	492	8	29	127	52	70	60	167	84
Homemade cheese sauce	1 cup	479	13	36	123	51	68	58	163	82
Alouette Horseradish Spread, cheese and chives	1 oz	85	1	8	22	9	12	10	29	14
Cheez Whiz Cheezin 'n Squeezin	2 tbsp	91	3	7	23	10	13	11	31	16
Cheez Whiz Light	2 tbsp	75	6	3	19	8	11	9	26	13
Cheez Whiz Squeezable	2 tbsp	100	4	8	26	11	14	12	34	17
Cracker Barrel Extra Sharp Cheddar Spread	2 tbsp	80	1	8	21	9	11	10	27	14
Mohawk Valley Limburger Cheese Spread	1 oz	70	0	6	18	7	10	9	24	12
Sargento Brick Cheese Spread	1 oz	100	1	9	26	11	14	12	34	17

FOOD	AMOUNT	CAL	CARBS	FAT	WALK	RUN	BIKE	SWIM	YOGA	DANCE
Velveeta Reduced Fat	1 oz	62	3	3	16	7	9	8	21	11
Velveeta Spread	1 oz	85	3	6	22	9	12	10	29	14
Cream										
Half-and-half	1 cup	315	10	28	81	34	45	38	107	54
Light coffee cream	1 cup	468	9	46	121	50	66	57	159	80
Light whipping cream	1 cup	350	4	37	90	37	50	43	119	60
Heavy whipping cream	1 cup	412	3	44	106	44	58	50	140	70
Whipped cream (pressurized)	1 cup	154	7	13	40	16	22	19	52	26
Dessert topping (pressurized)	1 cup	185	11	16	48	20	26	22	63	31
Frozen dessert topping, semi solid	1 cup	239	17	19	61	25	34	29	81	41
Fat-free half-and-half	1 cup	143	22	3	37	15	20	17	49	24
Reddi-wip Fat Free Dairy Whipped Topping	2 tbsp	10	2	0	3	1	1	1	3	2
Reddi-wip Original Whipped Light Cream	2 tbsp	15	<1	1	4	2	2	2	5	3
Sour Cream										
Sour cream	1 cup	492	10	48	127	52	70	60	167	84
Reduced-fat sour cream	1 cup	327	10	29	84	35	46	40	111	56
Imitation sour cream	1 cup	478	15	45	123	51	68	58	163	81
Tofutti Sour Supreme (imitation sour cream)	1 tbsp	25	1	3	6	3	4	3	9	4
Breakstone's Fat Free Sour Cream	2 tbsp	29	5	0	8	3	4	4	10	5
Breakstone's Reduced Fat Sour Cream	2 tbsp	47	2	4	12	5	7	6	16	8
Friendship Sour Cream	1 oz	55	1	5	14	6	8	7	19	9
Friendship Lite Delite Sour Cream	2 tbsp	35	2	2	9	4	5	4	12	6
Land O' Lakes Light Sour Cream	2 tbsp	40	4	2	10	4	6	5	14	7
Land O' Lakes Nonfat Sour Cream	2 tbsp	30	5	0	8	3	4	4	10	5
Weight Watchers Light Sour Cream	2 tbsp	35	2	2	9	4	5	4	12	6
Eggnog										
Eggnog	1 cup	343	34	19	88	37	49	42	117	58
Eggnog, prepared from mix with whole milk	1 cup	258	39	8	67	28	37	31	88	44

FOOD	AMOUNT	CAL	CARBS	FAT	WALK	RUN	BIKE	SWIM	YOGA	DANCE
Farmland Eggnog	.5 cup	180	20	9	46	19	26	22	61	31
Nondairy Creamer										
Cream substitute (liquid)	1 cup	326	27	24	84	35	46	40	111	56
Cream substitute (powder)	1 cup	513	52	33	132	55	73	62	175	87
Coffee-Mate Nonfat Nondairy Creamer, Liquid	1 tbsp	10	2	0	3	1	1	1	3	2
Coffee-Mate Nonfat Nondairy Creamer, Powder	1 tbsp	10	2	0	3	1	1	1	3	2
Coffee-Mate Nonfat Nondairy Liquid Creamer, Hazelnut/Butter Rum	1 tbsp	25	5	0	6	3	4	3	9	4
Coffee-Mate Nonfat Nondairy Liquid Creamer, Irish Creme/French Vanilla	1 tbsp	25	5	0	6	3	4	3	9	4
Cow's Milk										
Whole milk (3.25%)	1 cup	146	11	8	38	16	21	18	50	25
Reduced-fat milk (2%)	1 cup	122	11	5	31	13	17	15	41	21
Reduced-fat milk (2%), with nonfat milk solids and vitamin A	1 cup	125	12	5	32	13	18	15	43	21
Protein-fortified reduced-fat milk (2%), with vitamin A	1 cup	138	14	5	36	15	20	17	47	23
Reduced-fat milk (2%), with nonfat milk solids, without vitamin A	1 cup	137	13	5	35	15	19	17	47	23
Low-fat milk (1%)	1 cup	102	12	2	26	11	15	12	35	17
Low-fat milk (1%), with nonfat milk solids and vitamin A	1 cup	105	12	2	27	11	15	13	36	18
Protein-fortified reduced-fat milk (1%), with vitamin A	1 cup	118	14	3	30	13	17	14	40	20
Nonfat (skim) milk, with vitamin A	1 cup	83	12	0	21	9	12	10	28	14
Nonfat (skim) milk without vitamin A	1 cup	86	12	0	22	9	12	10	29	15
Nonfat (skim) milk, with nonfat milk solids and vitamin A	1 cup	91	12	1	23	10	13	11	31	15
Protein-fortified nonfat (skim) milk, with vitamin A	1 cup	101	14	1	26	11	14	12	34	17
Lactaid Fat Free Lactose-Free Milk	1 cup	80	13	0	21	9	11	10	27	14
Lactaid low-fat (1%) lactose-free milk	1 cup	110	13	3	28	12	16	13	37	19

FOOD	AMOUNT	CAL	CARBS	FAT	WALK	RUN	BIKE	SWIM	YOGA	DANCE
Low-sodium milk	1 cup	149	11	8	38	16	21	18	51	25
Buttermilk										
Reduced-fat buttermilk	1 cup	137	13	5	35	15	19	17	47	23
Low-fat buttermilk	1 cup	98	12	2	25	10	14	12	33	17
Chocolate Milk										
Chocolate milk	1 cup	208	26	8	53	22	29	25	71	35
Reduced-fat chocolate milk	1 cup	180	26	5	46	19	26	22	61	31
Low-fat chocolate milk	1 cup	158	26	3	41	17	22	19	54	27
Homemade hot cocoa	1 cup	193	27	6	50	21	27	23	65	33
Nestlé Nesquik Chocolate Milk	1 cup	230	31	8	59	24	33	28	78	39
Dry Milk										
Dry whole milk	.25 cup	159	12	9	41	17	23	19	54	27
Dry nonfat (skim) milk	.25 cup	109	16	0	28	12	15	13	37	19
Dry nonfat (skim) milk, reduced calcium	1 oz	100	15	0	26	11	14	12	34	17
Dry buttermilk	1 cup	464	59	7	120	49	66	56	158	79
Canned Milk										
Canned sweetened condensed milk	1 cup	982	166	27	253	105	139	119	334	167
Canned evaporated milk, without vitamin A	1 cup	338	25	19	87	36	48	41	115	58
Canned evaporated skim milk	1 cup	200	29	1	51	21	28	24	68	34
Carnation Sweetened Condensed Milk	2 tbsp	130	22	3	34	14	18	16	44	22
Carnation Evaporated Milk	2 tbsp	40	3	2	10	4	6	5	14	7
Carnation Low Fat Evaporated Milk	2 tbsp	25	3	1	6	3	4	3	9	4
Carnation Fat Free Evaporated Milk	2 tbsp	25	4	0	6	3	4	3	9	4
Goat Milk										
Goat milk	1 cup	168	11	10	43	18	24	20	57	29
Other Milks										
Soy milk	1 cup	127	12	5	33	14	18	15	43	22
Calcium-fortified soy milk	1 cup	98	8	4	25	10	14	12	33	17
Chocolate soy milk	1 cup	120	14	5	31	13	17	15	41	20
Rice Dream Original	1 cup	120	25	2	31	13	17	15	41	20
Rice Dream Vanilla	1 cup	130	28	2	34	14	18	16	44	22
Silk Vanilla Soymilk	1 cup	100	10	4	26	11	14	12	34	17

FOOD	AMOUNT	CAL	CARBS	FAT	WALK	RUN	BIKE	SWIM	YOGA	DANCE
Silk Chocolate Soymilk	1 cup	140	23	4	36	15	20	17	48	24
WestSoy Non Fat Soymilk Beverage	1 cup	80	15	0	21	9	11	10	27	14
WestSoy Low Fat Vanilla Soymilk Drink	1 cup	120	21	2	31	13	17	15	41	20
WestSoy Vanilla Soy Shake	1 cup	170	28	3	44	18	24	21	58	29
Milk Shakes										
Thick Chocolate milk shake	16 fl oz	541	96	12	139	58	77	66	184	92
Thick Vanilla milk shake	16 fl oz	509	81	14	131	54	72	62	173	87
Weight Watchers Chocolate Shake	1 serving	80	12	1	21	9	11	10	27	14
Whey										
Whey, acid	1 cup	59	13	0	15	6	8	7	20	10
Dry whey	1 cup	193	42	0	50	21	27	24	66	33
Sweet dried whey	1 cup	512	108	2	132	55	73	62	174	87
Sweet fluid whey	1 cup	66	13	1	17	7	9	8	23	11
Yogurt										
■ Plain										
Plain whole-milk	1 cup	149	11	8	39	16	21	18	51	25
Plain low-fat	1 cup	154	17	4	40	16	22	19	53	26
Plain nonfat	1 cup	137	19	0	35	15	19	17	47	23
Whole-milk, any flavor	1 cup	170	12	8	44	18	24	21	58	29
Dannon Plain	1 cup	170	14	8	44	18	24	21	58	29
Dannon Plain Nonfat	6 oz	90	14	0	23	10	13	11	31	15
Stonyfield Farm Plain Nonfat	1 cup	100	15	0	26	11	14	12	34	17
Stonyfield Farm Plain Low Fat	1 cup	120	17	2	31	13	17	15	41	20
■ Fruited Yogurt										
Breyer's 1% Mixed Berry	8 oz	230	43	3	59	24	33	28	78	39
Breyer's Light Nonfat Strawberry (with artificial sweetener)	1 container	125	22	0	32	13	18	15	42	21
Breyer's Light Peaches 'n Cream Nonfat	8 oz	120	22	0	31	13	17	15	41	20
Breyer's Low Fat Blueberry	8 oz	230	43	3	59	24	33	28	78	39
Breyer's Low Fat Blueberry Blended	4.4 oz	130	25	1	34	14	18	16	44	22

FOOD	AMOUNT	CAL	CARBS	FAT	WALK	RUN	BIKE	SWIM	YOGA	DANCE
Breyer's Low Fat Strawberry	1 container	218	41	2	56	23	31	27	74	37
Breyer's Low Fat Strawberry Banana	8 oz	240	44	3	62	26	34	29	82	41
Breyer's Nonfat Cherry Vanilla Cream	8 oz	120	22	0	31	13	17	15	41	20
Breyer's Smooth & Creamy Low Fat Strawberry (1%)	1 container	232	45	2	60	25	33	28	79	39
Breyer's Smooth & Creamy Peaches 'n Cream Low Fat	4.4 oz	130	25	1	34	14	18	16	44	22
Breyer's Smooth & Creamy Strawberry Banana Split Low Fat	8 oz	240	48	2	62	26	34	29	82	41
Dannon Fruit on the Bottom Low Fat Blueberry	8 oz	210	39	2	54	22	30	26	71	36
Dannon Fruit on the Bottom Low Fat Cherry	8 oz	210	40	2	54	22	30	26	71	36
Dannon Fruit on the Bottom Low Fat Peach	8 oz	210	40	2	54	22	30	26	71	36
Dannon Fruit on the Bottom Mixed Berries	8 oz	210	39	2	54	22	30	26	71	36
Dannon Light 'N Fit Cherry Vanilla	8 oz	120	24	0	31	13	17	15	41	20
Dannon Light 'N Fit Peach	8 oz	120	23	0	31	13	17	15	41	20
Dannon Light 'N Fit Strawberry Banana	8 oz	120	22	0	31	13	17	15	41	20
Dannon Light 'N Fit Blueberry	8 oz	120	23	0	31	13	17	15	41	20
Dannon Nonfat Peach Snack Packs	4 oz	100	20	0	26	11	14	12	34	17
Dannon Nonfat Raspberry Blended	4 oz	100	21	0	26	11	14	12	34	17
Dannon Nonfat Strawberry/ Banana Snack Packs	4 oz	100	21	0	26	11	14	12	34	17
Dannon Nonfat Strawberry/ Blueberry Snack Packs	4 oz	100	21	0	26	11	14	12	34	17
Light n' Lively Low Fat Blueberry	4.4 oz	130	25	1	34	14	18	16	44	22
Light n' Lively Nonfat Blueberry	4.4 oz	70	13	0	18	7	10	9	24	12
Light n' Lively Nonfat Peach	4.4 oz	70	12	0	18	7	10	9	24	12
Light n' Lively Strawberry (1%)	1 container	135	27	1	35	14	19	16	46	23

FOOD	AMOUNT	CAL	CARBS	FAT	WALK	RUN	BIKE	SWIM	YOGA	DANCE
Low-fat fruited	1 cup	243	46	3	63	26	34	30	83	41
Nonfat fruited	1 cup	230	47	1	59	25	33	28	78	39
Stonyfield Farm Low Fat Banana Blended	1 container	160	31	2	41	17	23	19	54	27
Stonyfield Farm Low Fat Blueberry	1 container	130	23	2	34	14	18	16	44	22
Stonyfield Farm Low Fat Peach Blended	6 oz	160	33	2	41	17	23	19	54	27
Stonyfield Farm Low Fat Raspberry Blended	1 container	160	30	2	41	17	23	19	54	27
Stonyfield Farm Low Fat Strawberry Banana	1 container	170	33	2	44	18	24	21	58	29
Stonyfield Farm Low Fat Strawberry Blended	1 container	160	32	2	41	17	23	19	54	27
Stonyfield Farm Nonfat Black Cherry	1 container	160	31	0	41	17	23	19	54	27
Stonyfield Farm Nonfat Blueberry	1 container	160	30	0	41	17	23	19	54	27
Stonyfield Farm Nonfat Cherry Vanilla	1 container	190	41	0	49	20	27	23	65	32
Stonyfield Farm Nonfat Mixed Berry	1 container	160	30	0	41	17	23	19	54	27
Stonyfield Farm Nonfat Peach	8 oz	150	30	0	39	16	21	18	51	26
Stonyfield Farm Nonfat Strawberry Banana	8 oz	160	32	0	41	17	23	19	54	27
Yoplait Light, all flavors	6 oz	100	17	0	26	11	14	12	34	17
■ **Coffee and Cappucino**										
Dannon Coffee	8 oz	220	37	4	57	23	31	27	75	37
Dannon Light 'N Fit Cappucino	8 oz	120	23	0	31	13	17	15	41	20
Stonyfield Farm Nonfat Cappucino	1 container	160	31	0	41	17	23	19	54	27
■ **Lemon**										
Dannon Lemon	8 oz	220	37	4	57	23	31	27	75	37
Dannon Light 'N Fit Nonfat Lemon Chiffon	6 oz	60	10	0	15	6	9	7	20	10
Dannon Low Fat Lemon Meringue Pie	6 oz	180	37	1	46	19	26	22	61	31
Stonyfield Farm Nonfat Lotsa Lemon	1 container	160	30	0	41	17	23	19	54	27

FOOD	AMOUNT	CAL	CARBS	FAT	WALK	RUN	BIKE	SWIM	YOGA	DANCE
Stonyfield Farm Low Fat Luscious Lemon	1 container	130	23	2	34	14	18	16	44	22
Yoplait Lemon	6 oz	180	36	2	46	19	26	22	61	31
■ **Vanilla and French Vanilla**										
Low-fat vanilla	1 cup	208	34	3	54	22	30	25	71	35
Dannon Fruit on the Bottom French Vanilla Raspberry	8 oz	240	43	3	62	26	34	29	82	41
Dannon Fruit on the Bottom French Vanilla Strawberry	8 oz	240	43	3	62	26	34	29	82	41
Stonyfield Farm Nonfat French Vanilla	1 container	160	30	0	41	17	23	19	54	27
Stonyfield Farm Whole Milk French Vanilla	1 container	170	23	6	44	18	24	21	58	29
■ **Soy Yogurt**										
Stonyfield Farm O'Soy Blueberry	6 oz	170	33	2	44	18	24	21	58	29
Stonyfield Farm O'Soy Peach	6 oz	170	32	2	44	18	24	21	58	29
Stonyfield Farm O'Soy Raspberry	6 oz	170	32	2	44	18	24	21	58	29
Stonyfield Farm O'Soy Strawberry	6 oz	170	32	2	44	18	24	21	58	29
■ **Yogurt With Add-Ons**										
Low Fat YoCrunch, with granola	1 container	210	40	3	54	22	30	26	71	36
Low Fat Yocrunch, with Nestlé Crunch	1 container	220	39	4	57	23	31	27	75	37
Low Fat Yocrunch, with Oreos	1 container	200	36	4	52	21	28	24	68	34
■ **Yogurt Drinks**										
Dannon Danimals Low Fat Cherry Cool	3.1 oz	90	16	2	23	10	13	11	31	15
Dannon Danimals Low Fat Rockin' Raspberry	3.1 oz	90	16	2	23	10	13	11	31	15
Dannon Danimals Low Fat Strawberry Explosion	3.1 oz	90	16	2	23	10	13	11	31	15
Dannon Banana Berry Frusion Smoothie	10 oz (1 bottle)	280	52	4	72	30	40	34	95	48
Dannon Strawberry Kiwi Frusion Smoothie	10 oz (1 bottle)	270	52	4	70	29	38	33	92	46
Stonyfield Farm Peach Smoothie	10 oz (1 bottle)	250	49	3	64	27	35	30	85	43

FOOD	AMOUNT	CAL	CARBS	FAT	WALK	RUN	BIKE	SWIM	YOGA	DANCE
Stonyfield Farm Vanilla Smoothie	10 oz (1 bottle)	250	46	3	64	27	35	30	85	43
Stonyfield Farm Light Strawberry Smoothie	10 oz (1 bottle)	130	41	0	34	14	18	16	44	22
Yoplait Nouriche Nonfat Strawberry Smoothie	11 oz (1 bottle)	290	60	0	75	31	41	35	99	49
Yoplait Go-Gurt	1 tube	80	13	2	21	9	11	10	27	14
Eggs										
■ General										
Whole raw egg	1 cup	357	2	24	92	38	51	43	122	61
Egg white, raw	1 cup	126	2	0	33	13	18	15	43	22
Egg yolk, raw	1 cup	782	9	64	202	83	111	95	266	133
Frozen egg yolk	.5 lb	688	3	58	177	73	98	84	234	117
Fried whole egg	1 large	92	0	7	24	10	13	11	31	16
Hard-boiled whole egg	1 cup, chopped	211	2	14	54	22	30	26	72	36
Poached whole egg	1 large	74	0	5	19	8	10	9	25	13
Scrambled whole egg	1 cup	365	5	27	94	39	52	44	124	62
■ Egg Substitute										
Frozen egg substitute	1 cup	384	8	27	99	41	54	47	131	65
Liquid egg substitute	1 cup	211	2	8	54	22	30	26	72	36
Powdered egg substitute	.35 oz	44	2	1	11	5	6	5	15	7
■ Dried Egg										
Dried whole egg	1 cup	505	4	35	130	54	72	61	172	86
Dried egg white flakes	.5 lb	797	9	0	205	85	113	97	271	136
Dried egg white powder	1 cup	402	5	0	104	43	57	49	137	69
Dried egg yolk	1 cup	446	2	37	115	48	63	54	152	76

Fruit

Fresh Fruit										
Raw apple	1 cup, quartered or chopped	72	19	0	19	8	10	9	24	12
Raw apricot	1 apricot	17	4	0	4	2	2	2	6	3
California avocado	.25 whole	72	4	7	19	8	10	9	24	12
Florida avocado	.25 whole	91	6	8	23	10	13	11	31	16

FOOD	AMOUNT	CAL	CARBS	FAT	WALK	RUN	BIKE	SWIM	YOGA	DANCE
Raw banana	1 large	121	31	0	31	13	17	15	41	21
Raw blackberries	1 cup	62	14	1	16	7	9	8	21	11
Raw blueberries	1 cup	83	21	0	21	9	12	10	28	14
Sour red cherries	1 cup, without pits	78	19	0	20	8	11	9	26	13
Sweet cherries	1 cup, without pits	91	23	0	23	10	13	11	31	16
Raw cranberries	1 cup, whole	44	0	0	11	5	6	5	15	7
Raw currants	1 cup	63	15	0	16	7	9	8	21	11
Dates	10 dates	234	62	0	60	25	33	28	80	40
Raw figs	1 large	47	12	0	12	5	7	6	16	8
Raw guava	1 fruit	37	8	1	10	4	5	5	13	6
Raw grapefruit (red, white, or pink)	1 medium	82	21	0	21	9	12	10	28	14
Red or green grapes	1 cup, seedless	110	29	0	28	12	16	13	38	19
Raw lemon	1 medium	24	8	0	6	3	3	3	8	4
Lemon peel	1 tbsp	3	1	0	1	0	0	0	1	0
Raw lime	1 fruit	20	7	0	5	2	3	2	7	3
Raw kiwi	1 large	56	13	0	14	6	8	7	19	10
Raw kumquat	1 fruit	13	3	0	3	1	2	2	5	2
Raw mango	1 fruit	135	35	1	35	14	19	16	46	23
Raw nectarine	1 fruit	60	14	0	15	6	9	7	20	10
Raw cantaloupe	.5 melon	138	33	1	36	15	20	17	47	24
Raw casaba melon	.5 melon	230	54	1	59	24	33	28	78	39
Raw honeydew melon	.5 melon	230	58	1	59	24	33	28	78	39
Raw orange (any variety)	1 large	86	22	0	22	9	12	10	29	15
Raw Florida orange	1 orange	69	17	0	18	7	10	8	23	12
Raw navel orange	1 orange	69	18	0	18	7	10	8	23	12
Raw Valencia orange	1 orange	59	14	0	15	6	8	7	20	10
Orange peel	1 tbsp	6	2	0	2	1	1	1	2	1
Raw papaya	1 large	148	37	1	38	16	21	18	50	25
Raw pear	1 large	121	32	0	31	13	17	15	41	21
Raw passionfruit	1 fruit	17	4	0	4	2	2	2	6	3
Raw plantain	1 medium	218	57	1	56	23	31	27	74	37

FOOD	AMOUNT	CAL	CARBS	FAT	WALK	RUN	BIKE	SWIM	YOGA	DANCE
Raw persimmon	1 fruit	118	31	0	30	13	17	14	40	20
Raw peaches	1 large	61	15	0	16	6	9	7	21	10
Raw pineapple	1 cup, diced	74	20	0	19	8	11	9	25	13
Raw plum	1 fruit	30	8	0	8	3	4	4	10	5
Raw pomegranate	1 fruit	105	26	0	27	11	15	13	36	18
Raw pummelo	.5 fruit	116	29	0	30	12	16	14	39	20
Raw prickly pear	1 pear	42	10	1	11	4	6	5	14	7
Raw Asian pear	1 pear	51	13	0	13	5	7	6	17	9
Raw quince	1 quince	52	14	0	14	6	7	6	18	9
Raw raspberries	1 cup	64	15	1	16	7	9	8	22	11
Raw rhubarb	1 cup, diced	26	6	0	7	3	4	3	9	4
Raw star fruit	1 medium	28	6	0	7	3	4	3	10	5
Raw strawberries	1 cup, whole	46	11	0	12	5	7	6	16	8
Raw tangerine	1 large	52	13	0	13	6	7	6	18	9
Raw watermelon	1 cup, diced	46	11	0	12	5	7	6	16	8
Canned Fruit										
Canned sweetened apple slices	1 cup, slices	137	34	1	35	15	19	17	46	23
Apricots canned in water	1 cup, whole, without pits	50	12	0	13	5	7	6	17	9
Apricots canned in juice	1 cup	117	30	0	30	12	17	14	40	20
Apricots canned in extra-light syrup	1 cup (halves)	121	31	0	31	13	17	15	41	21
Apricots canned in light syrup	1 cup (halves)	159	42	0	41	17	23	19	54	27
Apricots canned in heavy syrup	1 cup (halves)	214	55	0	55	23	30	26	73	36
Blackberries canned in heavy syrup	1 cup	236	59	0	61	25	33	29	80	40
Blueberries canned in heavy syrup	1 cup	225	56	1	58	24	32	27	77	38
Boysenberries canned in heavy syrup	1 cup	225	57	0	58	24	32	27	77	38
Sour red cherries canned in water	1 cup	88	22	0	23	9	12	11	30	15

FOOD	AMOUNT	CAL	CARBS	FAT	WALK	RUN	BIKE	SWIM	YOGA	DANCE
Sour red cherries canned in light syrup	1 cup	189	49	0	49	20	27	23	64	32
Sour red cherries canned in heavy syrup	1 cup	233	60	0	60	25	33	28	79	40
Sour red cherries canned in extra-heavy syrup	1 cup	298	76	0	77	32	42	36	101	51
Sweet cherries canned in water	1 cup	114	29	0	29	12	16	14	39	19
Sweet cherries canned in juice	1 cup	135	35	0	35	14	19	16	46	23
Sweet cherries canned in light syrup	1 cup	169	44	0	44	18	24	21	57	29
Sweet cherries canned in heavy syrup	1 cup	210	54	0	54	22	30	26	71	36
Sweet cherries canned in extra-heavy syrup	1 cup	266	69	0	69	28	38	32	91	45
Canned cranberry sauce	1 cup	418	108	0	108	45	59	51	142	71
Canned cranberry-orange relish	1 cup	490	127	0	126	52	69	60	166	83
Figs canned in water	1 cup	131	35	0	34	14	19	16	45	22
Figs canned in light syrup	1 cup	174	45	0	45	19	25	21	59	30
Figs canned in heavy syrup	1 cup	228	59	0	59	24	32	28	78	39
Figs canned in extra-heavy syrup	1 cup	279	73	0	72	30	40	34	95	48
Fruit cocktail canned in water	1 cup	76	20	0	20	8	11	9	26	13
Fruit cocktail canned in juice	1 cup	109	28	0	28	12	15	13	37	19
Fruit cocktail canned in extra-light syrup	1 cup	111	29	0	29	12	16	14	38	19
Fruit cocktail canned in light syrup	1 cup	138	36	0	36	15	20	17	47	23
Fruit cocktail canned in heavy syrup	1 cup	181	47	0	47	19	26	22	62	31
Fruit cocktail canned in extra-heavy syrup	1 cup	229	60	0	59	24	32	28	78	39
Fruit salad canned in water	1 cup	74	19	0	19	8	10	9	25	13
Fruit salad canned in juice	1 cup	124	32	0	32	13	18	15	42	21
Fruit salad canned in light syrup	1 cup	146	38	0	38	16	21	18	50	25
Fruit salad canned in heavy syrup	1 cup	186	49	0	48	20	26	23	63	32

FOOD	AMOUNT	CAL	CARBS	FAT	WALK	RUN	BIKE	SWIM	YOGA	DANCE
Fruit salad canned in extra-heavy syrup	1 cup	228	59	0	59	24	32	28	78	39
Canned gooseberries	1 cup	184	47	1	47	20	26	22	63	31
Grapefruit canned in water	1 cup	88	22	0	23	9	12	11	30	15
Grapefruit canned in juice	1 cup	92	23	0	24	10	13	11	31	16
Grapefruit canned in light syrup	1 cup	152	39	0	39	16	22	19	52	26
Grapes canned in water	1 cup	98	25	0	25	10	14	12	33	17
Grapes canned in heavy syrup	1 cup	187	50	0	48	20	27	23	64	32
Mandarin oranges canned in juice	1 cup	92	24	0	24	10	13	11	31	16
Mandarin oranges canned in light syrup	1 cup	154	41	0	40	16	22	19	52	26
Mixed fruit canned in heavy syrup	1 cup	184	48	0	47	20	26	22	62	31
Peaches canned in water	1 cup, halves or slices	59	15	0	15	6	8	7	20	10
Peaches canned in juice	1 cup, halves or slices	109	29	0	28	12	15	13	37	19
Peaches canned in extra-light syrup	1 cup, halves or slices	104	27	0	27	11	15	13	35	18
Peaches canned in light syrup	1 cup, halves or slices	136	37	0	35	14	19	16	46	23
Peaches canned in heavy syrup	1 cup	194	52	0	50	21	28	24	66	33
Peaches canned in extra-heavy syrup	1 cup, halves or slices	252	68	0	65	27	36	31	86	43
Pears canned in water	1 cup	71	19	0	18	8	10	9	24	12
Pears canned in juice	1 cup, halves	124	32	0	32	13	18	15	42	21
Pears canned in extra-light syrup	1 cup, halves	116	30	0	30	12	16	14	39	20
Pears canned in light syrup	1 cup	143	38	0	37	15	20	17	49	24
Pears canned in heavy syrup	1 cup	197	51	0	51	21	28	24	67	34
Pears canned in extra-heavy syrup	1 cup, halves	258	67	0	66	27	37	31	88	44

FOOD	AMOUNT	CAL	CARBS	FAT	WALK	RUN	BIKE	SWIM	YOGA	DANCE
Pineapple canned in water	1 cup, crushed, sliced, or chunked	79	20	0	20	8	11	10	27	13
Pineapple canned in juice	1 cup, crushed, sliced, or chunked	149	39	0	39	16	21	18	51	25
Pineapple canned in light syrup	1 cup, crushed, sliced, or chunked	131	34	0	34	14	19	16	45	22
Pineapple canned in heavy syrup	1 cup, crushed, sliced, or chunked	198	51	0	51	21	28	24	67	34
Pineapple canned in extra-heavy syrup	1 cup, crushed, sliced, or chunked	216	56	0	56	23	31	26	73	37
Plums canned in water	1 cup	102	27	0	26	11	14	12	35	17
Plums canned in juice	1 cup	146	38	0	38	16	21	18	50	25
Plums canned in light syrup	1 cup	159	41	0	41	17	23	19	54	27
Plums canned in heavy syrup	1 cup	230	60	0	59	24	33	28	78	39
Plums canned in extra-heavy syrup	1 cup	264	69	0	68	28	37	32	90	45
Prunes canned in heavy syrup	1 cup	246	65	0	63	26	35	30	84	42
Raspberries canned in heavy syrup	1 cup	233	60	0	60	25	33	28	79	40
Tropical fruit salad canned in heavy syrup	1 cup	221	57	0	57	24	31	27	75	38
Strawberries canned in heavy syrup	1 cup	234	60	1	60	25	33	28	79	40
Frozen Fruit										
Frozen unsweetened apple slices	1 cup, slices	83	21	1	21	9	12	10	28	14
Frozen sweetened apricots	1 cup	237	61	0	61	25	34	29	81	40
Frozen unsweetened boysenberries	1 cup, unthawed	66	16	0	17	7	9	8	22	11
Frozen unsweetened blackberries	1 cup, unthawed	97	24	1	25	10	14	12	33	16
Frozen unsweetened blueberries	1 cup, unthawed	79	19	1	20	8	11	10	27	13

FOOD	AMOUNT	CAL	CARBS	FAT	WALK	RUN	BIKE	SWIM	YOGA	DANCE
Frozen sweetened blueberries	1 cup, thawed	186	50	0	48	20	26	23	63	32
Frozen unsweetened sour red cherries	1 cup, unthawed	71	17	1	18	8	10	9	24	12
Frozen sweetened cherries	1 cup, thawed	231	58	0	59	25	33	28	78	39
Frozen melon balls	1 cup, unthawed	57	14	0	15	6	8	7	19	10
Mixed frozen sweetened fruit	1 cup, thawed	245	61	0	63	26	35	30	83	42
Frozen sweetened peach slices	1 cup, thawed	235	60	0	61	25	33	29	80	40
Frozen sweetened pineapple	1 cup, chunks	211	54	0	54	22	30	26	72	36
Frozen sweetened cooked rhubarb	1 cup	278	75	0	72	30	39	34	95	47
Frozen sweetened raspberries	1 cup, unthawed	258	65	0	66	27	37	31	88	44
Frozen sweetened strawberries	1 cup, slices	245	66	0	63	26	35	30	83	42
Frozen unsweetened strawberries	1 cup, unthawed	52	14	0	13	6	7	6	18	9
Olives										
Canned olives	7 large	35	2	3	9	4	5	4	12	6
Canned jumbo olives	7 olives	47	3	4	12	5	7	6	16	8
Canned pickled green olives	1 oz	41	1	4	11	4	6	5	14	7
Goya Spanish Olives	6 olives	30	1	3	8	3	4	4	10	5
Goya Olives, with pimento and capers	2 tbsp	25	1	3	6	3	4	3	9	4
Goya Stuffed Spanish Olives	4 olives	25	1	2	6	3	4	3	9	4
Dried Fruit and Nuts										
Dried apples	1 cup	208	56	0	54	22	29	25	71	35
Stewed dried apples	1 cup	143	38	0	37	15	20	17	49	24
Dried apricots	1 cup (halves)	313	81	1	81	33	44	38	107	53
Stewed dried apricots	1 cup (halves)	212	55	0	55	23	30	26	72	36
Stewed dried apricots, with sugar	1 cup (halves)	305	79	0	79	32	43	37	104	52
Dried sweetened cranberries	.33 cup	123	33	1	32	13	17	15	42	21

FOOD	AMOUNT	CAL	CARBS	FAT	WALK	RUN	BIKE	SWIM	YOGA	DANCE
Dried figs	1 cup	371	95	1	96	40	53	45	126	63
Stewed dried figs	1 cup	277	71	1	71	30	39	34	94	47
Mixed dried fruit	1 package (11 oz)	712	188	1	184	76	101	87	242	121
Dried peaches	1 cup, halves	382	98	1	98	41	54	46	130	65
Stewed dried peaches	1 cup	199	51	1	51	21	28	24	68	34
Stewed dried peaches, with sugar	1 cup	278	72	1	72	30	39	34	95	47
Dried pears	1 cup, halves	472	125	1	122	50	67	57	160	80
Stewed dried pears	1 cup, halves	324	86	1	83	34	46	39	110	55
Stewed dried pears, with sugar	1 cup, halves	392	104	1	101	42	56	48	133	67
Dried persimmon	1 fruit	93	25	0	24	10	13	11	32	16
Dried plums	1 cup, pitted	408	109	1	105	43	58	50	139	70
Stewed dried plums	1 cup, pitted	265	70	0	68	28	38	32	90	45
Stewed dried plums, with sugar	1 cup, pitted	308	82	1	79	33	44	37	105	52
Raisins	.5 cup	247	65	0	64	26	35	30	84	42
Cooked Fruit										
Cooked plantain	1 cup, mashed	232	62	0	60	25	33	28	79	40
Guava sauce (cooked)	1 cup	86	23	0	22	9	12	10	29	15
Microwaved apple	1 cup, slices	95	25	1	25	10	14	12	32	16
Sweetened applesauce	1 cup	194	51	0	50	21	27	24	66	33
Unsweetened applesauce	1 cup	105	28	0	27	11	15	13	36	18
Mott's Chunky or Homestyle Applesauce	.5 cup	90	23	0	23	10	13	11	31	15
Mott's Cinnamon Applesauce	.5 cup	120	29	0	31	13	17	15	41	20
Mott's Natural Applesauce	.5 cup	50	14	0	13	5	7	6	17	9
Mott's Original Applesauce	.5 cup	110	27	0	28	12	16	13	37	19
Candied Fruit										
Maraschino cherry	1 cherry	8	2	0	2	1	1	1	3	1
Raisinets	1 package (1.58 oz)	185	32	7	48	20	26	23	63	32

FOOD	AMOUNT	CAL	CARBS	FAT	WALK	RUN	BIKE	SWIM	YOGA	DANCE

Vegetables

Fresh Vegetables, Nonstarchy										
Raw artichoke	1 large	76	17	0	20	8	11	9	26	13
Raw arugula	1 cup	5	1	0	1	1	1	1	2	1
Raw asparagus	1 cup	27	5	0	7	3	4	3	9	5
Raw beets	1 cup	58	13	0	15	6	8	7	20	10
Raw broccoli	1 cup, chopped	31	6	0	8	3	4	4	11	5
Raw broccoli rabe	1 oz	6	1	0	2	1	1	1	2	1
Raw Brussels sprouts	1 cup	38	8	0	10	4	5	5	13	6
Raw cabbage	1 cup, shredded	17	4	0	4	2	2	2	6	3
Raw red cabbage	1 cup, shredded	22	5	0	6	2	3	3	7	4
Raw Chinese cabbage	1 cup, shredded	9	0	0	2	1	1	1	3	2
Raw Savoy cabbage	1 cup, shredded	19	4	0	5	2	3	2	6	3
Raw carrots	1 large	30	7	0	8	3	4	4	10	5
Raw baby carrots	1 cup	50	12	0	13	5	7	6	17	9
Raw cauliflower	1 cup	25	5	0	6	3	4	3	9	4
Raw celery	1 cup, chopped	14	3	0	4	2	2	2	5	2
Raw Swiss chard	1 cup	7	1	0	2	1	1	1	2	1
Raw chicory greens	1 cup, chopped	7	1	0	2	1	1	1	2	1
Raw chives	1 tbsp, chopped	1	0	0	0	0	0	0	0	0
Raw collard greens	1 cup, chopped	11	2	0	3	1	2	1	4	2
Raw cucumber	1 medium	24	4	0	6	3	3	3	8	4
Raw dandelion greens	1 cup, chopped	25	5	0	6	3	4	3	8	4
Raw eggplant	1 cup, cubes	20	5	0	5	2	3	2	7	3
Raw endive	1 cup	8	2	0	2	1	1	1	3	1
Raw fennel	1 cup, sliced	27	6	0	7	3	4	3	9	5

FOOD	AMOUNT	CAL	CARBS	FAT	WALK	RUN	BIKE	SWIM	YOGA	DANCE
Garlic	3 cloves	13	3	0	3	1	2	2	4	2
Ginger root	1 tsp	2	0	0	0	0	0	0	1	0
Raw grape leaves	1 leaf	3	1	0	1	0	0	0	1	1
Raw Jerusalem artichoke	1 cup, slices	114	26	0	29	12	16	14	39	19
Raw kale	1 cup, chopped	34	7	0	9	4	5	4	11	6
Raw kohlrabi	1 cup	36	8	0	9	4	5	4	12	6
Raw leeks	1 cup	54	13	0	14	6	8	7	18	9
Raw lettuce	1 cup, shredded	8	2	0	2	1	1	1	3	1
Raw romaine lettuce	1 cup, shredded	8	2	0	2	1	1	1	3	1
Raw mushrooms	1 cup, pieces or slices	15	2	0	4	2	2	2	5	3
Raw portobello mushrooms	1 cup, diced	22	4	0	6	2	3	3	7	4
Raw mustard greens	1 cup, chopped	15	3	0	4	2	2	2	5	2
Raw okra	1 cup	31	7	0	8	3	4	4	11	5
Raw onions	1 cup, chopped	67	16	0	17	7	10	8	23	11
Raw parsley	1 tbsp	1	0	0	0	0	0	0	0	0
Raw green pepper	1 large	33	8	0	9	4	5	4	11	6
Raw red pepper (sweet)	1 large	43	10	0	11	5	6	5	15	7
Raw radish	1 large	1	0	0	0	0	0	0	0	0
Raw daikon	1 radish	61	14	0	16	6	9	7	21	10
Raw radicchio	1 cup, shredded	9	2	0	2	1	1	1	3	2
Seaweed	10 sheets	9	1	0	2	1	1	1	3	2
Raw shallots	1 tbsp, chopped	7	2	0	2	1	1	1	2	1
Raw spinach	1 cup	7	1	0	2	1	1	1	2	1
Raw summer squash	1 cup, sliced	18	4	0	5	2	3	2	6	3
Raw taro leaves	1 cup	12	2	0	3	1	2	1	4	2
Raw turnips	1 large	51	12	0	13	5	7	6	17	9
Raw turnip greens	1 cup, chopped	18	4	0	5	2	2	2	6	3

FOOD	AMOUNT	CAL	CARBS	FAT	WALK	RUN	BIKE	SWIM	YOGA	DANCE
Raw tomatoes	1 medium	22	5	0	6	2	3	3	7	4
Raw green tomatoes	1 medium	28	6	0	7	3	4	3	10	5
Raw watercress	1 cup, chopped	4	0	0	1	0	1	0	1	1
Raw zucchini	1 large	52	11	1	13	6	7	6	18	9
Fresh Vegetables, Starchy										
Raw cassava	1 cup	330	78	1	85	35	47	40	112	56
Raw sweet corn	1 medium ear	77	17	1	20	8	11	9	26	13
Raw jicama	1 medium	250	58	1	64	27	35	30	85	43
Raw parsnip	1 cup, slices	100	24	0	26	11	14	12	34	17
Raw edible-pod peas	1 cup, whole	26	5	0	7	3	4	3	9	4
Raw pumpkin	1 cup	30	8	0	8	3	4	4	10	5
Raw rutabaga	1 large	278	63	2	72	30	39	34	95	47
Raw taro	1 cup, sliced	116	28	0	30	12	17	14	40	20
Raw wasabi root	1 cup, sliced	142	31	1	37	15	20	17	48	24
Cooked Vegetables										
Cooked artichoke	.5 cup	42	9	0	11	4	6	5	14	7
Cooked asparagus	.5 cup	20	4	0	5	2	3	2	7	3
Cooked bamboo shoots	1 cup	14	2	0	4	2	2	2	5	2
Cooked beets	.5 cup, slices	37	8	0	10	4	5	5	13	6
Cooked broccoli	.5 cup, chopped	22	4	0	6	2	3	3	7	4
Cooked broccoli rabe	1 bunch, cooked (437 g)	144	14	2	37	15	20	18	49	25
Cooked Brussels sprouts	.5 cup	32	7	0	8	3	5	4	11	5
Cooked cabbage	1 cup, shredded	33	7	1	9	4	5	4	11	6
Cooked Chinese cabbage	1 cup, shredded	20	3	0	5	2	3	2	7	3
Cooked red cabbage	1 cup, shredded	44	10	0	11	5	6	5	15	7
Cooked Savoy cabbage	1 cup, shredded	35	8	0	9	4	5	4	12	6

FOOD	AMOUNT	CAL	CARBS	FAT	WALK	RUN	BIKE	SWIM	YOGA	DANCE
Cooked carrots	.5 cup, slices	27	6	0	7	3	4	3	9	5
Cooked cauliflower	1 cup, pieces	29	5	1	7	3	4	4	10	5
Cooked celery	1 cup, diced	27	6	0	7	3	4	3	9	5
Cooked Swiss chard	1 cup, chopped	35	7	0	9	4	5	4	12	6
Red hot chili peppers in sauce	1 cup	51	10	1	13	5	7	6	17	9
Green immature hot chili peppers in sauce	1 cup	49	12	0	13	5	7	6	17	8
Cooked collard greens	1 cup, chopped	49	9	1	13	5	7	6	17	8
Cooked sweet corn	1 medium ear	111	26	1	29	12	16	14	38	19
Cooked daikon	1 cup, slices	25	5	0	6	3	4	3	9	4
Cooked dandelion greens	1 cup, chopped	35	7	1	9	4	5	4	12	6
Cooked eggplant	1 cup, cubes	35	9	0	9	4	5	4	12	6
Cooked jicama	3 oz	32	8	0	8	3	5	4	11	5
Cooked kale	1 cup, chopped	36	7	1	9	4	5	4	12	6
Cooked kohlrabi	1 cup, sliced	48	11	0	12	5	7	6	16	8
Cooked leeks	1 cup, chopped	32	8	0	8	3	5	4	11	5
Cooked mushrooms	1 cup, pieces	44	8	1	11	5	6	5	15	7
Grilled portobello mushrooms	2 oz	20	3	0	5	2	3	2	7	3
Cooked shiitake mushrooms	1 cup, pieces	80	21	0	21	8	11	10	27	14
Cooked mustard greens	1 cup, chopped	21	3	0	5	2	3	3	7	4
Cooked okra	.5 cup, slices	18	4	0	5	2	2	2	6	3
Cooked onions	1 cup	92	21	0	24	10	13	11	31	16
Baked breaded onion rings (from frozen)	10 medium rings	244	23	16	63	26	35	30	83	42

FOOD	AMOUNT	CAL	CARBS	FAT	WALK	RUN	BIKE	SWIM	YOGA	DANCE
Cooked parsnip	1 cup, slices	126	30	0	32	13	18	15	43	21
Cooked edible-pod peas	1 cup	67	11	0	17	7	10	8	23	11
Cooked green peas	1 cup	134	25	0	35	14	19	16	46	23
Cooked green pepper	1 cup, chopped	50	12	0	13	5	7	6	17	9
Sautéed green pepper	2 oz	71	2	7	18	8	10	9	24	12
Cooked red pepper (sweet)	1 cup, strips	38	9	0	10	4	5	5	13	6
Sautéed red pepper (sweet)	2 oz	81	4	7	21	9	11	10	28	14
Poi	1 cup	269	65	0	69	29	38	33	91	46
Baked potato skin	1 skin	115	27	0	30	12	16	14	39	20
Baked red potato	1 potato, large	266	59	0	69	28	38	32	90	45
Baked russet potato	1 potato, large	290	64	0	75	31	41	35	99	49
Baked white potato	1 potato, large	281	63	0	72	30	40	34	96	48
Boiled potatoes	1 cup	136	31	0	35	14	19	17	46	23
Homemade au gratin potatoes (with butter)	1 cup	323	28	19	83	34	46	39	110	55
Homemade hash browns	1 cup	413	55	20	107	44	59	50	141	70
Homemade mashed potatoes (with whole milk)	1 cup	174	37	1	45	19	25	21	59	30
Homemade mashed potatoes (with whole milk and butter)	1 cup	237	35	9	61	25	34	29	81	40
Homemade scalloped potatoes (with butter)	1 cup	211	26	9	54	22	30	26	72	36
Mashed potatoes, from flakes (with whole milk and butter)	1 cup	204	23	11	53	22	29	25	69	35
Cooked pumpkin	1 cup, mashed	49	12	0	13	5	7	6	17	8
Cooked rutabaga	1 cup, cubes	66	15	0	17	7	9	8	22	11
Cooked spinach	1 cup	41	7	0	11	4	6	5	14	7
Cooked summer squash	1 cup, slices	36	8	1	9	4	5	4	12	6
Cooked spaghetti squash	1 cup	42	10	0	11	4	6	5	14	7
Baked acorn squash	1 cup, cubes	115	30	0	30	12	16	14	39	20

FOOD	AMOUNT	CAL	CARBS	FAT	WALK	RUN	BIKE	SWIM	YOGA	DANCE
Mashed acorn squash	1 cup, mashed	83	22	0	21	9	12	10	28	14
Cooked butternut squash	1 cup, cubes	82	22	0	21	9	12	10	28	14
Succotash	1 cup	221	47	2	57	24	31	27	75	38
Baked sweet potato	1 large	162	37	0	42	17	23	20	55	28
Boiled sweet potato	1 cup, mashed	249	58	0	64	27	35	30	85	42
Candied sweet potato	3 oz	122	24	3	31	13	17	15	41	21
Cooked taro	1 cup, slices	187	46	0	48	20	27	23	64	32
Cooked taro leaves	1 cup	35	6	1	9	4	5	4	12	6
Cooked tomatoes	1 cup	43	10	0	11	5	6	5	15	7
Cooked turnips	1 cup	36	7	0	9	4	5	4	12	6
Cooked turnip greens	1 cup, chopped	29	6	0	7	3	4	4	10	5
Cooked yams	1 cup, cubes	158	38	0	41	17	22	19	54	27
Cooked zucchini	1 cup, slices	29	7	0	7	3	4	4	10	5
Homemade corn pudding	1 cup	328	43	13	85	35	47	40	112	56
Homemade spinach soufflé	1 cup	233	8	18	60	25	33	28	79	40
Kohinoor Sarson Ka Saag	⅓ pack (100 g)	123	8	9	32	13	17	15	42	21
Kohinoor Aloo Ki Sabzi	⅓ pack (100 g)	83	13	3	21	9	12	10	28	14
Canned Vegetables										
Canned asparagus	.5 cup	18	3	0	5	2	3	2	6	3
Canned bamboo shoots	1 cup	25	4	1	6	3	4	3	8	4
Canned beets	1 cup	74	18	0	19	8	10	9	25	13
Canned carrots	.5 cup, slices	28	7	0	7	3	4	3	10	5
Canned sweet corn	1 cup	164	39	1	42	17	23	20	56	28
Canned creamed sweet corn	1 cup	184	46	1	48	20	26	22	63	31
Canned corn with red and green peppers	1 cup	170	41	1	44	18	24	21	58	29
Canned mushrooms	1 cup	39	8	0	10	4	6	5	13	7
Canned onions	.5 cup	21	5	0	5	2	3	3	7	4
Canned hearts of palm	1 cup	41	7	1	11	4	6	5	14	7

FOOD	AMOUNT	CAL	CARBS	FAT	WALK	RUN	BIKE	SWIM	YOGA	DANCE
Canned green peas	1 cup	131	24	1	34	14	19	16	45	22
Canned peas and onions	1 cup	61	10	0	16	7	9	7	21	10
Canned peas and carrots	1 cup	97	22	1	25	10	14	12	33	17
Canned green pepper (sweet)	1 cup, halves	25	5	0	6	3	4	3	9	4
Canned hot chili peppers	1 cup, chopped or diced	29	7	0	7	3	4	4	10	5
Canned jalapeño peppers	1 cup, slices	28	5	1	7	3	4	3	10	5
Canned red pepper (sweet)	1 cup	25	5	0	6	3	4	3	9	4
Canned potatoes	1 cup, whole	132	30	0	34	14	19	16	45	22
Canned pumpkin	1 cup	83	20	1	21	9	12	10	28	14
Canned pumpkin pie mix	1 cup	281	71	0	72	30	40	34	96	48
Canned spinach	1 cup	44	7	1	11	5	6	5	15	8
Canned succotash (with cream-style corn)	1 cup	205	47	1	53	22	29	25	70	35
Canned succotash (with corn kernels)	1 cup	161	36	1	41	17	23	20	55	27
Canned summer squash	1 cup, diced	27	6	0	7	3	4	3	9	5
Canned sweet potatoes, in syrup	1 cup	203	48	0	52	22	29	25	69	35
Canned sweet potato	1 cup, cubes	182	42	0	47	19	26	22	62	31
Canned mashed sweet potato	1 cup	258	59	1	66	27	37	31	88	44
Canned stewed tomatoes	1 cup	66	16	0	17	7	9	8	23	11
Canned whole tomatoes	1 cup	41	9	0	11	4	6	5	14	7
Canned turnip greens	1 cup	33	6	1	9	4	5	4	11	6
Canned mixed vegetables	1 cup	88	17	1	23	9	13	11	30	15
Canned waterchestnuts	1 cup, slices	70	17	0	18	7	10	9	24	12
Canned crushed tomatoes	3 oz	27	6	0	7	3	4	3	9	5
Canned Italian-style zucchini	1 cup	66	16	0	17	7	9	8	22	11
Frozen Vegetables										
Frozen artichokes	1 package (9 oz)	97	20	1	25	10	14	12	33	17
Frozen asparagus	1 package (10 oz)	68	12	1	18	7	10	8	23	12

FOOD	AMOUNT	CAL	CARBS	FAT	WALK	RUN	BIKE	SWIM	YOGA	DANCE
Frozen chopped broccoli	1 package (10 oz)	74	14	1	19	8	10	9	25	13
Frozen broccoli spears	1 package (10 oz)	82	15	1	21	9	12	10	28	14
Frozen Brussels sprouts	1 package (10 oz)	116	22	1	30	12	17	14	40	20
Frozen carrots	.5 cup, slices	23	5	0	6	2	3	3	8	4
Frozen collard greens	1 package	94	18	1	24	10	13	11	32	16
Frozen cauliflower	1 package (10 oz)	68	13	1	18	7	10	8	23	12
Frozen sweet corn kernels	1 cup	144	34	1	37	15	20	18	49	25
Frozen sweet corn on the cob	1 ear	122	29	1	31	13	17	15	41	21
Frozen kale	1 package (10 oz)	80	14	1	20	8	11	10	27	14
Frozen mustard greens	1 cup, chopped	29	5	0	8	3	4	4	10	5
Frozen onions	1 package (10 oz)	99	24	0	26	11	14	12	34	17
Frozen okra	1 package (10 oz)	85	19	1	22	9	12	10	29	15
Frozen green peas	1 cup	111	20	1	29	12	16	14	38	19
Frozen edible-pod peas	1 cup	60	10	0	15	6	9	7	20	10
Frozen peas and carrots	1 cup	74	16	1	19	8	10	9	25	13
Frozen peas and onions	1 cup	97	19	0	25	10	14	12	33	17
Frozen hash browns	1 patty (1 oz)	63	8	3	16	7	9	8	22	11
Frozen hash browns (with butter sauce)	3 oz	151	21	7	39	16	21	18	51	26
Frozen potatoes O'Brien	3 oz	173	19	11	45	18	25	21	59	29
Frozen green pepper (sweet)	1 package (10 oz)	57	13	1	15	6	8	7	19	10
Frozen red pepper (sweet)	1 package (10 oz)	57	13	1	15	6	8	7	19	10
Frozen potato puffs	2 oz	98	15	4	25	10	14	12	33	17
Frozen whole potatoes	1 cup	142	32	0	37	15	20	17	48	24
Frozen French fries	10 strips	131	22	4	34	14	19	16	45	22
Frozen spinach	1 cup	48	7	1	12	5	7	6	16	8
Frozen butternut squash	1 package (12 oz)	194	49	0	50	21	27	24	66	33

FOOD	AMOUNT	CAL	CARBS	FAT	WALK	RUN	BIKE	SWIM	YOGA	DANCE
Frozen summer squash	1 cup, slices	26	6	0	7	3	4	3	9	4
Frozen succotash	1 cup	145	31	1	37	15	21	18	49	25
Frozen sweet potato	1 cup, cubes	169	39	0	44	18	24	21	57	29
Frozen turnips	1 package, mashed (10 oz)	45	8	0	12	5	6	6	15	8
Frozen turnip greens	1 cup, chopped or diced	36	7	1	9	4	5	4	12	6
Frozen mixed vegetables	1 package	182	38	1	47	19	26	22	62	31
Frozen zucchini	1 package	48	10	0	12	5	7	6	16	8
Dried Vegetables										
Dried daikon	.25 cup	79	18	0	20	8	11	10	27	13
Dried shiitake mushrooms	4 mushrooms (15 g)	44	11	0	11	5	6	5	15	7
Sun-dried tomatoes	1 cup	139	30	2	36	15	20	17	47	24
Sun-dried tomatoes, packed in oil	1 cup	234	26	15	60	25	33	29	80	40
Pickled vegetables										
Pickled beets	1 cup, slices	148	37	0	38	16	21	18	50	25
Dill pickles	5 spears	27	6	0	7	3	4	3	9	5
Sweet cucumber pickles	5 gherkins	146	40	0	38	16	21	18	50	25
Sour cucumber pickles	5 spears	16	3	0	4	2	2	2	5	3
Bread and butter pickles	1 cup	138	32	0	36	15	20	17	47	24
Canned pimento	1 tbsp	3	1	0	1	0	0	0	1	1
Pickle relish	1 tbsp	14	4	0	4	1	2	2	5	2
Sweet pickle relish	1 tbsp	20	5	0	5	2	3	2	7	3
Salads										
Homemade coleslaw	.5 cup	41	7	2	11	4	6	5	14	7
Homemade potato salad	1 cup	358	28	21	92	38	51	43	122	61
Canned sauerkraut	1 cup	27	6	0	7	3	4	3	9	5
Tomatoes / Tomato Products										
Raw green tomatoes	1 medium	28	6	0	7	3	4	3	10	5
Raw tomatoes	1 medium	22	5	0	6	2	3	3	7	4

FOOD	AMOUNT	CAL	CARBS	FAT	WALK	RUN	BIKE	SWIM	YOGA	DANCE
Tomato sauce	1 cup	78	18	1	20	8	11	10	27	13
Tomato sauce (with mushrooms)	1 cup	86	21	0	22	9	12	10	29	15
Tomato sauce (with onions)	1 cup	103	24	0	27	11	15	13	35	18
Tomato sauce (with cheese)	.5 cup	144	25	5	37	15	20	18	49	25
Canned crushed tomatoes	3 oz	27	6	0	7	3	4	3	9	5
Canned stewed tomatoes	1 cup	66	16	0	17	7	9	8	23	11
Canned whole tomatoes	1 cup	41	9	0	11	4	6	5	14	7
Cooked tomatoes	1 cup	43	10	0	11	5	6	5	15	7
Tomato juice	1 cup	41	10	0	11	4	6	5	14	7
Tomato paste	1 cup	215	50	1	55	23	30	26	73	37
Tomato puree	1 cup	95	22	1	24	10	13	12	32	16
Homemade catsup	1 tbsp	15	4	0	4	2	2	2	5	3
Heinz Ketchup	1 tbsp	15	4	0	4	2	2	2	5	3
Stewed tomatoes	1 cup	80	13	3	21	8	11	10	27	14
Potatoes										
Baked potato skin	1 skin	115	27	0	30	12	16	14	39	20
Baked red potato	1 large	266	59	0	69	28	38	32	90	45
Baked russet potato	1 large	290	64	0	75	31	41	35	99	49
Baked white potato	1 large	281	63	0	72	30	40	34	96	48
Boiled potatoes	1 cup	136	31	0	35	14	19	17	46	23
Canned potatoes	1 cup, whole	132	30	0	34	14	19	16	45	22
Homemade au gratin potatoes (with butter)	1 cup	323	28	19	83	34	46	39	110	55
Homemade hash browns	1 cup	413	55	20	107	44	59	50	141	70
Homemade mashed potatoes (with whole milk and butter)	1 cup	237	35	9	61	25	34	29	81	40
Homemade mashed potatoes (with whole milk)	1 cup	174	37	1	45	19	25	21	59	30
Homemade scalloped potatoes (with butter)	1 cup	211	26	9	54	22	30	26	72	36
Mashed potatoes, from flakes (with whole milk and butter)	1 cup	204	23	11	53	22	29	25	69	35
Frozen French fries	10 strips	131	22	4	34	14	19	16	45	22
Frozen potato puffs	2 oz	98	15	4	25	10	14	12	33	17
Frozen whole potatoes	1 cup	142	32	0	37	15	20	17	48	24
Baked sweet potato	1 large	162	37	0	42	17	23	20	55	28

FOOD	AMOUNT	CAL	CARBS	FAT	WALK	RUN	BIKE	SWIM	YOGA	DANCE
Boiled sweet potato	1 cup, mashed	249	58	0	64	27	35	30	85	42
Candied sweet potato	3 oz	122	24	3	31	13	17	15	41	21
Canned sweet potatoes in syrup	1 cup	203	48	0	52	22	29	25	69	35
Canned sweet potato	1 cup, cubes	182	42	0	47	19	26	22	62	31
Canned mashed sweet potato	1 cup	258	59	1	66	27	37	31	88	44
Frozen sweet potato	1 cup, cubes	169	39	0	44	18	24	21	57	29
Homemade potato pancakes	1 medium	100	10	5	26	11	14	12	34	17
Homemade potato salad	1 cup	358	28	21	92	38	51	43	122	61

Breakfast Foods

French toast										
Homemade French toast (with 2% milk)	1 slice (65 g)	149	16	7	38	16	21	18	51	25
Frozen French toast	1 slice (59 g)	126	19	4	32	13	18	15	43	21
French toast (with butter)	1 slice (67.5 g)	178	18	9	46	19	25	22	61	30
French toast sticks	5 sticks	513	58	29	132	55	73	62	174	87
Aunt Jemima Original French Toast	2 slices	240	39	6	62	26	34	29	82	41
Aunt Jemima Cinnamon French Toast	2 slices	220	34	6	57	23	31	27	75	37
Aunt Jemima Cinnamon French Toast Sticks	4 sticks	350	52	13	90	37	50	43	119	60
Pancakes										
Homemade plain pancakes	2 6" pancakes	350	44	15	90	37	50	43	119	60
Homemade buttermilk pancakes	2 6" pancakes	350	44	14	90	37	50	43	119	60
Homemade blueberry pancakes	2 6" pancakes	342	45	14	88	36	49	42	116	58
Plain pancakes (prepared from mix)	2 6" pancakes	336	45	12	87	36	48	41	114	57
Whole-wheat pancakes (prepared from mix)	2 6" pancakes	537	76	17	138	57	76	65	183	91

FOOD	AMOUNT	CAL	CARBS	FAT	WALK	RUN	BIKE	SWIM	YOGA	DANCE
Frozen pancakes	2 6" pancakes	328	57	8	85	35	47	40	112	56
Aunt Jemima Original Pancakes	3 pancakes	210	40	4	54	22	30	26	71	36
Aunt Jemima Buttermilk Pancakes	3 pancakes	210	40	4	54	22	30	26	71	36
Aunt Jemima Mini Pancakes	13 pancakes	240	46	4	62	26	34	29	82	41
Kellogg's Eggo Pancakes	3 pancakes	270	44	8	70	29	38	33	92	46
Krusteaz Frozen Mini Buttermilk Pancakes	1 serving	116	22	2	30	12	16	14	39	20
Maple and Pancake Syrup										
Pancake syrup	.25 cup	184	48	0	47	20	26	22	63	31
Pancake syrup (with 2% maple)	.25 cup	209	55	0	54	22	30	25	71	36
Reduced-calorie pancake syrup	.25 cup	98	27	0	25	10	14	12	33	17
Maple syrup	.25 cup	210	54	0	54	22	30	26	71	36
Eggo Original Syrup	.25 cup	240	60	0	62	26	34	29	82	41
Aunt Jemima Pancake and Waffle Syrup	.25 cup	210	52	0	54	22	30	26	71	36
Aunt Jemima Lite Syrup	.25 cup	100	26	0	26	11	14	12	34	17
Aunt Jemima Butter Rich Syrup	.25 cup	210	52	0	54	22	30	26	71	36
Aunt Jemima Butter Lite Syrup	.25 cup	100	26	0	26	11	14	12	34	17
Maple Grove Farms Pure Maple Syrup	.25 cup	200	53	0	52	21	28	24	68	34
Log Cabin Original Syrup	.25 cup	210	53	0	54	22	30	26	71	36
Mrs. Butterworth Original Syrup	.25 cup	220	55	0	57	23	31	27	75	37
Waffles										
Homemade waffles	1 7" round waffle	218	25	11	56	23	31	27	74	37
Aunt Jemima Original Waffles	1 serving	197	30	6	51	21	28	24	67	34
Belgian Chef Low Fat Waffles	2 waffles	180	34	2	46	19	26	22	61	31
Eggo Homestyle Waffles	2 waffles	190	29	7	49	20	27	23	65	32
Eggo Mini Homestyle Waffles	12 mini waffles	260	38	9	67	28	37	32	88	44
Eggo Nutri-Grain Whole Wheat Waffles	2 waffles	170	28	5	44	18	24	21	58	29

FOOD	AMOUNT	CAL	CARBS	FAT	WALK	RUN	BIKE	SWIM	YOGA	DANCE
Eggo Special K Fat Free Waffles	2 waffles	120	26	0	31	13	17	15	41	20
Eggo Buttermilk Waffles	2 waffles	190	28	7	49	20	27	23	65	32
Eggo Blueberry Waffles	2 waffles	190	30	7	49	20	27	23	65	32
Eggo Strawberry Waffles	2 waffles	200	30	7	52	21	28	24	68	34
Eggo Banana Bread Waffles	2 waffles	212	32	7	55	23	30	26	72	36
Eggo Golden Oat Waffles	2 waffles	139	26	2	36	15	20	17	47	24
Eggo Chocolate Chip Waffles	2 waffles	200	32	7	52	21	28	24	68	34
Eggo Cinnamon Toast Waffles	12 mini waffles	290	46	20	75	31	41	35	99	49
Eggs										
Egg white	1 large	17	0	0	4	2	2	2	6	3
Hard-boiled whole egg	1 cup, chopped	211	2	14	54	22	30	26	72	36
Poached whole egg	1 large	74	0	5	19	8	10	9	25	13
Scrambled whole egg	1 large	101	1	7	26	11	14	12	34	17
Fleischmann's Egg Beaters	.25 cup	30	1	0	8	3	4	4	10	5
Health Is Wealth Egg Whites & Cheese Breakfast Munchees	2 Munchees	70	9	4	18	7	10	9	24	12
Bacon and Sausage										
Morningstar Farms Breakfast Sausage Links	2 links	80	3	3	21	9	11	10	27	14
Swift Premium Brown 'n Serve Beef Sausage Links	3 links	230	1	22	59	24	33	28	78	39
Swift Premium Brown 'n Serve Maple Sausage Links	3 links	210	2	19	54	22	30	26	71	36
Health Is Wealth Egg Whites, Meatless Ham & Cheese Breakfast Munchees	2 Munchees	70	9	3	18	7	10	9	24	12
Jones Golden Brown Patties	1 patty	150	1	14	39	16	21	18	51	26
Toaster Pastries										
Fruit-filled toaster pastry	1 pastry	204	37	5	53	22	29	25	69	35
Brown sugar and cinnamon toaster pastry	1 pastry	206	34	7	53	22	29	25	70	35
Pop-Tarts										
Apple cinnamon Pop Tarts	1 pastry	205	37	5	53	22	29	25	70	35
Blueberry Pop Tarts	1 pastry	212	36	7	55	23	30	26	72	36
Cherry Pop Tarts	1 pastry	204	37	5	53	22	29	25	69	35
Frosted blueberry Pop Tarts	1 pastry	203	37	5	52	22	29	25	69	35

FOOD	AMOUNT	CAL	CARBS	FAT	WALK	RUN	BIKE	SWIM	YOGA	DANCE
Frosted cherry Pop Tarts	1 pastry	204	37	5	53	22	29	25	69	35
Frosted chocolate fudge Pop Tarts	1 pastry	201	37	5	52	21	29	24	68	34
Frosted chocolate vanilla crème Pop Tarts	1 pastry	203	37	5	52	22	29	25	69	35
Milk chocolate Pop Tarts	1 pastry	205	36	6	53	22	29	25	70	35
Strawberry Pop Tarts	1 pastry	200	37	5	52	21	28	24	68	34
Frosted brown sugar cinnamon Pop Tarts	1 pastry	210	34	7	54	22	30	26	71	36
Frosted strawberry with sprinkles Pop Tarts	1 pastry	200	38	5	52	21	28	24	68	34
S'mores Pop Tarts	1 pastry	200	36	6	52	21	28	24	68	34

Cereals

Basic Cereals										
Basic 4	1 cup	200	42	3	52	21	28	24	68	34
Cheerios	1 cup	110	22	2	28	12	16	13	37	19
Cinnamon Oatmeal Squares	1 cup	227	48	3	58	24	32	28	77	39
Corn Chex	1 cup	110	25	1	28	12	16	13	37	19
Corn Flakes	1 cup	100	24	0	26	11	14	12	34	17
Crispix	1 cup	110	25	0	28	12	16	13	37	19
Fiber One	.5 cup	60	24	1	15	6	9	7	20	10
General Mills Raisin Nut Bran	1.25 cup	200	44	3	52	21	28	24	68	34
Grape Nuts	.5 cup	210	47	1	54	22	30	26	71	36
Grape Nuts Flakes	.75 cup	110	24	1	28	12	16	13	37	19
Health Valley Organic Fiber 7 Multigrain Flakes	.75 cup	100	0	24	26	11	14	12	34	17
Honey Puffed Kashi	1 cup	120	25	1	31	13	17	15	41	20
Kashi GoLean	1 cup	140	30	1	36	15	20	17	48	24
Kashi GoLean Crunch	1 cup	190	36	3	49	20	27	23	65	32
Kashi Good Friends	1 cup	170	43	2	44	18	24	21	58	29
Kashi Heart To Heart	.75 cup	110	25	2	28	12	16	13	37	19
Kellogg's Fruit Harvest Strawberry Blueberry	.75 cup	110	24	2	28	12	16	13	37	19
Kellogg's Just Right Fruit and Nut	.75 cup	200	43	2	52	21	28	24	68	34
Kellogg's Raisin Bran	1 cup	190	45	2	49	20	27	23	65	32

FOOD	AMOUNT	CAL	CARBS	FAT	WALK	RUN	BIKE	SWIM	YOGA	DANCE
Kellogg's Raisin Bran Crunch	1 cup	190	45	1	49	20	27	23	65	32
Kellogg's Special K, with Red Berries	1 cup	110	25	0	28	12	16	13	37	19
Life	.75 cup	120	25	2	31	13	17	15	41	20
Mother's Peanut Butter Bumpers	1 cup	130	26	3	34	14	18	16	44	22
Multi-Grain Cheerios	1 cup	110	24	1	28	12	16	13	37	19
Oatmeal Crisp, Raisin	1 cup	210	44	2	54	22	30	26	71	36
Oatmeal Crisp with Almonds	1 cup	220	42	5	57	23	31	27	75	37
Oatmeal Squares	1 cup	210	44	3	54	22	30	26	71	36
Para Su Familia Raisin Bran	1.33 cup	170	42	1	44	18	24	21	58	29
Post Banana Nut Crunch Cereal	1 cup	240	44	6	62	26	34	29	82	41
Post Frosted Shredded Wheat	1 cup	180	43	1	46	19	26	22	61	31
Product 19	1 cup	100	25	0	26	11	14	12	34	17
Puffed Kashi	1 cup	70	13	1	18	7	10	9	24	12
Quaker Puffed Rice	1 cup	54	12	0	14	6	8	7	18	9
Quaker Puffed Wheat	1.25 cup	55	11	0	14	6	8	7	19	9
Quaker Uncle Sam Cereal	1 cup	237	36	6	61	25	34	29	81	40
Rice Chex	1.25 cup	120	27	0	31	13	17	15	41	20
Rice Krispies	1.25 cup	120	29	0	31	13	17	15	41	20
Smart Start	1 cup	180	43	1	46	19	26	22	61	31
Smart Start Soy Protein	1 cup	202	40	1	52	21	29	25	69	34
Special K	1 cup	110	22	0	28	12	16	13	37	19
Total Corn Flakes	1.333 cup	112	26	0	29	12	16	14	38	19
Total Raisin Bran	1 cup	170	41	1	44	18	24	21	58	29
Wheat Chex	1 cup	180	40	1	46	19	26	22	61	31
Wheaties	1 cup	110	24	1	28	12	16	13	37	19
Whole Grain Total	.75 cup	97	23	1	25	10	14	12	33	17
Kids Cereals										
Alpha-Bits	1 cup	110	22	2	28	12	16	13	37	19
Apple Cinnamon Cheerios	.75 cup	118	25	2	30	13	17	14	40	20
Apple Jacks	1 cup	130	30	1	34	14	18	16	44	22
Berry Berry Kix	.75 cup	118	26	1	30	13	17	14	40	20
Brown Sugar and Oat Total	.75 cup	102	23	1	26	11	14	12	35	17
Cap'N Crunch	.75 cup	110	23	2	28	12	16	13	37	19
Cap'N Crunch with Crunchberries	.75 cup	104	22	1	27	11	15	13	35	18

FOOD	AMOUNT	CAL	CARBS	FAT	WALK	RUN	BIKE	SWIM	YOGA	DANCE
Cinnamon Crunch Crispix	.75 cup	120	26	1	31	13	17	15	41	20
Cinnamon Life	.75 cup	120	25	2	31	13	17	15	41	20
Cinnamon Toast Crunch	.75 cup	130	24	4	34	14	18	16	44	22
Cinna-Raisin Crunch	1 cup	165	41	1	43	18	23	20	56	28
Cocoa Krispies	.75 cup	120	27	1	31	13	17	15	41	20
Cocoa Pebbles	.75 cup	120	25	2	31	13	17	15	41	20
Cocoa Puffs	1 cup	120	26	1	31	13	17	15	41	20
Cookie Crisp	1 cup	117	26	1	30	12	17	14	40	20
Corn Pops	1 cup	120	28	0	31	13	17	15	41	20
French Toast Crunch	.75 cup	120	26	2	31	13	17	15	41	20
Froot Loops	1 cup	120	28	1	31	13	17	15	41	20
Frosted Cheerios	1 cup	120	25	1	31	13	17	15	41	20
Frosted Flakes	.75 cup	120	28	0	31	13	17	15	41	20
Frosted Mini-Wheats	24 biscuits (59 g)	200	48	1	52	21	28	24	68	34
Fruity Pebbles	.75 cup	110	24	1	28	12	16	13	37	19
Golden Crisp	.75 cup	107	25	0	28	11	15	13	37	18
Golden Grahams	.75 cup	120	25	1	31	13	17	15	41	20
Honey Bunches of Oats	.75 cup	120	25	2	31	13	17	15	41	20
Honey Bunches of Oats with Almonds	.75 cup	130	24	3	34	14	18	16	44	22
Honey Graham Oh!s	.75 cup	110	23	2	28	12	16	13	37	19
Honey Nut Cheerios	1 cup	110	22	2	28	12	16	13	37	19
Honey Nut Clusters	1 cup	210	46	3	54	22	30	26	71	36
Honeycomb	1.333 cup	110	26	1	28	12	16	13	37	19
Honey-Nut Chex	.75 cup	120	26	1	31	13	17	15	41	20
Kellogg's Pokemon	1 cup	116	30	12	16	14	39	20		
Kellogg's Rice Krispies Treats	.75 cup	120	26	2	31	13	17	15	41	20
Kix	1.333 cup	120	26	1	31	13	17	15	41	20
Lucky Charms	1 cup	120	25	1	31	13	17	15	41	20
Malt-O-Meal Berry Colossal Crunch	.75 cup	120	26	2	31	13	17	15	41	20
Malt-O-Meal Coco Roos	.75 cup	119	27	1	31	13	17	14	40	20
Malt-O-Meal Colossal Crunch	.75 cup	124	26	2	32	13	18	15	42	21
Malt-O-Meal Crispy Rice	1 cup	126	29	0	32	13	18	15	43	21
Malt-O-Meal Honey Nut Toasty O's	1 cup	110	24	2	28	12	16	13	37	19

FOOD	AMOUNT	CAL	CARBS	FAT	WALK	RUN	BIKE	SWIM	YOGA	DANCE
Malt-O-Meal Marshmallow Mateys	1 cup	120	25	1	31	13	17	15	41	20
Malt-O-Meal Tootie Fruities	1 cup	130	28	1	34	14	18	16	44	22
Marshmallow Blasted Froot Loops	1 cup	118	27	1	30	13	17	14	40	20
Mother's Cinnamon Oat Crunch	1 cup	230	48	3	59	24	33	28	78	39
Mother's Groovy Grahams	.75 cup	100	24	1	26	11	14	12	34	17
Oreo O's	.75 cup	110	22	2	28	12	16	13	37	19
Quisp	1 cup	109	23	2	28	12	16	13	37	19
Reese's Puffs	.75 cup	130	23	4	34	14	18	16	44	22
Smacks	.75 cup	100	24	1	26	11	14	12	34	17
Trix	1 cup	120	27	1	31	13	17	15	41	20
Bran Cereals										
All-Bran Bran Buds	.333 cup	75	24	1	19	8	11	9	26	13
All-Bran	.5 cup	80	23	1	21	9	11	10	27	14
All-Bran with Extra Fiber	.5 cup	50	20	1	13	5	7	6	17	9
Cracklin' Oat Bran	.75 cup	200	35	7	52	21	28	24	68	34
Kellogg's Complete Oat Bran Flakes	.75 cup	110	23	1	28	12	16	13	37	19
Kellogg's Wheat Bran Flakes	.75 cup	90	23	1	23	10	13	11	31	15
Kretschmer Toasted Wheat Bran	.25 cup (16 g)	30	10	1	8	3	4	4	10	5
Kretschmer Wheat Germ	2 tbsp	50	6	1	13	5	7	6	17	9
Mother's Toasted Oat Bran	.75 cup	120	25	1	31	13	17	15	41	20
Multi-Bran Chex	1 cup	200	49	2	52	21	28	24	68	34
Post 100% Bran Cereal	.333 cup	80	22	1	21	9	11	10	27	14
Post Bran Flakes	.75 cup	100	24	1	26	11	14	12	34	17
Post Raisin Bran	1 cup	190	46	1	49	20	27	23	65	32
Post Shredded Wheat 'n Bran	1.25 cup	200	47	1	52	21	28	24	68	34
Post Shredded Wheat 'n Bran Spoon Size	1 cup	170	40	1	44	18	24	21	58	29
Quaker Crunchy Corn Bran	.75 cup	90	23	1	23	10	13	11	31	15
Granola and Mueslix										
Homemade granola	1 cup	598	65	30	154	64	85	73	203	102
Back to Nature Classic Granola	.5 cup	180	36	3	46	19	26	22	61	31
Back to Nature Raisin Granola	.5 cup	190	38	2	49	20	27	23	65	32
Kellogg's Low Fat Granola	.5 cup	190	39	3	49	20	27	23	65	32

OOD	AMOUNT	CAL	CARBS	FAT	WALK	RUN	BIKE	SWIM	YOGA	DANCE
Kellogg's Low Fat Granola with Raisins	.667 cup	220	48	3	57	23	31	27	75	37
Quaker 100% Natural Granola with Oats, Honey, and Raisins	.5 cup	237	38	10	61	25	34	29	81	40
Quaker 100% Natural Oats and Honey Granola	.5 cup	232	34	10	60	25	33	28	79	40
Quaker Low Fat 100% Natural Granola with Raisins	.5 cup	195	41	3	50	21	28	24	66	33
Mueslix	.667 cup	200	40	3	52	21	28	24	68	34
Hot Cereals										
Cream of rice (prepared with water)	1 cup	127	28	0	33	14	18	15	43	22
Dry oats (regular, quick, and instant)	1 cup	311	54	5	80	33	44	38	106	53
Farina (prepared with water)	1 cup	112	24	0	29	12	16	14	38	19
Flavored cream of wheat (apple, banana, or maple; prepared with water)	1 packet	132	29	0	34	14	19	16	45	22
Fortified instant oatmeal (prepared with water)	1 packet	97	17	2	25	10	14	12	33	17
Fortified instant raisins and spice oatmeal (prepared with water)	1 packet	158	32	2	41	17	22	19	54	27
Instant cheddar cheese-flavored corn grits (prepared with water)	1 packet	102	20	2	26	11	14	12	35	17
Instant corn grits (prepared with water)	1 cup	167	37	0	43	18	24	20	57	28
Instant corn grits, with bacon bits (prepared with water)	1 packet	97	21	0	25	10	14	12	33	17
Instant cream of wheat (prepared with water)	1 cup	149	32	1	39	16	21	18	51	25
Maltex (prepared with water)	1 cup	189	39	1	49	20	27	23	64	32
Malt-O-Meal (plain and chocolate; prepared with water)	1 cup	130	27	1	34	14	18	16	44	22
Mother's Oat Bran, dry	.5 cup	150	25	3	39	16	21	18	51	26
Oats (regular, quick, and Instant; prepared with water)	1 cup	145	25	2	37	15	21	18	49	25
Quaker Instant Apple Cinnamon Oatmeal (prepared with water)	1 packet	130	27	2	33	14	18	16	44	22
Quaker Instant Fruit & Cream Oatmeal (prepared with water)	1 packet	140	27	3	36	15	20	17	48	24

FOOD	AMOUNT	CAL	CARBS	FAT	WALK	RUN	BIKE	SWIM	YOGA	DANCE
Quaker Instant Maple Brown Sugar Oatmeal (prepared with water)	1 packet	160	33	2	41	17	23	19	54	27
Quaker Instant Oatmeal	1 packet	100	19	2	26	11	14	12	34	17
Quaker Instant Raisins and Spice Oatmeal (prepared with water)	1 packet	150	33	2	39	16	21	18	51	26
Quaker Instant Lower Sugar Apples & Cinnamon Oatmeal	1 packet	110	22	2	28	12	16	13	37	19
Quaker Oat Bran	.5 cup	150	25	3	39	16	21	18	51	26
Quaker Quick Oats, Dry	.5 cup	150	27	3	39	16	21	18	51	26
Quick cream of wheat (prepared with water)	1 cup	129	27	0	33	14	18	16	44	22
Wheatena (prepared with water)	1 cup	136	29	1	35	14	19	17	46	23
White or yellow corn grits, quick and regular (prepared with water)	1 cup	143	31	0	37	15	20	17	49	24

Breads

Bagels

FOOD	AMOUNT	CAL	CARBS	FAT	WALK	RUN	BIKE	SWIM	YOGA	DANCE
Cinnamon raisin bagel (3 ½" diameter)	1 bagel	194	0	1	50	21	28	24	66	33
Cinnamon raisin mini bagel (2 ½" diameter)	1 mini-bagel	71	14	0	18	8	10	9	24	12
Cinnamon raisin New York-style bagel (4 ½" diameter)	1 bagel	322	65	2	83	34	46	39	110	55
Egg bagel (3 ½" diameter)	1 bagel	292	56	2	75	31	41	36	99	50
Egg mini bagel (2 ½" diameter)	1 mini-bagel	72	14	1	19	8	10	9	24	12
Egg New York-style bagel (4 ½" diameter)	1 bagel	364	69	3	94	39	52	44	124	62
Oat bran bagel (3 ½" diameter)	1 bagel	181	38	1	47	19	26	22	62	31
Oat bran mini bagel (2 ½" diameter)	1 mini-bagel	66	14	0	17	7	9	8	22	11
Oat bran New York-style bagel (4 ½" diameter)	1 bagel	280	59	1	72	30	40	34	95	48
Plain bagel (3 ½" diameter)	1 bagel	289	56	2	74	31	41	35	98	49
Plain mini bagel (2 ½" diameter)	1 mini-bagel	72	14	0	19	8	10	9	24	12

FOOD	AMOUNT	CAL	CARBS	FAT	WALK	RUN	BIKE	SWIM	YOGA	DANCE
Plain New York-style bagel (4 ½" diameter)	1 bagel	360	70	2	93	38	51	44	122	61

■ Packaged Bagels

FOOD	AMOUNT	CAL	CARBS	FAT	WALK	RUN	BIKE	SWIM	YOGA	DANCE
Just Bagels Plain Bagel	1 bagel	280	62	0	72	30	40	34	95	48
Just Bagels Onion Bagel	1 bagel	280	62	1	72	30	40	34	95	48
Just Bagels Everything Bagel	1 bagel	280	62	1	72	30	40	34	95	48
Just Bagels Cinnamon Raisin Bagel	1 bagel	280	64	0	72	30	40	34	95	48
Just Bagels Poppy Bagel	1 bagel	280	62	1	72	30	40	34	95	48
Just Bagels Sesame Bagel	1 bagel	280	62	1	72	30	40	34	95	48
Lender's Plain Bagel	1 bagel	150	30	1	39	16	21	18	51	26
Lender's Plain Bagelettes	1 bagel	130	26	1	34	14	18	16	44	22
Lender's Cinnamon Raisin Bagel	1 bagel	160	32	1	41	17	23	19	54	27
Lender's Onion Bagel	1 bagel	150	30	1	39	16	21	18	51	26
Lender's Big 'N Crusty Blueberry Bagel	1 serving	214	46	1	55	23	30	26	73	36
Lender's Premium Refrigerated Blueberry Bagel	1 bagel	209	42	1	54	22	30	25	71	36
Lender's Bagel Shop Blueberry Bagel	1 bagel	264	53	2	68	28	37	32	90	45
Thomas' Mini Bagel	1 mini-bagel	130	26	1	34	14	18	16	44	22
Thomas' Whole Wheat Bagel	1 bagel	270	55	2	70	29	38	33	92	46

■ Takeout Bagels

FOOD	AMOUNT	CAL	CARBS	FAT	WALK	RUN	BIKE	SWIM	YOGA	DANCE
Dunkin' Donuts Cinnamon Raisin Bagel	1 bagel	330	65	3	85	35	47	40	112	56
Dunkin' Donuts Plain Bagel	1 bagel	320	62	3	82	34	45	39	109	55
Dunkin' Donuts Sesame Bagel	1 bagel	380	64	8	98	40	54	46	129	65
Dunkin' Donuts Poppyseed Bagel	1 bagel	370	65	7	95	39	52	45	126	63
Dunkin' Donuts Onion Bagel	1 bagel	320	61	4	82	34	45	39	109	55
Dunkin' Donuts Wheat Bagel	1 bagel	330	62	4	85	35	47	40	112	56
Dunkin' Donuts Multigrain Bagel	1 bagel	380	68	6	98	40	54	46	129	65
Dunkin' Donuts Everything Bagel	1 bagel	370	67	6	95	39	52	45	126	63
Dunkin' Donuts Blueberry Bagel	1 bagel	330	66	3	85	35	47	40	112	56
Dunkin' Donuts Salsa Bagel	1 bagel	310	60	3	80	33	44	38	105	53

FOOD	AMOUNT	CAL	CARBS	FAT	WALK	RUN	BIKE	SWIM	YOGA	DANCE
Dunkin' Donuts Harvest Bagel	1 bagel	350	61	6	90	37	50	43	119	60
Dunkin' Donuts Reduced Carb Bagel with Cheese	1 bagel	380	45	12	98	40	54	46	129	65
Dunkin' Donuts Salt Bagel	1 bagel	320	62	3	82	34	45	39	109	55
Einstein Bros. Plain Bagel	1 bagel	320	71	1	82	34	45	39	109	55
Einstein Bros. Jalapeño Bagel	1 bagel	310	68	1	80	33	44	38	105	53
Einstein Bros. Asiago Bagel	1 bagel	360	71	3	93	38	51	44	122	61
Einstein Bros. Chopped Onion Bagel	1 bagel	330	71	1	85	35	47	40	112	56
Einstein Bros. Everything Bagel	1 bagel	340	75	2	88	36	48	41	116	58
Einstein Bros. Potato Bagel	1 bagel	350	69	5	90	37	50	43	119	60
Einstein Bros. Cinnamon Raisin Swirl Bagel	1 bagel	350	78	1	90	37	50	43	119	60
Einstein Bros. Cinnamon Sugar Bagel	1 bagel	500	72	21	129	53	71	61	170	85
Einstein Bros. Powerbagel	1 bagel	410	81	5	106	44	58	50	139	70
Einstein Bros. Chocolate Chip Bagel	1 bagel	370	76	3	95	39	52	45	126	63
Einstein Bros. Poppy Dip Bagel	1 bagel	350	74	2	90	37	50	43	119	60
Einstein Bros. Wild Blueberry Bagel	1 bagel	350	77	1	90	37	50	43	119	60
Einstein Bros. Egg Bagel	1 bagel	340	69	3	88	36	48	41	116	58
Einstein Bros. Salt Bagel	1 bagel	330	73	1	85	35	47	40	112	56
Einstein Bros. Sesame Dipped Bagel	1 bagel	380	75	5	98	40	54	46	129	65
Einstein Bros. Pumpernickel Bagel	1 bagel	320	68	1	82	34	45	39	109	55
Einstein Bros. Cranberry Bagel	1 bagel	350	78	1	90	37	50	43	119	60
Einstein Bros. Sun-Dried Tomato Bagel	1 bagel	320	69	1	82	34	45	39	109	55
Einstein Bros. Honey Whole Wheat Bagel	1 bagel	320	71	1	82	34	45	39	109	55
Panera Bread Plain Bagel	1 bagel	290	61	1	75	31	41	35	99	49
Panera Bread Whole Grain Bagel	1 bagel	340	66	3	88	36	48	41	116	58
Panera Bread Everything Bagel	1 bagel	300	60	2	77	32	43	36	102	51
Panera Bread Sesame Bagel	1 bagel	310	59	4	80	33	44	38	105	53
Panera Bread French Toast Bagel	1 bagel	380	73	5	98	40	54	46	129	65

FOOD	AMOUNT	CAL	CARBS	FAT	WALK	RUN	BIKE	SWIM	YOGA	DANCE
Panera Bread Dutch Apple & Raisin Bagel	1 bagel	370	78	3	95	39	52	45	126	63
Panera Bread Asiago Cheese Bagel	1 bagel	350	60	6	90	37	50	43	119	60
Panera Bread Blueberry Bagel	1 bagel	330	69	2	85	35	47	40	112	56
Panera Bread Choc-O-Nut Bagel	1 bagel	440	76	11	113	47	62	54	150	75
Panera Bread Cinnamon Crunch Bagel	1 bagel	410	74	8	106	44	58	50	139	70
Panera Bread Cranberry Walnut Bagel	1 bagel	360	68	5	93	38	51	44	122	61
Starbucks Plain Bagel	1 bagel	430	92	1	111	46	61	52	146	73
Starbucks Cinnamon Raisin Bagel	1 bagel	440	96	1	113	47	62	54	150	75
Starbucks Sesame Bagel	1 bagel	440	92	3	113	47	62	54	150	75
Biscuits										
Biscuits made from low-fat refrigerated dough	1 biscuit (2 ¼" diameter)	63	12	1	16	7	9	8	21	11
Biscuits made from refrigerated dough	1 biscuit (2 ½" diameter)	94	13	4	24	10	13	11	32	16
Homemade biscuits	1 biscuit (2 ½" diameter)	212	27	10	55	23	30	26	72	36
Plain or buttermilk biscuit	1 biscuit (2 ½" diameter)	128	17	6	33	14	18	16	44	22
Plain or buttermilk biscuit (prepared from mix)	1 biscuit (2 ½" diameter)	117	17	4	30	12	17	14	40	20
Dunkin' Donuts Biscuit	1 biscuit	250	29	13	64	27	35	30	85	43
Pillsbury Buttermilk Biscuits	1 biscuit (34 g)	100	14	5	26	11	14	12	34	17
Pillsbury Grands Flaky Biscuits	1 biscuit (61 g)	200	25	9	52	21	28	24	68	34
Pillsbury Grands Flaky Buttermilk Biscuits	1 biscuit (58 g)	190	23	9	49	20	27	23	65	32
Pillsbury Grands Homestyle Biscuits	1 biscuit (58 g)	180	24	8	46	19	26	22	61	31
Pillsbury Hungry Jack Buttermilk Biscuits	1 biscuit (34 g)	100	14	5	26	11	14	12	34	17

FOOD	AMOUNT	CAL	CARBS	FAT	WALK	RUN	BIKE	SWIM	YOGA	DANCE
White bread										
White bread	1 large slice (30 g)	80	15	1	21	9	11	10	27	14
Reduced-calorie white bread	1 slice (23 g)	48	10	1	12	5	7	6	16	8
Homemade white bread (made with 2% milk)	1 slice (42 g)	120	21	2	31	13	17	15	41	20
Homemade white bread (made with nonfat milk)	1slice (44 g)	121	24	1	31	13	17	15	41	21
Arnold Brick Oven White Bread	2 slices (48 g)	140	25	3	36	15	20	17	48	24
Arnold Country White Bread	1 slice (38 g)	110	20	2	28	12	16	13	37	19
Dutch Country Stroehmann Honey White Bread	1 slice (35 g)	90	18	1	23	10	13	11	31	15
Pepperidge Farm White Sandwich Bread	2 slices	130	23	3	34	14	18	16	44	22
Wonder White Bread	2 slices (43 g)	110	20	2	28	12	16	13	37	19
Whole-Wheat Bread										
Whole-wheat bread	1 slice (28 g)	69	13	1	18	7	10	8	23	12
Homemade Whole-wheat bread	1 slice (46 g)	128	24	2	33	14	18	16	44	22
Arnold Stoneground 100% Whole Wheat Bread	1 slice (27 g)	60	12	1	15	6	9	7	20	10
Arnold Carb Counting Whole Wheat Bread	1 slice (27 g)	60	9	2	15	6	9	7	20	10
Arnold Bakery Light Whole Wheat Bread	2 slices (43 g)	80	19	1	21	9	11	10	27	14
Arnold Natural Whole Wheat Bread	1 slice (38 g)	90	16	1	23	10	13	11	31	15
Arnold Hearty Whole Wheat Bread	1 slice (38 g)	90	18	1	23	10	13	11	31	15
Dutch Country Stroehmann 100% Whole Wheat Bread	1 slice (38 g)	90	17	2	23	10	13	11	31	15
Pepperidge Farm 100% Whole Wheat Natural Whole Grain	1 slice	110	20	2	28	12	16	13	37	19
Pepperidge Farm Very Thin Sliced 100% Whole Wheat	3 slices	110	20	2	28	12	16	13	37	19

FOOD	AMOUNT	CAL	CARBS	FAT	WALK	RUN	BIKE	SWIM	YOGA	DANCE
Vermont Bread Company Soft Whole Wheat Bread	1 slice (38 g)	70	15	1	18	7	10	9	24	12
Vermont Bread Company Sour Dough Whole Wheat Bread	1 slice (33 g)	70	15	0	18	7	10	9	24	12
Wheat Bread										
Wheat bread	1 slice (25 g)	65	12	102	17	7	9	8	22	11
Reduced-calorie wheat bread	1 slice (23 g)	46	10	1	12	5	7	6	16	8
Cracked wheat bread	1 slice (25 g)	65	12	1	17	7	9	8	22	11
Dutch Country Stroehmann Honey Cracked Wheat Bread	1 slice (35 g)	90	18	1	23	10	13	11	31	15
Home Pride Wheat Bread	1 slice (28 g)	80	14	1	21	9	11	10	27	14
Pepperidge Farm Light Soft Wheat	1 slice	45	9	1	12	5	6	5	15	8
Vermont Bread Company Organic Wheat Bread	1 slice (31 g)	70	15	0	18	7	10	9	24	12
Grain Bread										
Mixed-grain bread	1 slice (32 g)	80	15	1	21	9	11	10	27	14
Homemade multigrain bread	1 slice (37 g)	110	21	1	28	12	16	13	37	19
Arnold Carb Counting Multi Grain Bread	1 slice (27 g)	60	9	2	15	6	9	7	20	10
Arnold 12 Grain Bread	1 slice (38 g)	110	19	2	28	12	16	13	37	19
Arnold Healthy Multi Grain Bread	1 slice (49 g)	120	23	2	31	13	17	15	41	20
Dutch Country Stroehmann 12 Grain Bread	1 slice (35 g)	90	18	1	23	10	13	11	31	15
Food for Life Organic Sprouted 7-Grain Bread	1 slice (34 g)	80	15	1	21	9	11	10	27	14
Food for Life Ezekiel 4:9 Sprouted Grain Bread	1 slice (34 g)	80	15	1	21	9	11	10	27	14
Food for Life Organic Ezekiel 4:9 Sprouted Grain Bread	1 slice (34 g)	80	15	1	21	9	11	10	27	14
Food for Life Ezekiel 4:9 Cinnamon Raisin Sprouted Grain Bread	1 slice (34 g)	80	18	1	21	9	11	10	27	14

FOOD	AMOUNT	CAL	CARBS	FAT	WALK	RUN	BIKE	SWIM	YOGA	DANCE
Mestemacher 3 Grain Bread	1 slice (72 g)	120	24	2	31	13	17	15	41	20
Pepperidge Farm Light 7 Grain	1 slice	45	9	0	12	5	6	5	15	8
Pepperidge Farm 15 Grain Whole Grain blend	1 slice	120	20	2	31	13	17	15	41	20
Vermont Bread Company Organic Multigrain Bread	1 slice (31 g)	70	15	0	18	7	10	9	24	12
Oat Bread										
Oatmeal bread	1 slice (27 g)	73	13	1	19	8	10	9	25	12
Reduced-calorie oatmeal bread	1 slice (23 g)	48	10	1	12	5	7	6	16	8
Oat bran bread	1 slice (30 g)	71	12	1	18	8	10	9	24	12
Reduced-calorie oat bran bread	1 slice (23 g)	46	10	1	12	5	7	6	16	8
Rye Bread										
Rye bread	1 slice (32 g)	83	15	1	21	9	12	10	28	14
Reduced-calorie rye bread	1 slice (23 g)	47	9	1	12	5	7	6	16	8
Rye bread, with caraway seeds	1 thick slice (51 g)	120	24	2	31	13	17	15	41	20
Beefsteak Soft Rye Bread Without Seeds	1 slice (28 g)	70	14	1	18	7	10	9	24	12
Levy's Real Jewish Seedless Rye Bread	1 slice (32 g)	90	17	2	23	10	13	11	31	15
Mestemacher Whole Rye Bread	1 slice (72 g)	120	24	1	31	13	17	15	41	20
French Bread										
French bread	1 large slice (96 g)	263	50	3	68	28	37	32	89	45
French bread baguette	1 large slice (48 g)	120	23	1	31	13	17	15	41	20
Pillsbury Refrigerated Crusty French Loaf Dough	1 serving	154	29	2	40	16	22	19	53	26
Italian Bread										
Italian bread	1 slice (30 g)	81	15	1	21	9	11	10	28	14

FOOD	AMOUNT	CAL	CARBS	FAT	WALK	RUN	BIKE	SWIM	YOGA	DANCE
Garlic Bread										
Campione D'Italia Frozen Garlic Bread	1 serving	101	12	5	26	11	14	12	34	17
Pepperidge Farm Crusty Italian Garlic Bread	1 serving	186	21	10	48	20	26	23	63	32
Corn Bread										
Corn bread (prepared from mix)	1 slice (60 g)	188	29	6	48	20	27	23	64	32
Homemade corn bread	1 slice (65 g)	173	28	5	45	18	25	21	59	29
Hush puppies	1 hush puppy (22 g)	74	10	3	19	8	10	9	25	13
Fast food hush puppies	5 puppies (78 g)	257	35	12	66	27	36	31	87	44
Pumpernickel Bread										
Pumpernickel bread	1 slice (26 g)	65	12	1	17	7	9	8	22	11
Pumpernickel rye bread	1 slice (50 g)	120	23	2	31	13	17	15	41	20
Homemade pumpernickel bread	1 slice (45 g)	100	19	2	26	11	14	12	34	17
Mestemacher Pumpernickel Bread	1 slice (72 g)	115	23	1	30	12	16	14	39	20
Other Breads										
Banana bread	1 slice (60 g)	196	33	3	51	21	28	24	67	33
Boston brown bread	1 slice (45 g)	88	19	1	23	9	12	11	30	15
Raisin bread	1 slice (32 g)	88	17	1	23	9	12	11	30	15
Egg bread	1 slice (40 g)	113	19	2	29	12	16	14	38	19
Irish soda bread	1 slice (28 g)	82	16	1	21	9	12	10	28	14
High protein bread	1 slice (19 g)	47	8	0	12	5	7	6	16	8
Pepperidge Farm Raisin Cinnamon Swirl Bread	1 slice	80	15	2	21	9	11	10	27	14

FOOD	AMOUNT	CAL	CARBS	FAT	WALK	RUN	BIKE	SWIM	YOGA	DANCE
Restaurant/Bakery Breads										
■ **Breadsmith**										
100% Whole Wheat	1 slice (1 oz)	70	14	0	18	7	10	9	24	12
Austrian Pumpernickel	1 slice (1 oz)	53	13	1	14	6	8	6	18	9
Banana Dessert	1 slice (1 oz)	76	12	3	20	8	11	9	26	13
Banana Chocolate Chip	1 slice (1 oz)	86	14	3	22	9	12	10	29	15
Banana Chocolate Chip Walnut	1 slice (1 oz)	89	14	4	23	9	13	11	30	15
Banana Walnut	1 slice (1 oz)	79	12	3	20	8	11	10	27	13
Beer Bread	1 slice (1 oz)	72	15	0	19	8	10	9	24	12
Blueberry Cornbread	1 slice (1 oz)	72	15	0	19	8	10	9	24	12
Blueberry Corn Dessert	1 slice (1 oz)	91	14	3	23	10	13	11	31	16
Blueberry Lemon	1 slice (1 oz)	69	15	0	18	7	10	8	23	12
Cheddar Jalapeño Sourdough	1 slice (1 oz)	61	10	1	16	6	9	7	21	10
Cheddar Sourdough	1 slice (1 oz)	61	10	1	16	6	9	7	21	10
Cherry Walnut	1 slice (1 oz)	67	14	0	17	7	10	8	23	11
Chocolate Bread	1 slice (1 oz)	84	16	2	22	9	12	10	29	14
Chocolate Cherry	1 slice (1 oz)	81	15	1	21	9	11	10	28	14
Chocolate Dessert	1 slice (1 oz)	102	15	4	26	11	14	12	35	17
Ciabatta	1 slice (1 oz)	65	13	0	17	7	9	8	22	11
Cinnamon Spice	1 slice (1 oz)	79	17	0	20	8	11	10	27	13
Cornbread	1 slice (1 oz)	73	16	0	19	8	10	9	25	12
Country Buttertop	1 slice (1 oz)	57	10	1	15	6	8	7	19	10

FOOD	AMOUNT	CAL	CARBS	FAT	WALK	RUN	BIKE	SWIM	YOGA	DANCE
Country Sourdough	1 slice (1 oz)	66	14	0	17	7	9	8	22	11
Cranberry Cornbread	1 slice (1 oz)	72	15	0	19	8	10	9	24	12
Cranberry Orange	1 slice (1 oz)	68	14	0	18	7	10	8	23	12
Cranberry Orange Dessert	1 slice (1 oz)	86	13	3	22	9	12	10	29	15
Cranberry Sourdough Whole Grain	1 slice (1 oz)	68	14	0	18	7	10	8	23	12
Cranberry Walnut Sourdough	1 slice (1 oz)	66	13	0	17	7	9	8	22	11
Dark Rye	1 slice (1 oz)	58	13	0	15	6	8	7	20	10
Dark Rye with Caraway Seeds	1 slice (1 oz)	59	13	0	15	6	8	7	20	10
Dark Rye with Golden Raisins	1 slice (1 oz)	71	15	0	18	8	10	9	24	12
Egg	1 slice (1 oz)	89	15	2	23	9	13	11	30	15
English Muffin	1 slice (1 oz)	70	13	1	18	7	10	9	24	12
Farmer's Wheat	1 slice (1 oz)	70	13	1	18	7	10	9	24	12
Flax Seed	1 slice (1 oz)	73	14	1	19	8	10	9	25	12
Focaccia	1 slice (1 oz)	74	14	1	19	8	10	9	25	13
Freedom	1 slice (1 oz)	93	20	0	24	10	13	11	32	16
French	1 slice (1 oz)	68	14	0	18	7	10	8	23	12
French Peasant	1 slice (1 oz)	69	14	0	18	7	10	8	23	12
Frontier	1 slice (1 oz)	74	15	0	19	8	10	9	25	13
Fruit Bread	1 slice (1 oz)	65	14	0	17	7	9	8	22	11
Garlic Onion	1 slice (1 oz)	67	14	0	17	7	10	8	23	11
Garlic Onion Parmesan	1 slice (1 oz)	71	13	1	18	8	10	9	24	12

FOOD	AMOUNT	CAL	CARBS	FAT	WALK	RUN	BIKE	SWIM	YOGA	DANCE
Gluten Free	1 slice (1 oz)	74	10	3	19	8	10	9	25	13
Greek Olive	1 slice (1 oz)	67	13	1	17	7	10	8	23	11
Greek Olive Ciabatta	1 slice (1 oz)	61	12	1	16	6	9	7	21	10
Hamburger Buns	1 bun	300	56	4	77	32	43	36	102	51
Honey Oat Bran	1 slice (1 oz)	72	15	0	19	8	10	9	24	12
Honey Oat Bran with Blueberries	1 slice (1 oz)	69	14	0	18	7	10	8	23	12
Honey Oat Bran with Cranberries	1 slice (1 oz)	67	14	0	17	7	10	8	23	11
Honey Raisin	1 slice (1 oz)	75	17	0	19	8	11	9	26	13
Honey Raisin Pecan	1 slice (1 oz)	78	16	1	20	8	11	9	27	13
Honey Sunflower Whole Wheat	1 slice (1 oz)	71	13	1	18	8	10	9	24	12
Honey Wheat	1 slice (1 oz)	71	15	0	18	8	10	9	24	12
Honey Wheat with Blueberries	1 slice (1 oz)	69	14	1	18	7	10	8	23	12
Honey Wheat with Cranberries	1 slice (1 oz)	67	14	0	17	7	10	8	23	11
Honey White	1 slice (1 oz)	72	15	0	19	8	10	9	24	12
Honey Whole Wheat	1 slice (1 oz)	64	13	0	16	7	9	8	22	11
Icelandic Brown	1 slice (1 oz)	84	16	2	22	9	12	10	29	14
Irish Oat Bran	1 slice (1 oz)	67	14	0	17	7	10	8	23	11
Irish Soda Bread	1 slice (1 oz)	94	16	2	24	10	13	11	32	16
Jalapeño Cornbread	1 slice (1 oz)	73	16	0	19	8	10	9	25	12
Jalapeño Cheddar Cornbread	1 slice (1 oz)	77	14	1	20	8	11	9	26	13
Lemon Poppyseed Dessert	1 slice (1 oz)	89	13	3	23	9	13	11	30	15
Light Rye	1 slice (1 oz)	69	15	0	18	7	10	8	23	12

FOOD	AMOUNT	CAL	CARBS	FAT	WALK	RUN	BIKE	SWIM	YOGA	DANCE
Light Rye with Caraway Seeds	1 slice (1 oz)	69	15	0	18	7	10	8	23	12
Maple Walnut	1 slice (1 oz)	94	19	1	24	10	13	11	32	16
Marathon Multigrain	1 slice (1 oz)	74	13	1	19	8	10	9	25	13
Mediterranean Herb	1 slice (1 oz)	68	14	0	18	7	10	8	23	12
Multigrain	1 slice (1 oz)	64	13	1	16	7	9	8	22	11
Multigrain Light	1 slice (1 oz)	69	14	1	18	7	10	8	23	12
Multigrain Light with Rosemary	1 slice (1 oz)	67	14	1	17	7	10	8	23	11
Multigrain Whole Wheat	1 slice (1 oz)	70	14	1	18	7	10	9	24	12
Norwegian Rye	1 slice (1 oz)	62	15	0	16	7	9	8	21	11
Onion Rye	1 slice (1 oz)	59	14	0	15	6	8	7	20	10
Panettone	1 slice (1 oz)	80	14	2	21	9	11	10	27	14
Pecan Sourdough Whole Grain	1 slice (1 oz)	68	12	1	18	7	10	8	23	12
Peppercorn Swiss	1 slice (1 oz)	77	12	2	20	8	11	9	26	13
Pepperoni Bread	1 slice (1 oz)	77	11	2	20	8	11	9	26	13
Pesto	1 slice (1 oz)	70	14	0	18	7	10	9	24	12
Potato Cheddar Chive	1 slice (1 oz)	64	12	1	16	7	9	8	22	11
Potato Flake Roll	1 roll	224	47	1	58	24	32	27	76	38
Pretzel	1 slice (1 oz)	84	15	2	22	9	12	10	29	14
Pumpernickel Brick	1 slice (1 oz)	46	12	1	12	5	7	6	16	8
Pumpkin Dessert	1 slice (1 oz)	85	14	3	22	9	12	10	29	14
Pumpkin Chocolate Chip Dessert	1 slice (1 oz)	95	15	4	24	10	13	12	32	16
Pumpkin Chocolate Chip and Walnut Dessert	1 slice (1 oz)	97	15	4	25	10	14	12	33	17

FOOD	AMOUNT	CAL	CARBS	FAT	WALK	RUN	BIKE	SWIM	YOGA	DANCE
Pumpkin and Walnut Dessert	1 slice (1 oz)	88	14	3	23	9	12	11	30	15
Raisin Cinnamon	1 slice (1 oz)	73	16	0	19	8	10	9	25	12
Raisin Cinnamon Walnut	1 slice (1 oz)	70	14	1	18	7	10	9	24	12
Raisin Cinnamon Whole Wheat	1 slice (1 oz)	70	15	0	18	7	10	9	24	12
Raisin Sunflower	1 slice (1 oz)	73	15	1	19	8	10	9	25	12
Raisin Walnut	1 slice (1 oz)	71	14	1	18	8	10	9	24	12
Reduced Carb Multigrain	1 slice (1 oz)	57	10	2	15	6	8	7	19	10
Reduced Carb Raisin Cinnamon	1 slice (1 oz)	59	11	1	15	6	8	7	20	10
Reduced Carb Wheat	1 slice (1 oz)	49	8	1	13	5	7	6	17	8
Reduced Carb White	1 slice (1 oz)	49	8	1	13	5	7	6	17	8
Rosemary Country	1 slice (1 oz)	69	14	0	18	7	10	8	23	12
Rosemary Focaccia	1 slice (1 oz)	73	14	1	19	8	10	9	25	12
Rosemary Fougasse	1 slice (1 oz)	72	14	1	19	8	10	9	24	12
Rosemary Garlic Ciabatta	1 slice (1 oz)	65	13	0	17	7	9	8	22	11
Russian Rye	1 slice (1 oz)	78	15	1	20	8	11	9	27	13
Rustic Italian	1 slice (1 oz)	69	14	0	18	7	10	8	23	12
Semolina	1 slice (1 oz)	70	14	0	18	7	10	9	24	12
Soft Onion Buns	1 bun	277	50	5	71	29	39	34	94	47
Soft Rye Buns	1 bun	249	45	5	64	26	35	30	85	42
Soft Tomato Basil Buns	1 bun	273	49	5	70	29	39	33	93	47
Soft Wheat Buns	1 bun	273	47	6	70	29	39	33	93	47
Sourdough	1 slice (1 oz)	70	14	0	18	7	10	9	24	12
Sourdough Rye	1 slice (1 oz)	66	15	0	17	7	9	8	22	11

FOOD	AMOUNT	CAL	CARBS	FAT	WALK	RUN	BIKE	SWIM	YOGA	DANCE
Sourdough Whole Grain	1 slice (1 oz)	65	13	0	17	7	9	8	22	11
Stollen	1 slice (1 oz)	93	16	3	24	10	13	11	32	16
Stoneground Wheat	1 slice (1 oz)	67	14	0	17	7	10	8	23	11
Swedish Limpa Rye	1 slice (1 oz)	78	17	0	20	8	11	9	27	13
Sweet Bellagio	1 slice (1 oz)	70	14	1	18	7	10	9	24	12
Toasted Onion Sourdough Whole Grain	1 slice (1 oz)	67	13	0	17	7	10	8	23	11
Tomato Basil	1 slice (1 oz)	70	14	0	18	7	10	9	24	12
Traditional Rye	1 slice (1 oz)	63	15	0	16	7	9	8	21	11
Tuscan Herb Formaggio	1 slice (1 oz)	71	13	1	18	8	10	9	24	12
Tuscan Rustica	1 slice (1 oz)	67	14	0	17	7	10	8	23	11
Vanilla Egg (Challah)	1 slice (1 oz)	77	16	0	20	8	11	9	26	13
Wheat Flax Seed	1 slice (1 oz)	73	14	1	19	8	10	9	25	12
Zucchini Dessert	1 slice (1 oz)	101	15	4	26	11	14	12	34	17
■ **Panera Bread**										
Artisan Country Demi	2 oz	130	27	0	34	14	18	16	44	22
Artisan Country Loaf	2 oz	130	27	0	34	14	18	16	44	22
Artisan Country Miche	2 oz	120	25	0	31	13	17	15	41	20
Artisan French Baguette	2 oz	140	28	0	36	15	20	17	48	24
Artisan French Miche	2 oz	120	25	0	31	13	17	15	41	20
Artisan Multigrain Loaf	2 oz	130	27	1	34	14	18	16	44	22
Artisan Sesame Semolina Loaf	2 oz	130	26	1	34	14	18	16	44	22
Artisan Sesame Semolina Miche	2 oz	120	25	1	31	13	17	15	41	20
Artisan Stone-Milled Rye Loaf	2 oz	120	25	0	31	13	17	15	41	20
Artisan Stone-Milled Rye Miche	2 oz	120	24	0	31	13	17	15	41	20
Artisan Three Cheese Demi	2 oz	140	25	3	36	15	20	17	48	24

FOOD	AMOUNT	CAL	CARBS	FAT	WALK	RUN	BIKE	SWIM	YOGA	DANCE
Artisan Three Cheese Loaf	2 oz	140	24	2	36	15	20	17	48	24
Artisan Three Cheese Miche	2 oz	130	23	2	34	14	18	16	44	22
Artisan Three Seed Demi	2 oz	130	27	0	34	14	18	16	44	22
Asiago Cheese Demi Loaf	2 oz	150	22	4	39	16	21	18	51	26
Asiago Cheese Focaccia	2 oz	160	21	6	41	17	23	19	54	27
Basil Pesto Focaccia	2 oz	160	22	6	41	17	23	19	54	27
Ciabatta	2 oz	500	82	12	129	53	71	61	170	85
Cinnamon Raisin Loaf	2 oz	170	31	3	44	18	24	21	58	29
French Baguette	2 oz	150	30	1	39	16	21	18	51	26
French XL Loaf	2 oz	140	28	1	36	15	20	17	48	24
French Roll	2.25 oz	170	34	1	44	18	24	21	58	29
Honey Wheat Loaf	2 oz	160	29	3	41	17	23	19	54	27
Lower-Carb Italian Herb Loaf	1.1 oz slice	80	10	1	21	9	11	10	27	14
Lower-Carb Pumpkin Seed Loaf	1.1 oz slice	90	9	3	23	10	13	11	31	15
Nine Grain Loaf	2 oz	160	29	3	41	17	23	19	54	27
Rosemary and Onion Focaccia	2 oz	150	21	5	39	16	21	18	51	26
Rye Loaf	2 oz	160	28	3	41	17	23	19	54	27
Sourdough Baguette	2 oz	150	30	0	39	16	21	18	51	26
Sourdough XL Loaf	2 oz	130	27	0	34	14	18	16	44	22
Sourdough roll	2.5 oz	190	38	1	49	20	27	23	65	32
Sourdough Bread Bowl	8 oz	560	115	2	144	60	79	68	190	95
Sunflower Loaf	2 oz	180	27	6	46	19	26	22	61	31
Tomato Basil XL Loaf	2 oz	130	27	1	34	14	18	16	44	22
Whole Grain Baguette	2 oz	140	28	1	36	15	20	17	48	24
Whole Grain Loaf, Miche	2 oz	150	28	1	39	16	21	18	51	26
Pita										
White (4" diameter)	1 pita	77	16	0	20	8	11	9	26	13
White (6 ½" diameter)	1 pita	165	33	1	43	18	23	20	56	28
Whole wheat (4" diameter)	1 pita	74	15	1	19	8	10	9	25	13
Whole wheat (6 ½" diameter)	1 pita	170	35	2	44	18	24	21	58	29
Challah										
Atlanta Bread Company Challah	2 oz slice	160	29	3	41	17	23	19	54	27
Kineret Ready-to-Bake Whole Wheat Challah	⅛ loaf	130	25	1	34	14	18	16	44	22

FOOD	AMOUNT	CAL	CARBS	FAT	WALK	RUN	BIKE	SWIM	YOGA	DANCE
Croutons										
Plain croutons	.5 cup	61	11	1	16	6	9	7	21	10
Seasoned croutons	.5 cup	93	13	4	24	10	13	11	32	16
Pepperidge Farm Seasoned Classic Croutons	1 serving	33	4	1	8	3	5	4	11	6
Hidden Valley Italian Style Parmesan Croutons	1 serving	30	5	1	8	3	4	4	10	5
Bread Crumbs										
Plain bread crumbs	1 cup	427	78	5	110	45	61	52	145	73
Soft white bread crumbs	1 cup	120	23	1	31	13	17	15	41	20
Seasoned bread crumbs	1 cup	460	82	7	119	49	65	56	156	78
Progresso Italian Style Bread crumbs	.25 cup	110	20	2	28	12	16	13	37	19
Kellogg's Corn Flake Crumbs	6 tbsp	120	29	0	31	13	17	15	41	20
Shake 'n Bake Original Recipe	1 serving	106	22	1	27	11	15	13	36	18
Breadsticks										
Breadsticks	1 stick (7-⅝" x ⅝")	41	7	1	11	4	6	5	14	7
Aladdin Garlic Breadsticks	3 sticks	80	11	3	21	9	11	10	27	14
Aladdin Sesame Breadsticks	3 sticks	80	11	3	21	9	11	10	27	14
Aladdin Wheat Breadsticks	3 sticks	80	11	3	21	9	11	10	27	14
Grissini Plain Breadsticks	5 sticks	110	26	2	28	12	16	13	37	19
Grissini Whole Wheat Breadsticks	5 sticks	100	20	2	26	11	14	12	34	17
Pepperidge Farm Sesame Snack Sticks	12 sticks	140	20	6	36	15	20	17	48	24
Pizza Hut Breadsticks	1 stick	150	20	6	39	16	21	18	51	26
Pizza Hut Cheese Breadsticks	1 stick	200	21	10	52	21	28	24	68	34
Stella D'oro Sesame Breadsticks	1 stick	50	7	2	13	5	7	6	17	9
Flatbread										
Aladdin Whole Wheat Flatbread	1 flatbread	210	37	5	54	22	30	26	71	36
Kavli Five Grain Crispbread	1 crispbread	40	9	0	10	4	6	5	14	7
Stuffing										
Corn bread stuffing (prepared from mix)	.5 cup	179	22	9	46	19	25	22	61	30

FOOD	AMOUNT	CAL	CARBS	FAT	WALK	RUN	BIKE	SWIM	YOGA	DANCE
Bread Stuffing (prepared from mix)	.5 cup	178	22	9	46	19	25	22	61	30
Brownberry Sage and Onion Stuffing Mix	1 serving	255	47	3	66	27	36	31	87	43
Stove Top Chicken Stuffing (prepared)	.5 cup	110	20	1	28	12	16	13	37	19
Stove Top Turkey Stuffing (prepared)	.5 cup	110	20	1	28	12	16	13	37	19
Rolls										
Dinner roll	1 small	84	14	2	22	9	12	10	29	14
Homemade dinner roll	1 large (3-½" diameter)	136	23	3	35	14	19	17	46	23
Oat bran dinner roll	1 roll	78	13	2	20	8	11	9	27	13
Rye dinner roll	1 large	123	23	1	32	13	17	15	42	21
Wheat dinner roll	1 roll	76	13	2	20	8	11	9	26	13
Whole wheat dinner roll	1 roll	96	18	2	25	10	14	12	33	16
Egg dinner roll	1 roll	107	18	2	28	11	15	13	36	18
Pumpernickel roll	1 roll	100	19	1	26	11	14	12	34	17
Hard roll	1 roll	167	30	2	43	18	24	20	57	28
French roll	1 roll	105	19	2	27	11	15	13	36	18
Hamburger or hot dog roll	1 roll	129	22	3	33	14	18	16	44	22
Mixed-grain hamburger or hot dog roll	1 roll	113	19	3	29	12	16	14	38	19
Reduced-calorie hamburger or hot dog roll	1 roll	84	18	1	22	9	12	10	29	14
Arnold Wheat Sandwich Rolls	1 roll	160	29	3	41	17	23	19	54	27
Arnold Soft Multigrain Kaiser Rolls	1 roll	180	36	2	46	19	26	22	61	31
Pillsbury Hot Roll	1 serving	130	21	3	34	14	18	16	44	22
Pillsbury Butterflake Dinner Roll	1 serving	130	19	5	34	14	18	16	44	22
Wonder Brown and Serve Dinner Roll	1 serving	80	13	2	21	9	11	10	27	14
Wonder 4" Hamburger Roll	1 bun	110	21	2	28	12	16	13	37	19
Wonder Bread Hot Dog Bun	1 bun	110	21	2	28	12	16	13	37	19
English muffin										
Plain English muffin	1 muffin (57 g)	134	26	1	35	14	19	16	46	23

FOOD	AMOUNT	CAL	CARBS	FAT	WALK	RUN	BIKE	SWIM	YOGA	DANCE
Mixed-grain English muffin	1 muffin (66 g)	155	31	1	40	17	22	19	53	26
Cinnamon raisin English muffin	1 muffin (57 g)	137	27	1	35	15	19	17	47	23
Wheat English muffin	1 muffin (57 g)	127	26	1	33	14	18	15	43	22
Whole-wheat English muffin	1 muffin (66 g)	134	27	1	35	14	19	16	46	23
English muffin, with butter	1 serving (63 g)	189	30	6	49	20	27	23	64	32
English muffin, with cheese and sausage	1 serving (115 g)	393	29	24	101	42	56	48	134	67
English muffin, with egg, cheese, and Canadian bacon	1 serving (137 g)	289	27	13	74	31	41	35	98	49
English muffin, with egg, cheese, and sausage	1 serving (165 g)	487	31	31	126	52	69	59	166	83
Thomas' Original	1 muffin	120	25	1	31	13	17	15	41	20
Thomas' 100% Whole Wheat	1 muffin	120	23	1	31	13	17	15	41	20
Thomas' Multi Grain	1 muffin	150	27	2	39	16	21	18	51	26
Thomas' Light Multi Grain	1 muffin	100	22	1	26	11	14	12	34	17
Thomas' Super Size	1 muffin	190	38	2	49	20	27	23	65	32
Tortillas and Taco Shells										
Baked taco shells	1 large shell	98	13	5	25	10	14	12	33	17
Ready-to-bake flour tortilla	12"	356	59	9	92	38	50	43	121	61
Ready-to-bake flour tortilla	6"	104	18	2	27	11	15	13	35	18
Ready-to-bake corn tortilla	6"	58	12	1	15	6	8	7	20	10
Food for Life Organic Ezekiel 4:9 Sprouted Grain Tortilla	1 tortilla	150	24	4	39	16	21	18	51	26
Gebhardt Taco Shell	1 shell	52	6	3	13	6	7	6	18	9
La Tortilla Factory 99% Fat Free Burrito Sized Flour Tortilla	1 serving	120	25	1	31	13	17	15	41	20
La Tortilla Factory Nonfat Flour Tortilla	1 serving	60	13	0	15	6	9	7	20	10
La Tortilla Factory 99% Fat Free Whole Wheat Tortilla	1 serving	60	12	0	15	6	9	7	20	10
La Tortilla Factory Low Fat Gordita	1 serving	150	29	3	39	16	21	18	51	26
Mission Flour Tortilla	Fajita size	100	17	3	26	11	14	12	34	17

FOOD	AMOUNT	CAL	CARBS	FAT	WALK	RUN	BIKE	SWIM	YOGA	DANCE
Mission Flour Tortilla	Soft taco size	140	24	3	36	15	20	17	48	24
Mission Corn Tortilla	2 tortillas	90	18	2	23	10	13	11	31	15
Old El Paso Taco Dinner Kit	2 shells	130	18	5	34	14	18	16	44	22
Old El Paso Super Taco Shell	2 shells	190	21	12	49	20	27	23	65	32
Richfood Flour Tortilla	1 tortilla	160	29	3	41	17	23	19	54	27
Rosarita Taco Shell	1 serving	52	6	3	13	6	7	6	18	9
Rosarita Tostada Shell	1 serving	63	9	2	16	7	9	8	21	11
Thomas' Sahara 100% Whole Wheat Wrap	1 wrap	170	27	5	44	18	24	21	58	29

Crackers

Snack Crackers										
Snack crackers	5 round	75	9	4	19	8	11	9	26	13
Gamesa Sabrosas	11 crackers	150	20	6	39	16	21	18	51	26
Goldfish Crackers, Original	55 crackers	150	20	6	39	16	21	18	51	26
Goldfish Crackers, Parmesan	60 crackers	130	20	4	34	14	18	16	44	22
Goldfish Crackers, Cheddar	55 crackers	140	20	5	36	15	20	17	48	24
Goldfish Crackers, Made with Whole Grains	55 crackers	140	19	5	36	15	20	17	48	24
Goldfish Crackers, Pizza	55 crackers	140	20	5	36	15	20	17	48	24
Goldfish Crackers, Colors	55 crackers	140	20	5	36	15	20	17	48	24
Goldfish Crackers, Queso Jalapeño	51 crackers	150	17	7	39	16	21	18	51	26
Goldfish Crackers, Giant	14 crackers	140	19	6	36	15	20	17	48	24
Goldfish Mini Sandwich Crackers, Peanut Butter	11 sandwiches	140	18	6	36	15	20	17	48	24
Keebler Town House Crackers	5 crackers	80	9	5	21	9	11	10	27	14
Keebler Reduced Fat Town House Crackers	6 crackers	60	11	2	15	6	9	7	20	10
Keebler Original Club Crackers	4 crackers	70	9	3	18	7	10	9	24	12

FOOD	AMOUNT	CAL	CARBS	FAT	WALK	RUN	BIKE	SWIM	YOGA	DANCE
Ritz Crackers	5 crackers	80	10	4	21	9	11	10	27	14
Ritz Original Chips	13 chips	130	21	5	34	14	18	16	44	22
Ritz Garlic and Butter Chips	5 crackers	80	10	4	21	9	11	10	27	14
Triscuits, Original	6 crackers	120	19	5	31	13	17	15	41	20
Triscuits, Reduced Fat	7 crackers	120	21	3	31	13	17	15	41	20
Triscuits, Garden Herb	6 crackers	120	20	4	31	13	17	15	41	20
Triscuits, Rosemary and Olive Oil	6 crackers	120	20	4	31	13	17	15	41	20
Wheat Thins	16 crackers	150	21	6	39	16	21	18	51	26
Wheat Thins, Big	11 crackers	150	21	6	39	16	21	18	51	26
Wheat Thins, Harvest 5 Grain	13 crackers	130	23	4	34	14	18	16	44	22
Wheat Thins, Reduced Fat	16 crackers	130	21	4	34	14	18	16	44	22
Wheat Thins, Multi-Grain	17 crackers	130	22	5	34	14	18	16	44	22
Wheat Thins, Ranch	14 crackers	140	19	6	36	15	20	17	48	24
Cheese Crackers										
Cheese crackers	10 crackers	50	6	3	13	5	7	6	17	9
Bitesize cheese crackers	.5 cup	156	18	8	40	17	22	19	53	27
Cheese sandwich crackers	6 crackers	191	23	10	49	20	27	23	65	33
Peanut butter cheese crackers	6 crackers	193	22	10	50	21	27	23	66	33
Cheese Nips 4 cheese	16 crackers	150	18	7	39	16	21	18	51	26
Cheese Nips Chips Bold Cheddar	13 chips	140	20	5	36	15	20	17	48	24
Cheez-It Baked Snack Crackers	27 crackers	160	18	8	41	17	23	19	54	27
Cheez-It Reduced Fat Snack Crackers	29 crackers	130	20	4	34	14	18	16	44	22
Cheez-It Party Mix	.5 cup	120	21	5	31	13	17	15	41	20
Cheez-It White Cheddar Baked Snack Crackers	25 crackers	150	18	8	39	16	21	18	51	26
Cheez-It Hot and Spicy Baked Snack Crackers	25 crackers	150	18	8	39	16	21	18	51	26

FOOD	AMOUNT	CAL	CARBS	FAT	WALK	RUN	BIKE	SWIM	YOGA	DANCE
Cheetos Bacon Cheddar on Cheese Flavored Crackers	1 oz	190	24	10	49	20	27	23	65	32
Cheetos Cheddar Cheese on Golden Toast Crackers	1 oz	210	22	13	54	22	30	26	71	36
Combos Cheddar Cheese Crackers	1 oz	140	18	6	36	15	20	17	48	24
Doritos Jalapeño Cheese on Golden Toast Crackers	1 oz	200	23	11	52	21	28	24	68	34
Doritos Nacho Cheesier on Golden Toast Crackers	1 oz	210	22	12	54	22	30	26	71	36
Frito-Lay Peanut Butter on Cheese Flavored Crackers	1 oz	190	24	9	49	20	27	23	65	32
Ritz Bits Cheese Sandwiches	12 sandwiches	150	16	9	39	16	21	18	51	26
Snackwell's Zesty Cheese Crackers	1 oz	129	23	3	33	14	18	16	44	22
Graham Crackers										
Plain	8 crackers (2 sheets)	118	22	3	30	13	17	14	40	20
Gamesa Ricanelas Cinnamon Graham Cookies	8 cookies	140	24	4	36	15	20	17	48	24
Keebler Low Fat Honey Grahams	8 crackers	110	22	2	28	12	16	13	37	19
Keebler Honey Grahams	8 crackers	140	23	4	36	15	20	17	48	24
Keebler Original Grahams	8 crackers	130	22	4	34	14	18	16	44	22
Keebler Cinnamon Crisp Grahams	8 crackers	130	22	4	34	14	18	16	44	22
Nabisco Graham Crackers	1 serving	119	21	3	31	13	17	14	40	20
Teddy Grahams, Honey	24 pieces	130	23	4	34	14	18	16	44	22
Teddy Grahams, Cinnamon	24 pieces	130	23	4	34	14	18	16	44	22
Teddy Grahams, Chocolate	24 pieces	130	22	5	34	14	18	16	44	22
Teddy Grahams, Chocolatey Chip	24 pieces	130	23	5	34	14	18	16	44	22
Wheat crackers										
Wheat crackers	12 crackers	114	16	5	29	12	16	14	39	19
Whole-wheat crackers	12 crackers	213	33	8	55	23	30	26	72	36
Carr's Whole Wheat Crackers	2 crackers	80	11	4	21	9	11	10	27	14
Health Valley Nonfat Whole Wheat Crackers	5 crackers	50	11	0	13	5	7	6	17	9

FOOD	AMOUNT	CAL	CARBS	FAT	WALK	RUN	BIKE	SWIM	YOGA	DANCE
Health Valley Nonfat Whole Wheat Herb Crackers	5 crackers	50	11	0	13	5	7	6	17	9
Health Valley Nonfat Whole Wheat Onion Crackers	5 crackers	50	11	0	13	5	7	6	17	9
Health Valley Nonfat Whole Wheat Vegetable Crackers	5 crackers	50	11	0	13	5	7	6	17	9
Keebler Toasted Wheats	5 crackers	80	10	4	21	9	11	10	27	14
Snackwell's Wheat Crackers	1 serving	62	12	2	16	7	9	8	21	11
Snackwell's Nonfat Wheat Crackers	5 crackers	60	12	0	15	6	9	7	20	10
South Beach Diet Wheat Crackers	1 pack	100	116	4	26	11	14	12	34	17
Wheatables Low Fat	19 crackers	140	22	4	36	15	20	17	48	24
Wasa										
Original	1 cracker	35	7	0	9	4	5	4	12	6
Sesam	1 cracker	55	9	2	14	6	8	7	19	9
Delikatess	1 cracker	26	5	0	7	3	4	3	9	4
Fibre	1 cracker	32	5	1	8	3	5	4	11	5
Wheat Dore	1 cracker	51	9	1	13	5	7	6	17	9
Runda	1 cracker	55	9	1	14	6	8	7	19	9
Matzo										
Matzo	1 matzo	111	23	0	29	12	16	14	38	19
Egg matzo	1 matzo	109	22	1	28	12	15	13	37	19
Egg and onion matzo	1 matzo	109	22	1	28	12	15	13	37	19
Whole-wheat matzo	1 matzo	98	22	0	25	10	14	12	33	17
Other Crackers										
Plain rye wafers	3 crackers	110	27	0	28	12	16	13	37	19
Seasoned rye wafers	1 triple cracker	84	16	2	22	9	12	10	29	14
Milk crackers	5 crackers	250	38	9	64	27	35	30	85	43
Cracker meal	1 cup	440	93	2	113	47	62	54	150	75
Oyster crackers	1 cup	193	32	5	50	21	27	23	66	33
Melba toast	10 rounds	117	23	1	30	12	17	14	40	20
Rye melba toast	10 crackers	194	39	2	50	21	28	24	66	33
Wheat melba toast	10 crackers	187	38	1	48	20	27	23	64	32

FOOD	AMOUNT	CAL	CARBS	FAT	WALK	RUN	BIKE	SWIM	YOGA	DANCE
Frito-Lay Peanut Butter on Golden Toast Crackers	1 oz	200	24	10	52	21	28	24	68	34
Saltines	8 crackers	103	17	3	27	11	15	13	35	18
Nabisco Premium Saltines	5 crackers	60	11	2	15	6	9	7	20	10
Snackwell's salsa snack cracker	1 serving	128	23	3	33	14	18	16	44	22
Snackwell's Italian ranch snack cracker	1 serving	128	23	3	33	14	18	16	44	22
Snackwell's French onion snack cracker	1 serving	128	23	3	33	14	18	16	44	22
Snackwell's cracked pepper cracker	1 serving	61	10	2	16	7	9	7	21	10

Donuts, Muffins, and Brownies

Donuts

■ General

FOOD	AMOUNT	CAL	CARBS	FAT	WALK	RUN	BIKE	SWIM	YOGA	DANCE
Chocolate coated or frosted cake donut	1 donut	204	21	13	53	22	29	25	69	35
Cream filled yeast donut	1 donut	307	26	21	79	33	44	37	104	52
French cruller	1 cruller	169	24	8	44	18	24	21	57	29
Jelly filled yeast donut	1 donut	289	33	16	74	31	41	35	98	49
Plain cake donut	1 donut	198	23	11	51	21	28	24	67	34
Plain yeast donut	1 donut	242	27	14	62	26	34	29	82	41
Sugared cake donut	1 donut	175	24	8	45	19	25	21	60	30
Wheat cake donut	1 donut	162	0	9	42	17	23	20	55	28

Dunkin' Donuts

■ Donuts

FOOD	AMOUNT	CAL	CARBS	FAT	WALK	RUN	BIKE	SWIM	YOGA	DANCE
Apple Crumb Donut	1 donut	230	34	10	59	24	33	28	78	39
Apple Crumb Cake Donut	1 donut	290	41	15	75	31	41	35	99	49
Apple n' Spice Donut	1 donut	200	29	8	52	21	28	24	68	34
Apple Raspberry Donut	1 donut	210	32	8	54	22	30	26	71	36
Bavarian Kreme Donut	1 donut	210	30	9	54	22	30	26	71	36
Boston Kreme Donut	1 donut	240	36	9	62	26	34	29	82	41
Blueberry Cake Donut	1 donut	290	35	16	75	31	41	35	99	49
Blueberry Crumb Donut	1 donut	240	36	10	62	26	34	29	82	41
Chocolate Coconut Cake Donut	1 donut	300	31	19	77	32	43	36	102	51

FOOD	AMOUNT	CAL	CARBS	FAT	WALK	RUN	BIKE	SWIM	YOGA	DANCE
Chocolate Frosted Cake Donut	1 donut	360	40	20	93	38	51	44	122	61
Chocolate Frosted Donut	1 donut	200	29	9	52	21	28	24	68	34
Chocolate Glazed Cake Donut	1 donut	290	33	16	75	31	41	35	99	49
Chocolate Kreme Filled Donut	1 donut	270	35	13	70	29	38	33	92	46
Cinnamon Cake Donut	1 donut	330	34	20	85	35	47	40	112	56
Double Chocolate Cake Donut	1 donut	310	37	17	80	33	44	38	105	53
French Cruller	1 cruller	150	17	8	39	16	21	18	51	26
Glazed Gingerbread Cake Donut	1 donut	260	35	11	67	28	37	32	88	44
Glazed Donut	1 donut	180	25	8	46	19	26	22	61	31
Glazed Cake Donut	1 donut	350	41	19	90	37	50	43	119	60
Jelly Filled Donut	1 donut	210	32	8	54	22	30	26	71	36
Frosted Lemon Cake Donut	1 donut	240	28	14	62	26	34	29	82	41
Glazed Lemon Cake Donut	1 donut	240	28	14	62	26	34	29	82	41
Lemon Burst Donut	1 donut	300	35	14	77	32	43	36	102	51
Maple Frosted Donut	1 donut	210	30	9	54	22	30	26	71	36
Marble Frosted Donut	1 donut	200	29	9	52	21	28	24	68	34
Old Fashioned Cake Donut	1 donut	300	28	19	77	32	43	36	102	51
Powdered Cake Donut	1 donut	330	36	19	85	35	47	40	112	56
Strawberry Donut	1 donut	210	32	8	54	22	30	26	71	36
Strawberry Frosted Donut	1 donut	210	30	9	54	22	30	26	71	36
Sugar Raised Donut	1 donut	170	22	8	44	18	24	21	58	29
Vanilla Kreme Filled Donut	1 donut	270	36	13	70	29	38	33	92	46
Whole Wheat Glazed Cake Donut	1 donut	310	32	19	80	33	44	38	105	53
■ **Fancies**										
Chocolate Iced Bismark	1 bismark	340	50	15	88	36	48	41	116	58
Bow Tie Donut	1 donut	300	34	17	77	32	43	36	102	51
Éclair	1 éclair	270	39	11	70	29	38	33	92	46
Apple Fritter	1 fritter	300	41	14	77	32	43	36	102	51
Glazed Fritter	1 fritter	260	31	14	67	28	37	32	88	44
Chocolate Frosted Coffee Roll	1 roll	290	36	15	75	31	41	35	99	49
Coffee Roll	1 roll	270	33	14	70	29	38	33	92	46
Maple Frosted Coffee Roll	1 roll	290	36	14	75	31	41	35	99	49
Vanilla Frosted Coffee Roll	1 roll	290	36	14	75	31	41	35	99	49

FOOD	AMOUNT	CAL	CARBS	FAT	WALK	RUN	BIKE	SWIM	YOGA	DANCE
■ Munchkins										
Cinnamon Cake Munchkins	4 munchkins	270	31	15	70	29	38	33	92	46
Glazed Cake Munchkins	3 munchkins	280	38	13	72	30	40	34	95	48
Plain Cake Munchkins	4 munchkins	270	27	16	70	29	38	33	92	46
Powdered Cake Munchkins	4 munchkins	270	31	14	70	29	38	33	92	46
Glazed Chocolate Cake Munchkins	3 munchkins	200	26	10	52	21	28	24	68	34
Glazed Munchkins	5 munchkins	200	27	9	52	21	28	24	68	34
Jelly Filled Munchkins	5 munchkins	210	30	9	54	22	30	26	71	36
Lemon Filled Munchkins	4 munchkins	170	23	8	44	18	24	21	58	29
Sugar Raised Munchkins	7 munchkins	220	26	12	57	23	31	27	75	37
■ Sticks										
Plain Cake Stick	1 stick	420	35	29	108	45	60	51	143	72
Glazed Cake Stick	1 stick	490	51	29	126	52	70	60	167	83
Jelly Stick	1 stick	530	61	29	137	56	75	64	180	90
Powdered Cake Stick	1 stick	450	42	29	116	48	64	55	153	77
Cinnamon Cake Stick	1 stick	450	42	30	116	48	64	55	153	77
Glazed Chocolate Cake Stick	1 stick	470	49	29	121	50	67	57	160	80
Krispy Kreme										
■ Doughnuts										
Original Glazed	1 doughnut	200	22	12	52	21	28	24	68	34
Chocolate Iced Glazed	1 doughnut	250	33	12	64	27	35	30	85	43
Chocolate Iced with Sprinkles	1 doughnut	260	38	12	67	28	37	32	88	44
Chocolate Iced, Kreme Filled	1 doughnut	350	38	20	90	37	50	43	119	60
Chocolate Iced, Custard Filled	1 doughnut	300	35	17	77	32	43	36	102	51
Glazed Lemon Filled	1 doughnut	290	35	16	75	31	41	35	99	49

FOOD	AMOUNT	CAL	CARBS	FAT	WALK	RUN	BIKE	SWIM	YOGA	DANCE
Glazed Raspberry Filled	1 doughnut	300	39	16	77	32	43	36	102	51
Glazed Cruller	1 cruller	240	26	14	62	26	34	29	82	41
Cinnamon Apple Filled	1 doughnut	290	32	16	75	31	41	35	99	49
New York Cheesecake	1 doughnut	320	35	19	82	34	45	39	109	55
Caramel Kreme Crunch	1 doughnut	350	43	19	90	37	50	43	119	60
Key Lime Pie	1 doughnut	320	40	17	82	34	45	39	109	55
Glazed Chocolate Cake	1 doughnut	300	41	15	77	32	43	36	102	51
Traditional Cake	1 doughnut	230	25	13	59	24	33	28	78	39
Glazed Kreme Filled	1 doughnut	340	38	20	88	36	48	41	116	58
Glazed Blueberry	1 doughnut	330	43	17	85	35	47	40	112	56
Glazed Cinnamon	1 doughnut	210	24	12	54	22	30	26	71	36
Cinnamon Bun	1 doughnut	260	28	16	67	28	37	32	88	44
Cinnamon Twist	1 twist	230	33	9	59	24	33	28	78	39
Maple Iced Glazed	1 doughnut	240	32	12	62	26	34	29	82	41
Glazed Sour Cream	1 doughnut	340	42	18	88	36	48	41	116	58
Sugar	1 doughnut	200	21	12	52	21	28	24	68	34
Powdered, Blueberry Filled	1 doughnut	290	33	16	75	31	41	35	99	49
Powdered, Strawberry Filled	1 doughnut	290	33	16	75	31	41	35	99	49
Powdered Cake	1 doughnut	280	37	14	72	30	40	34	95	48
Chocolate Iced Cake	1 doughnut	270	36	14	70	29	38	33	92	46
Chocolate Glazed Cruller	1 doughnut	290	37	15	75	31	41	35	99	49
Dulce de Leche	1 doughnut	290	30	18	75	31	41	35	99	49

FOOD	AMOUNT	CAL	CARBS	FAT	WALK	RUN	BIKE	SWIM	YOGA	DANCE
Apple Fritter	1 fritter	400	43	24	103	43	57	49	136	68
■ **Doughnut Holes**										
Original Glazed	5 holes	200	24	11	52	21	28	24	68	34
Glazed Blueberry	4 holes	220	26	12	57	23	31	27	75	37
Glazed Cake	4 holes	210	28	11	54	22	30	26	71	36
Glazed Chocolate Cake	4 holes	210	28	11	54	22	30	26	71	36
Entenmann's										
■ **Donuts**										
Plain	1 donut	180	20	11	46	19	26	22	61	31
Powdered	1 donut	220	27	11	57	23	31	27	75	37
Frosted	1 donut	320	29	22	82	34	45	39	109	55
Devil's Food Crumb	1 donut	250	35	12	64	27	35	30	85	43
Devil's Food	1 donut	310	36	19	80	33	44	38	105	53
Crumb Topped	1 donut	260	36	12	67	28	37	32	88	44
Rich Frosted	1 donut	350	29	26	90	37	50	43	119	60
■ **Popems**										
Glazed Popems	4 Popems	220	30	10	57	23	31	27	75	37
Holiday Popems	4 Popems	210	33	9	54	22	30	26	71	36
Little Bites Glazed Holes	1 pouch	220	29	11	57	23	31	27	75	37
Little Bites Softee Powdered Poppettes	1 pouch	240	30	14	62	26	34	29	82	41
Softee Powdered Popems	4 Popems	250	31	13	64	27	35	30	85	43
Muffins (and Scones)										
■ **General**										
Plain homemade muffin	1 muffin (2 oz)	169	24	7	44	18	24	21	57	29
Wheat bran toaster muffin	1 toaster muffin	106	19	3	27	11	15	13	36	18
Store-bought oat bran muffin	1 extra large muffin (6 oz)	454	81	12	117	48	64	55	154	77
Homemade corn muffin	1 muffin (2 oz)	180	25	7	46	19	26	22	61	31
Store-bought corn muffin	1 extra large muffin (6 oz)	512	86	14	132	55	73	62	174	87
Homemade blueberry muffin	1 muffin (2 oz)	162	23	6	42	17	23	20	55	28

FOOD	AMOUNT	CAL	CARBS	FAT	WALK	RUN	BIKE	SWIM	YOGA	DANCE
Store-bought blueberry muffin	1 extra large muffin (6 oz)	465	81	11	120	50	66	57	158	79
Hostess Low Fat Blueberry Muffin	1 serving	230	47	3	59	24	33	28	78	39
Thomas' Corn Muffin Toaster Cake	1 cake	100	18	4	26	11	14	12	34	17
Weight Watchers Honey Harvest Muffin	1 serving	220	42	5	57	23	31	27	75	37
Weight Watchers Chocolate Chip Muffin	1 muffin	200	39	4	52	21	28	24	68	34
Weight Watchers Blueberry Muffin	1 muffin	180	33	4	46	19	26	22	61	31
■ **Muffin Mix**										
Betty Crocker Banana Nut Muffin Mix (prepared)	3 tbsp	170	27	6	44	18	24	21	58	29
Betty Crocker Wild Blueberry Muffin Mix (prepared)	.25 cup	170	28	5	44	18	24	21	58	29
Duncan Hines All Bran Blueberry Muffin Mix (prepared)	.08 pkg	140	25	5	36	15	20	17	48	24
■ **Dunkin' Donuts**										
Blueberry	1 muffin	470	73	17	121	50	67	57	160	80
Reduced Fat Blueberry	1 muffin	400	78	5	103	43	57	49	136	68
Cranberry Orange	1 muffin	440	66	17	113	47	62	54	150	75
Banana Walnut	1 muffin	540	69	25	139	58	77	66	184	92
Chocolate Chip	1 muffin	630	89	26	162	67	89	77	214	107
Coffee Cake	1 muffin	580	78	19	149	62	82	71	197	99
Corn	1 muffin	510	77	18	131	54	72	62	173	87
Honey Bran Raisin	1 muffin	480	79	15	124	51	68	58	163	82
English Muffin	1 muffin	160	31	2	41	17	23	19	54	27
■ **Panera Bread**										
Banana Nut Muffie	1 Muffie	220	33	8	57	23	31	27	75	37
Chocolate Chip Muffie	1 Muffie	240	36	10	62	26	34	29	82	41
Pumpkin Muffie	1 Muffie	340	49	7	88	36	48	41	116	58
Banana Nut Muffin	1 muffin	410	63	15	106	44	58	50	139	70
Blueberry Muffin	1 muffin	530	85	18	137	56	75	64	180	90
Chocolate Chip Muffin	1 muffin	540	83	22	139	58	77	66	184	92
Low-Fat Tripleberry Muffin	1 muffin	300	63	3	77	32	43	36	102	51
Pumpkin Muffin	1 muffin	640	93	13	165	68	91	78	218	109

FOOD	AMOUNT	CAL	CARBS	FAT	WALK	RUN	BIKE	SWIM	YOGA	DANCE
■ **Entenmann's**										
Corn Muffin	1 muffin	240	35	9	62	26	34	29	82	41
Holiday Golden Cupcake	1 cupcake	290	40	14	75	31	41	35	99	49
Little Bites Fudge Brownie	1 pouch	270	34	15	70	29	38	33	92	46
Little Bites Blueberry Muffin	1 pouch	210	28	10	54	22	30	26	71	36
Little Bites Chocolate Chip Muffin	1 pouch	210	28	10	54	22	30	26	71	36
■ **Au Bon Pain**										
Apple Spice	1 muffin	420	65	15	108	45	60	51	143	72
Banana Walnut	1 muffin	440	60	19	113	47	62	54	150	75
Blueberry	1 muffin	510	76	19	131	54	72	62	173	87
Carrot Nut	1 muffin	520	66	25	134	55	74	63	177	89
Chocolate Chunk	1 muffin	590	83	20	152	63	84	72	201	101
Corn	1 muffin	460	69	16	119	49	65	56	156	78
Cranberry Blueberry	1 muffin	520	76	20	134	55	74	63	177	89
Cranberry Walnut	1 muffin	500	61	24	129	53	71	61	170	85
Low Fat Chocolate Cake	1 muffin	320	74	2	82	34	45	39	109	55
Low Fat Triple Berry	1 muffin	290	61	2	75	31	41	35	99	49
Milk Chocolate Chip	1 muffin	570	81	23	147	61	81	69	194	97
Pumpkin	1 muffin	470	66	14	121	50	67	57	160	80
Raisin Bran	1 muffin	410	74	9	106	44	58	50	139	70
■ **Starbucks muffins and scones**										
Blueberry Muffin	1 serving (101 g)	380	49	19	98	40	54	46	129	65
Morning Surprise Muffin	1 serving (110 g)	330	54	12	85	35	47	40	112	56
Cranberry Orange Muffin	1 serving (110 g)	410	53	20	106	44	58	50	139	70
Cinnamon Chip Scone with icing	1 serving (128 g)	510	71	23	131	54	72	62	173	87
Butterscotch Pecan Scone	1 serving (120 g)	520	64	27	134	55	74	63	177	89
Brownies										
■ **General**										
Homemade brownie	2″ square	112	12	7	29	12	16	14	38	19
Fast food brownie	2″ square	243	39	10	63	26	34	30	83	41
Store-bought brownie	2 oz	227	36	9	59	24	32	28	77	39

FOOD	AMOUNT	CAL	CARBS	FAT	WALK	RUN	BIKE	SWIM	YOGA	DANCE
■ Brownie Mix										
Betty Crocker Fudge Brownie Mix (prepared)	.05 pkg	170	23	7	44	18	24	21	58	29
Betty Crocker Original Supreme Brownie Mix (prepared)	.05 pkg	160	27	6	41	17	23	19	54	27
Betty Crocker Turtle Supreme Brownie Mix (prepared)	.05 pkg	170	23	8	44	18	24	21	58	29
Betty Crocker Walnut Supreme Brownie Mix (prepared)	.05 pkg	180	22	9	46	19	26	22	61	31
Duncan Hines Chocolate Lovers Brownie Mix (prepared)	.25 pkg	150	22	7	39	16	21	18	51	26
Duncan Hines Milk Chocolate Chunk Brownie Mix (prepared)	.25 cup	160	23	7	41	17	23	19	54	27
Duncan Hines Turtle Brownie Mix (prepared)	.25 cup	150	20	8	39	16	21	18	51	26
Duncan Hines Walnut Brownie Mix (prepared)	.25 cup	160	20	9	41	17	23	19	54	27
■ Weight Watchers										
Weight Watchers Brownie à la Mode	1 serving	190	34	4	49	20	27	23	65	32
Weight Watchers Brownie Cheesecake	1 serving	200	33	6	52	21	28	24	68	34
Weight Watchers Chocolate Frosted Brownie	1 serving	100	22	3	26	11	14	12	34	17
■ Little Debbie										
Little Debbie Fudge Brownie	1 brownie	270	39	13	70	29	38	33	92	46
■ Panera Bread										
Caramel Pecan Brownie	1 brownie	470	60	24	121	50	67	57	160	80
Chocolate Raspberry Brownie	1 brownie	450	66	18	116	48	64	55	153	77
Very Chocolate Brownie	1 brownie	460	62	21	119	49	65	56	156	78
■ Au Bon Pain										
Cheesecake Brownie	1 brownie	470	55	26	121	50	67	57	160	80
Chocolate Chip Brownie	1 brownie	480	61	25	124	51	68	58	163	82
Pecan Brownie	1 brownie	510	55	31	131	54	72	62	173	87
Rocky Road Brownie	1 brownie	550	49	33	142	59	78	67	187	94
Blondie with Nuts	1 brownie	570	57	36	147	61	81	69	194	97

FOOD	AMOUNT	CAL	CARBS	FAT	WALK	RUN	BIKE	SWIM	YOGA	DANCE

Bakery Goods

General

■ Danishes and Sweet Rolls

FOOD	AMOUNT	CAL	CARBS	FAT	WALK	RUN	BIKE	SWIM	YOGA	DANCE
Cheese danish	1 pastry	266	26	16	69	28	38	32	90	45
Cinnamon danish	1 pastry	262	29	15	68	28	37	32	89	45
Cream puffs, unfilled	1 puff	239	15	17	62	25	34	29	81	41
Cream puffs, filled with cream	1 puff	335	30	20	86	36	48	41	114	57
Éclair	1 éclair	262	24	16	68	28	37	32	89	45
Fruit-filled danish	1 pastry	263	34	13	68	28	37	32	89	45
Nut danish	1 pastry	280	30	16	72	30	40	34	95	48
Apple strudel	1 piece (71 g)	195	29	8	50	21	28	24	66	33
Cheese sweet Roll	1 roll	238	29	12	61	25	34	29	81	41
Cinnamon roll (made from refrigerated dough)	1 roll	109	17	4	28	12	15	13	37	19
Cinnamon raisin sweet roll	1 roll (2 ¾" square)	223	31	10	57	24	32	27	76	38
Entenmann's Apple Puffs	1 puff	290	39	14	75	31	41	35	99	49
Entenmann's Apple Strudel	¼ strudel	360	53	15	93	38	51	44	122	61
Entenmann's Butter Twist	⅛ danish	230	29	11	59	24	33	28	78	39
Entenmann's Cheese Buns	1 bun	320	40	15	82	34	45	39	109	55
Entenmann's Cinnamon Hazelnut Ring	⅛ danish	270	27	16	70	29	38	33	92	46
Entenmann's Cinnamon Raising Swirl Buns	1 bun	320	45	13	82	34	45	39	109	55
Entenmann's Éclairs	1 éclair	260	46	9	67	28	37	32	88	44
Entenmann's Guava Cheese Puffs	1 puff	310	34	18	80	33	44	38	105	53
Entenmann's Pecan Danish Ring	⅛ danish	250	33	16	64	27	35	30	85	43
Entenmann's Raspberry Danish Twist	⅛ danish	220	28	11	57	23	31	27	75	37
Entenmann's Turtle Sundae Twist	⅛ danish	220	26	12	57	23	31	27	75	37
Entenmann's Ultimate Sugar Honey Buns	1 bun	660	96	26	170	70	94	80	224	112
Hostess Cinnamon Sweet Roll Snack Cake	1 serving	210	34	7	54	22	30	26	71	36

FOOD	AMOUNT	CAL	CARBS	FAT	WALK	RUN	BIKE	SWIM	YOGA	DANCE
Pepperidge Farm Apple Turnovers	1 serving	284	31	16	73	30	40	35	97	48
Pillsbury Cinnamon Raisin Sweet Roll with Icing	1 serving	180	26	7	46	19	26	22	61	31
Pillsbury Refrigerated Iced Cinnamon Roll Dough	1 serving	150	24	5	39	16	21	18	51	26
Weight Watchers Glazed Cinnamon Roll	1 serving	200	33	5	52	21	28	24	68	34
■ Croissants										
Apple croissant	1 medium	145	21	5	37	15	21	18	49	25
Cheese croissant	1 medium	236	27	12	61	25	33	29	80	40
Butter croissant	1 medium	231	26	12	60	25	33	28	79	39
Panera Bread										
French Croissant	1 croissant	270	29	15	70	29	38	33	92	46
Cinnamon Roll	1 roll	590	81	26	152	63	84	72	201	101
Pecan Roll	1 roll	530	62	30	137	56	75	64	180	90
Cinnamon Chip Scone	1 scone	570	69	29	147	61	81	69	194	97
Orange Scone	1 scone	430	54	21	111	46	61	52	146	73
Apple Raisin Strudel	1 serving	390	45	22	101	42	55	47	133	66
Bear Claw	1 serving	440	46	25	113	47	62	54	150	75
Carrot Walnut Mini Bundt Cake	1 serving	430	51	21	111	46	61	52	146	73
Cheese Pastry	1 serving	340	35	20	88	36	48	41	116	58
Cherry Pastry	1 serving	410	53	20	106	44	58	50	139	70
Cherry Strudel	1 serving	400	42	24	103	43	57	49	136	68
Chocolate Pastry	1 serving	400	46	23	103	43	57	49	136	68
Cobblestone	1 serving	590	107	12	152	63	84	72	201	101
Cherry Cheese Coffee Cake	1 serving	210	25	11	54	22	30	26	71	36
Fresh Apple Pastry	1 serving	320	37	17	82	34	45	39	109	55
Fresh Strawberries & Cream Pastry	1 serving	320	35	18	82	34	45	39	109	55
Lemon Poppyseed Mini Bundt Cake	1 serving	460	63	20	119	49	65	56	156	78
Pineapple Upside-Down Mini Bundt Cake	1 serving	520	74	25	134	55	74	63	177	89
Dunkin' Donuts										
Biscuit	1 biscuit	250	29	13	64	27	35	30	85	43
Croissant	1 croissant	330	37	18	85	35	47	40	112	56
Apple Danish	1 danish	330	32	20	85	35	47	40	112	56

FOOD	AMOUNT	CAL	CARBS	FAT	WALK	RUN	BIKE	SWIM	YOGA	DANCE
Cheese Danish	1 danish	340	30	22	88	36	48	41	116	58
Strawberry Danish	1 danish	320	31	20	82	34	45	39	109	55
Breadsmith										
Almond Chocolate Stick	1 stick	344	33	21	89	37	49	42	117	59
Babka	1 slice (1 oz)	102	16	3	26	11	14	12	35	17
Bostock	1 bostock	407	62	15	105	43	58	50	138	69
Brioche	1 slice (1 oz)	118	13	6	30	13	17	14	40	20
Brownie	1 brownie (4 oz)	492	68	24	127	52	70	60	167	84
Brownie with Walnuts	1 brownie (4 oz)	448	59	23	115	48	64	55	152	76
Cinnamon Bun	1 bun	798	133	24	206	85	113	97	271	136
Cinnamon Bun with Icing	1 bun	846	133	29	218	90	120	103	288	144
Cinnamon Claw	1 claw	251	48	4	65	27	36	31	85	43
Coffee Cake	1 serving (2 oz)	194	36	5	50	21	28	24	66	33
Individual Coffee Cake	1 cake	864	160	22	223	92	123	105	294	147
Hot cross Buns	1 bun	504	112	1	130	54	71	61	171	86
Scone	1 scone	424	60	16	109	45	60	52	144	72
Chocolate Chip Scone	1 scone	484	65	22	125	52	69	59	165	82
Currant Scone	1 scone	420	68	14	108	45	60	51	143	72
Pecan Scone	1 scone	420	68	14	108	45	60	51	143	72
Shortbread Tart, Caramel Cinnamon Apple	1 serving (2 oz)	267	34	13	69	28	38	32	91	45
Shortbread Tart, Cherry Almond	1 serving (2 oz)	248	31	12	64	26	35	30	84	42
Shortbread Tart, Key Lime	1 serving (2 oz)	269	34	14	69	29	38	33	91	46
Shortbread Tart, Strawberry Rhubarb	1 serving (2 oz)	251	33	12	65	27	36	31	85	43
Au Bon Pain										
Raspberry Crumb Cake	1 serving	770	94	41	198	82	109	94	262	131
Cinnamon Scone	1 scone	420	53	23	108	45	60	51	143	72
Orange Scone	1 scone	380	48	19	98	40	54	46	129	65
Apple Crumble Cake	1 serving	540	62	30	139	58	77	66	184	92
Butter Crumb Cake	1 serving	790	96	42	204	84	112	96	269	135

FOOD	AMOUNT	CAL	CARBS	FAT	WALK	RUN	BIKE	SWIM	YOGA	DANCE
Apple Strudel	1 serving	410	56	18	106	44	58	50	139	70
Cherry Strudel	1 serving	390	49	19	101	42	55	47	133	66
Cherry Danish	1 serving	410	52	19	106	44	58	50	139	70
Lemon Danish	1 serving	430	57	20	111	46	61	52	146	73
Sweet Cheese Danish	1 serving	470	54	26	121	50	67	57	160	80
Cinnamon Roll	1 serving	300	39	13	77	32	43	36	102	51
Pecan Roll	1 serving	520	61	28	134	55	74	63	177	89
Creme de Fleur	1 serving	550	71	26	142	59	78	67	187	94
Plain Croissant	1 croissant	270	28	15	70	29	38	33	92	46
Almond Croissant	1 croissant	510	63	25	131	54	72	62	173	87
Apple Strudel Croissant	1 croissant	330	36	20	85	35	47	40	112	56
Cherry Strudel Croissant	1 croissant	330	34	20	85	35	47	40	112	56
Chocolate Croissant	1 croissant	340	42	17	88	36	48	41	116	58
Cinnamon Raisin Croissant	1 croissant	340	69	5	88	36	48	41	116	58
Raspberry Croissant	1 croissant	340	39	18	88	36	48	41	116	58
Sweet Cheese Croissant	1 croissant	350	35	21	90	37	50	43	119	60
Starbucks										
Classic Coffee Cake	1 serving (139 g)	570	75	28	147	61	81	69	194	97
Crumb Cake	1 serving (163 g)	670	89	32	173	71	95	82	228	114
Iced Lemon Pound Cake	1 serving (142 g)	500	69	23	129	53	71	61	170	85
Zucchini Pound Cake	1 serving (113 g)	370	47	19	95	39	52	45	126	63
Sour Cream Coffee Cake	1 serving (90 g)	420	43	25	108	45	60	51	143	72
Blueberry Walnut Coffee Cake	1 serving (88 g)	340	43	18	88	36	48	41	116	58
Butter Croissant with Apricot Glaze	1 serving (85 g)	320	37	17	82	34	45	39	109	55
Chocolate Filled Croissant	1 serving (92 g)	350	43	19	90	37	50	43	119	60
Raspberry and Cream Cheese Filled Croissant	1 serving (92 g)	260	34	12	67	28	37	32	88	44
Almond Filled Croissant	1 serving (92 g)	330	39	18	85	35	47	40	112	56
Caramel Pecan Sticky Roll	1 serving (184 g)	730	75	40	188	78	104	89	248	124

FOOD	AMOUNT	CAL	CARBS	FAT	WALK†	RUN	BIKE	SWIM	YOGA	DANCE
Cinnamon Roll	1 serving (170 g)	620	80	29	160	66	88	75	211	106
Cinnamon Twist	1 serving (85 g)	320	37	17	82	34	45	39	109	55
Cheese Danish with Mocha Swirls	1 serving (120 g)	460	44	28	119	49	65	56	156	78
TJ Cinnamons										
Original Roll	5.25 oz	510	73	10	131	54	72	62	173	87
Original Roll with Cream Cheese Icing	6.5 oz	650	95	17	168	69	92	79	221	111
Pecan Sticky Roll	6.5 oz	690	91	22	178	73	98	84	235	118
Cinnachips	10 oz bag	1130	157	50	291	120	160	137	384	193
Cinnamon Twist	2.5 oz	260	33	13	67	28	37	32	88	44
Chocolate Twist	2.5 oz	250	34	12	64	27	35	30	85	43
Twists with Icing (on side)	1 oz	120	18	5	31	13	17	15	41	20

Cookies (and Bars)

General										
■ **Animal Crackers**										
Animal Crackers	12 crackers	130	22	3	34	14	18	16	44	22
Barnum's	8 crackers	120	22	4	31	13	17	15	41	20
Ernie's Animal Crackers	1 box	250	41	9	64	27	35	30	85	43
Gamesa Animalitos	14 cookies	110	25	1	28	12	16	13	37	19
Grandma's Tiny Bites Animal Crackers	11 cookies	260	42	9	67	28	37	32	88	44
■ **Chocolate Chip Cookies**										
Homemade	1 cookie (2 ¼″ diameter)	78	9	5	20	8	11	9	27	13
Store-bought	1 cookie	48	7	2	12	5	7	6	16	8
Reduced Fat	1 cookie	45	7	2	12	5	6	5	15	8
Soft	1 cookie	69	9	4	18	7	10	8	23	12
From refrigerated dough	1 cookie	59	8	3	15	6	8	7	20	10
Nestlé Chocolate Chip Cookie Dough with Toll House Morsels	2 tbsp	140	20	6	36	15	20	17	48	24
Nestlé Toll House Break and Bake Chocolate Chunk	1 cookie	110	15	5	28	12	16	13	37	19

FOOD	AMOUNT	CAL	CARBS	FAT	WALK	RUN	BIKE	SWIM	YOGA	DANCE
Pillsbury Chocolate Chip Cookie Dough	1 oz	140	17	7	36	15	20	17	48	24

■ Coconut Cookies

FOOD	AMOUNT	CAL	CARBS	FAT	WALK	RUN	BIKE	SWIM	YOGA	DANCE
Coconut macaroon	1 cookie (2" diameter)	97	17	3	25	10	14	12	33	17
Archway Coconut Macaroon	1 cookie	80	12	5	21	9	11	10	27	14
Gamesa Barras de CoCo Coconut	5 cookies	120	21	4	31	13	17	15	41	20
Gamesa Hawaianas Coconut	3 cookies	130	22	4	34	14	18	16	44	22

■ Fruit Bars

FOOD	AMOUNT	CAL	CARBS	FAT	WALK	RUN	BIKE	SWIM	YOGA	DANCE
Fig bars	1 cookie	56	11	1	14	6	8	7	19	10
Fig Newtons	2 cookies	110	22	2	28	12	16	13	37	19
Fat Free Fig Newtons	2 cookies	90	22	0	23	10	13	11	31	15
Whole Grain Fig Newtons	2 cookies	110	22	2	28	12	16	13	37	19
Archway Fruit Filled Raspberry	1 cookie	90	15	3	23	10	13	11	31	15
Archway Fruit Filled Strawberry	1 cookie	90	15	3	23	10	13	11	31	15
Archway Fruit and Honey Bar	1 cookie	160	28	5	41	17	23	19	54	27
Archway Fruit Filled Apple Oatmeal	1 cookie	90	15	3	23	10	13	11	31	15
Archway Fruit Filled Apricot	1 cookie	90	15	3	23	10	13	11	31	15
Archway Fruit Filled Cherry	1 cookie	100	16	3	26	11	14	12	34	17
Archway Fruit Filled Oatmeal Date	1 cookie	99	17	3	25	11	14	12	34	17

■ Fudge Cookies

FOOD	AMOUNT	CAL	CARBS	FAT	WALK	RUN	BIKE	SWIM	YOGA	DANCE
Fudge cookie	1 cookie	73	16	1	19	8	10	9	25	12
Stella D'oro Swiss Fudge	3 cookies	170	22	9	44	18	24	21	58	29
Keebler Fudge Shop Grasshopper	4 cookies	140	19	7	36	15	20	17	48	24
Keebler Fudge Shop Deluxe Grahams	3 cookies	140	17	7	36	15	20	17	48	24
Keebler Fudge Shop Fudge Stripes	3 cookies	160	21	8	41	17	23	19	54	27
Keebler Fudge Shop Fudge Sticks	3 cookies	150	19	8	39	16	21	18	51	26

■ Ginger Cookies

FOOD	AMOUNT	CAL	CARBS	FAT	WALK	RUN	BIKE	SWIM	YOGA	DANCE
Ginger men	4 cookies	130	21	4	34	14	18	16	44	22
Ginger snap	1 cookie	29	5	1	7	3	4	4	10	5

FOOD	AMOUNT	CAL	CARBS	FAT	WALK	RUN	BIKE	SWIM	YOGA	DANCE
Nabisco Ginger Snaps	4 cookies	120	23	3	31	13	17	15	41	20
■ Oatmeal Cookies										
Homemade	1 cookie (2 ⅝" diameter)	67	10	3	17	7	10	8	23	11
Homemade with raisins	1 cookie (2 ⅝" diameter)	65	10	2	17	7	9	8	22	11
Store-bought	1 large	81	12	3	21	9	11	10	28	14
Store-bought, soft style	1 cookie	61	10	2	16	6	9	7	21	10
From refrigerated dough	1 cookie	57	8	3	15	6	8	7	19	10
Store-bought, fat free	1 cookie	61	10	2	16	6	9	7	21	10
Archway Ruth's Golden Oatmeal	1 cookie	120	18	5	31	13	17	15	41	20
Archway Oatmeal	1 cookie	110	17	4	28	12	16	13	37	19
Archway Oatmeal Raisin Bran	1 cookie	110	18	4	28	12	16	13	37	19
Entenmann's Soft Baked Oatmeal Raisin	1 cookie	160	26	6	41	17	23	19	54	27
Famous Amos Oatmeal Raisin	4 cookies	140	20	6	36	15	20	17	48	24
Keebler Country Style Oatmeal Raisin	2 cookies	130	18	6	34	14	18	16	44	22
Little Debbie's Oatmeal Crème Pies	1 cookie	170	26	7	44	18	24	21	58	29
Murray's Sugar-Free Oatmeal	3 cookies	150	21	7	39	16	21	18	51	26
Pepperidge Farm Soft Baked Oatmeal Raisin	1 cookie	130	23	5	34	14	18	16	44	22
■ Marshmallow Cookies										
Chocolate-coated marshmallow cookie	1 cookie	55	9	2	14	6	8	7	19	9
Gamesa Arcoiris Merengue	6 cookies	200	43	3	52	21	28	24	68	34
Gamesa Arcoiris	6 cookies	220	44	4	57	23	31	27	75	37
Gamesa Chocolate Arcoiris with Nuts	2 cookies	120	18	5	31	13	17	15	41	20
Little Debbie Marshmallow Pies	1 cookie	180	30	6	46	19	26	22	61	31
Little Debbie Marshmallow Supreme	1 cookie	140	22	5	36	15	20	17	48	24
■ Nutter Butter										
Nutter Butter	2 cookies	130	19	6	34	14	18	16	44	22
Milk Chocolate Covered Nutter Butter	1 cookie	90	12	5	23	10	13	11	31	15

FOOD	AMOUNT	CAL	CARBS	FAT	WALK	RUN	BIKE	SWIM	YOGA	DANCE
■ Peanut Butter Cookies										
Homemade	1 cookie (3″ diameter)	95	12	5	24	10	13	12	32	16
From refrigerated dough	1 cookie	60	7	3	15	6	9	7	20	10
Store-bought, soft style	1 cookie	69	9	4	18	7	10	8	23	12
Store-bought	1 cookie	72	9	4	19	8	10	9	24	12
Murray's Sugar Free Peanut Butter	3 cookies	150	17	9	39	16	21	18	51	26
Nutter Butter	2 cookies	130	19	6	34	14	18	16	44	22
Milk Chocolate Covered Nutter Butter	1 cookie	90	12	5	23	10	13	11	31	15
■ Shortbread Cookies										
Store-bought shortbread cookie	1 cookie (1 ⅝″ square)	40	5	2	10	4	6	5	14	7
Keebler Sandies Pecan Shortbread	1 cookie	80	9	5	21	9	11	10	27	14
Keebler Sandies Simply Shortbread	1 cookie	80	10	5	21	9	11	10	27	14
Keebler Sandies Reduced Fat Pecan Shortbread	1 cookie	80	10	4	21	9	11	10	27	14
Lorna Doone Shortbread	4 cookies	150	19	7	39	16	21	18	51	26
Pepperidge Farm Shortbread	2 cookies	140	16	7	36	15	20	17	48	24
■ Sugar cookies										
Homemade	1 cookie (3″ diameter)	66	8	3	17	7	9	8	22	11
From refrigerated dough	1 cookie	111	15	5	29	12	16	14	38	19
Store-bought	1 cookie	72	10	3	19	8	10	9	24	12
Sugar wafer with Crème Filling	1 wafer	138	19	7	36	15	20	17	47	24
Pepperidge Farm Soft Baked Sugar	1 cookie	140	22	5	36	15	20	17	48	24
Pepperidge Farm Sugar	3 cookies	140	20	6	36	15	20	17	48	24
■ Wafers										
Chocolate wafers	3 wafers	78	13	3	20	8	11	9	27	13
Gamesa Chocolate Sugar Wafers	3 cookies	160	23	7	41	17	23	19	54	27
Gamesa Strawberry Sugar Wafers	3 cookies	160	24	6	41	17	23	19	54	27

FOOD	AMOUNT	CAL	CARBS	FAT	WALK	RUN	BIKE	SWIM	YOGA	DANCE
Gamesa Vanilla Sugar Wafers	3 cookies	160	25	7	41	17	23	19	54	27
■ **Other Cookies**										
Tea biscuits	5 biscuits	160	30	5	41	17	23	19	54	27
Arrowroot	5 cookies	109	18	3	28	12	15	13	37	19
Molasses	1 oz	64	11	2	16	7	9	8	22	11
Ladyfingers	1 ladyfinger	40	7	1	10	4	6	5	14	7
Fortune	1 cookie	30	7	22	8	3	4	4	10	5
Danish Butter	4 cookies	165	21	8	43	18	23	20	56	28
Gamesa Roscas Cinnamon	3 cookies	130	4	22	34	14	18	16	44	22
Storebought Cookies										
■ **Archway**										
Aunt Bea's Pound Cake	1 cookie	105	16	4	27	11	15	13	36	18
Black Walnut Icebox	1 cookie	119	15	6	31	13	17	15	41	20
Chocolate Chip	1 cookie	130	18	6	34	14	18	16	44	22
Chocolate Chip Drop	1 cookie	101	16	4	26	11	14	12	34	17
Chocolate Chip Icebox	1 cookie	117	15	6	30	12	17	14	40	20
Cinnamon Apple	1 cookie	106	17	4	27	11	15	13	36	18
Dark Molasses	1 cookie	115	20	3	30	12	16	14	39	20
Dutch Cocoa	1 cookie	100	17	4	26	11	14	12	34	17
Frosty Lemon	1 cookie	112	17	4	29	12	16	14	38	19
Frosty Orange	1 cookie	113	17	5	29	12	16	14	38	19
Gourmet Apple n' Raisin	1 cookie	111	17	4	28	12	16	13	38	19
Gourmet Carrot Cake	1 cookie	120	18	5	31	13	17	15	41	21
Gourmet Chocolate Chip n' Toffee	1 cookie	131	18	6	34	14	19	16	45	22
Gourmet Oatmeal Pecan	1 cookie	134	16	7	34	14	19	16	45	23
Gourmet Old Fashioned Peanut Butter	1 cookie	117	15	6	30	12	17	14	40	20
Gourmet Rocky Road	1 cookie	127	18	6	33	14	18	15	43	22
Iced Ginger Snaps	1 cookie	172	26	7	44	18	24	21	59	29
Iced Molasses	1 cookie	114	20	4	29	12	16	14	39	19
Iced Oatmeal	1 cookie	123	18	5	32	13	17	15	42	21
Lemon Drop	1 cookie	93	15	3	24	10	13	11	32	16
Lemon Snaps	1 cookie	152	20	7	39	16	22	18	52	26
Molasses	1 cookie	103	18	3	27	11	15	13	35	18
Mud Pie	1 cookie	107	15	5	28	11	15	13	36	18

FOOD	AMOUNT	CAL	CARBS	FAT	WALK	RUN	BIKE	SWIM	YOGA	DANCE
Oatmeal	1 cookie	110	17	4	28	12	16	13	37	19
Oatmeal Raisin	1 cookie	120	20	4	31	13	17	15	41	20
Oatmeal Raisin Bran	1 cookie	110	18	4	28	12	16	13	37	19
Old Fashioned Molasses	1 cookie	105	18	3	27	11	15	13	36	18
Old Fashioned Windmill	1 cookie	91	14	3	23	10	13	11	31	16
Peanut Butter	1 cookie	101	12	5	26	11	14	12	34	17
Peanut Jumble	1 cookie	116	13	6	30	12	16	14	40	20
Pecan Icebox	1 cookie	120	15	6	31	13	17	15	41	20
Reduced Fat Ginger Snaps	1 cookie	136	25	4	35	14	19	17	46	23
Rocky Road with Walnuts	1 cookie	120	18	5	31	13	17	15	41	20
Ruth's Golden Oatmeal	1 cookie	120	18	5	31	13	17	15	41	20
Sugar	1 cookie	98	17	3	25	10	14	12	33	17
■ Chips Ahoy										
Chips Ahoy Chocolate Chip	3 cookies	160	22	8	41	17	23	19	54	27
Chips Ahoy Candy Blasts	1 cookie	80	10	4	21	9	11	10	27	14
Bite Size Chips Ahoy Chocolate Chip	5 cookies	150	21	7	39	16	21	18	51	26
Chips Ahoy White Fudge Chunky	1 cookie	80	11	4	21	9	11	10	27	14
Chips Ahoy Chunky Chocolate Chip	1 cookie	80	11	4	21	9	11	10	27	14
■ Entenmann's Cookies										
Coconut	2 cookies	120	16	7	31	13	17	15	41	20
Holiday Collection	2 cookies	120	15	7	31	13	17	15	41	20
Original Recipe Chocolate Chip	3 cookies	140	20	7	36	15	20	17	48	24
Soft Baked Oatmeal Raisin	1 cookie	160	26	6	41	17	23	19	54	27
■ Famous Amos										
Famous Amos Oatmeal Raisin	4 cookies	140	20	6	36	15	20	17	48	24
Famous Amos Chocolate Chip	4 cookies	140	19	7	36	15	20	17	48	24
Famous Amos Chocolate Chip and Pecan	4 cookies	150	18	8	39	16	21	18	51	26
■ Grandma's										
Tiny Bites Mini Chocolate Chip	12 cookies	280	38	12	72	30	40	34	95	48
Homestyle Fudge Chocolate Chip	1 cookie	190	28	7	49	20	27	23	65	32
Mini Fudge	9 cookies	150	21	7	39	16	21	18	51	26
Fudge Vanilla Sandwich Cookie	3 cookies	120	21	4	31	13	17	15	41	20

FOOD	AMOUNT	CAL	CARBS	FAT	WALK	RUN	BIKE	SWIM	YOGA	DANCE
Homestyle Molasses	1 cookie	160	29	4	41	17	23	19	54	27
Homestyle Oatmeal Raisin	1 cookie	180	30	6	46	19	26	22	61	31
Mini Peanut Butter	9 cookies	150	21	7	39	16	21	18	51	26
Homestyle Peanut Butter	1 cookie	200	24	10	52	21	28	24	68	34
Tiny Bite Sugar	12 cookies	280	38	13	72	30	40	34	95	48
Vanilla Sandwich	5 cookies	210	30	10	54	22	30	26	71	36
Mini Vanilla	9 cookies	150	22	7	39	16	21	18	51	26
■ Hershey's Cookies										
Almond Joy	2 cookies	150	17	9	39	16	21	18	51	26
Hershey's Caramel	1 package (56 g)	270	12	38	70	29	38	33	92	46
Hershey's Cookies 'n' Crème	1 package (56 g)	300	33	17	77	32	43	36	102	51
Hershey's Miniature Chocolate Cookie Mix	6 pieces	220	25	12	57	23	31	27	75	37
Hershey's with Almonds	2 cookies	150	16	9	39	16	21	18	51	26
Mauna Loa Chocolate Chip	4 cookies	150	16	9	39	16	21	18	51	26
Mauna Loa Toffee Crunch	4 cookies	150	16	9	39	16	21	18	51	26
Mauna Loa White Chocolate Chip	4 cookies	150	16	9	39	16	21	18	51	26
Reese's	2 cookies	150	17	8	39	16	21	18	51	26
York	2 cookies	160	17	9	41	17	23	19	54	27
■ Keebler										
Keebler Chips Deluxe Original	1 cookie	80	9	5	21	9	11	10	27	14
Keebler Chips Deluxe Rainbow	1 cookie	80	10	4	21	9	11	10	27	14
Keebler Chips Deluxe Chocolate Lovers	1 cookie	80	10	5	21	9	11	10	27	14
Keebler Chips Deluxe Soft 'n Chewy	1 cookie	70	11	3	18	7	10	9	24	12
Keebler Sandies Pecan Shortbread	1 cookie	80	9	5	21	9	11	10	27	14
Keebler Sandies Simply Shortbread	1 cookie	80	10	5	21	9	11	10	27	14
Keebler Sandies Reduced Fat Pecan Shortbread	1 cookie	80	10	4	21	9	11	10	27	14
Keebler Country Style Oatmeal Raisin	2 cookies	130	18	6	34	14	18	16	44	22
Keebler Soft Batch Chocolate Chip	1 cookie	80	11	4	21	9	11	10	27	14

FOOD	AMOUNT	CAL	CARBS	FAT	WALK	RUN	BIKE	SWIM	YOGA	DANCE
■ Nabisco										
Lorna Doone Shortbread	4 cookies	150	19	7	39	16	21	18	51	26
Mallomars	2 cookies	120	18	5	31	13	17	15	41	20
Nabisco Nilla Wafers	8 wafers	110	24	2	28	12	16	13	37	19
Nabisco Ginger Snaps	4 cookies	120	23	3	31	13	17	15	41	20
Nabisco Social Tea Biscuits	6 cookies	140	24	4	36	15	20	17	48	24
■ Pepperidge Farm										
Pepperidge Farm White Chocolate Chunk Macadamia Tahoe Crispy	1 cookie	130	17	6	34	14	18	16	44	22
Pepperidge Farm Milk Chocolate Macadamia Sausalito Crispy	1 cookie	140	16	8	36	15	20	17	48	24
Pepperidge Farm Dark Chocolate Pecan Chesapeake Crispy	1 cookie	140	15	8	36	15	20	17	48	24
Pepperidge Farm Dark Chocolate Nantucket Crispy	1 cookie	140	16	7	36	15	20	17	48	24
Pepperidge Farm Dark Chocolate Crispy	1 cookie	140	18	7	36	15	20	17	48	24
Pepperidge Farm Soft Baked Oatmeal Raisin	1 cookie	130	23	5	34	14	18	16	44	22
Pepperidge Farm Soft Baked Oatmeal Cranberry	1 cookie	130	22	4	34	14	18	16	44	22
Pepperidge Farm Soft Baked Dark Chocolate Brownie	1 cookie	140	22	5	36	15	20	17	48	24
Pepperidge Farm Soft Baked Milk Chocolate Caramel	1 cookie	140	21	6	36	15	20	17	48	24
Pepperidge Farm Milk Chocolate Cashew Stowe Crispy	1 cookie	130	17	6	34	14	18	16	44	22
Pepperidge Farm Soft Baked Snickerdoodle	1 cookie	140	22	5	36	15	20	17	48	24
Pepperidge Farm Soft Baked Dark Chocolate Nantucket	1 cookie	150	20	8	39	16	21	18	51	26
Pepperidge Farm Soft Baked Chocolate Dipped Dark Chocolate Brownie	1 cookie	160	22	7	41	17	23	19	54	27
Pepperidge Farm Soft Baked Chocolate Dipped Dark Chocolate	1 cookie	150	20	8	39	16	21	18	51	26
Pepperidge Farm Chocolate Dipped Chessmen	3 cookies	170	23	7	44	18	24	21	58	29
Ginger Men	4 cookies	130	21	4	34	14	18	16	44	22

FOOD	AMOUNT	CAL	CARBS	FAT	WALK	RUN	BIKE	SWIM	YOGA	DANCE
Shortbread	2 cookies	140	16	7	36	15	20	17	48	24
Apricot Raspberry Verona	3 cookies	140	22	5	36	15	20	17	48	24
Strawberry Verona	3 cookies	140	22	5	36	15	20	17	48	24
Raspberry Chantilly	2 cookies	120	23	3	31	13	17	15	41	20
Chessmen	3 cookies	120	18	5	31	13	17	15	41	20
Lido	1 cookie	90	10	5	23	10	13	11	31	15
Brussels	3 cookies	150	20	7	39	16	21	18	51	26
Geneva	3 cookies	160	19	9	41	17	23	19	54	27
Bordeaux	4 cookies	130	19	5	34	14	18	16	44	22
Chocolate Hazelnut Crème Filled Pirouette	2 cookies	130	20	5	34	14	18	16	44	22
Chocolate Fudge Crème Filled Pirouette	2 cookies	130	20	5	34	14	18	16	44	22
French Vanilla Cream Filled Pirouette	2 cookies	140	18	6	36	15	20	17	48	24
■ **Snackwell's**										
Snackwell's Black Forest Cookie Cakes	1 cookie	50	12	1	13	5	7	6	17	9
Snackwell's Fat Free Devil's Food Cookie Cakes	1 cookie	50	12	0	13	5	7	6	17	9
Snackwell's Chocolate Mint Cookie Cakes	1 cookie	50	12	1	13	5	7	6	17	9
Snackwell's Chocolate Sandwich	2 cookies	110	20	3	28	12	16	13	37	19
Snackwell's Coconut Crème	2 cookies	110	19	4	28	12	16	13	37	19
Snackwell's Crème Sandwich	2 cookies	110	20	3	28	12	16	13	37	19
Snackwell's Mint Crème	2 cookies	110	19	4	28	12	16	13	37	19
Snackwell's Reduced Fat Chocolate Chip	13 cookies	130	22	4	34	14	18	16	44	22
Snackwell's Reduced Fat Oatmeal Cookies with Raisins	2 cookies	110	20	3	28	12	16	13	37	19
Snackwell's Caramel Delight	1 serving	69	13	2	18	7	10	8	23	12
■ **Stella D'oro Cookies**										
Original	1 cookie	90	14	3	23	10	13	11	31	15
Lady Stella	3 cookies	130	19	5	34	14	18	16	44	22
Viennese Cinnamon	1 cookie	90	15	3	23	10	13	11	31	15
Margherite Cookies	2 cookies	130	20	5	34	14	18	16	44	22
Margherite Combination	2 cookies	130	20	5	34	14	18	16	44	22
Almond Biscotti	1 cookie	90	13	4	23	10	13	11	31	15

FOOD	AMOUNT	CAL	CARBS	FAT	WALK	RUN	BIKE	SWIM	YOGA	DANCE
Chocolate Almond Biscotti	1 cookie	90	14	4	23	10	13	11	31	15
Chocolate Chunk Biscotti	1 cookie	90	15	4	23	10	13	11	31	15
Anisette Sponge	2 cookies	90	18	1	23	10	13	11	31	15
Anisette Toast	3 cookies	130	27	1	34	14	18	16	44	22
Angel Wings	3 cookies	160	16	10	41	17	23	19	54	27
Roman Egg Biscuits	1 biscuit	130	19	5	34	14	18	16	44	22
Almond Delight	1 cookie	160	18	8	41	17	23	19	54	27
Almond Toast	2 cookies	100	20	2	26	11	14	12	34	17
Restaurant Cookies										
■ Au Bon Pain Cookies										
Chocolate Chip	1 cookie	260	37	11	67	28	37	32	88	44
Chocolate Dipped Cranberry Almond Macaroon	1 cookie	320	42	16	82	34	45	39	109	55
Chocolate Dipped Shortbread	1 cookie	300	52	10	77	32	43	36	102	51
Confetti Cookie with M&Ms	1 cookie	310	42	14	80	33	44	38	105	53
English Toffee Cookie	1 cookie	210	26	11	54	22	30	26	71	36
Oatmeal Raisin	1 cookie	230	37	8	59	24	33	28	78	39
Shortbread	1 cookie	310	34	18	80	33	44	38	105	53
Shortbread Heart with Chocolate	1 cookie	360	37	23	93	38	51	44	122	61
■ Breadsmith Cookies										
Chocolate Chip	1 cookie (2 oz)	310	40	16	80	33	44	38	105	53
Chocolate Chocolate Chip	1 cookie (2 oz)	258	39	12	66	27	37	31	88	44
Ginger Cookie	1 cookie (2 oz)	256	36	12	66	27	36	31	87	44
Oatmeal	1 cookie (2 oz)	276	34	14	71	29	39	34	94	47
Oatmeal Chocolate Chip	1 cookie (2 oz)	290	35	16	75	31	41	35	99	49
Oatmeal Cranberry	1 cookie (2 oz)	238	30	12	61	25	34	29	81	41
Oatmeal Raisin	1 cookie (2 oz)	262	37	12	68	28	37	32	89	45
Peanut Butter	1 cookie (2 oz)	312	31	19	80	33	44	38	106	53
■ Dunkin' Donuts Cookies										
Chocolate Chunk	2 cookies	220	28	11	57	23	31	27	75	37

FOOD	AMOUNT	CAL	CARBS	FAT	WALK	RUN	BIKE	SWIM	YOGA	DANCE
Chocolate Chunk with Walnuts	2 cookies	230	27	12	59	24	33	28	78	39
Chocolate White Chocolate Chunk	2 cookies	230	28	12	59	24	33	28	78	39
Oatmeal Raisin Pecan	2 cookies	220	29	10	57	23	31	27	75	37
■ **Panera Bread Cookies**										
Chocolate Chipper	1 cookie	410	55	20	106	44	58	50	139	70
Chocolate Duet Cookie with Walnuts	1 cookie	400	52	22	103	43	57	49	136	68
Nutty Chocolate Chipper	1 cookie	430	51	24	111	46	61	52	146	73
Nutty Oatmeal Raisin	1 cookie	340	50	14	88	36	48	41	116	58
Shortbread	1 cookie	350	36	21	90	37	50	43	119	60
■ **Starbucks Cookies (and Bars)**										
Black and White	1 serving (113 g)	430	68	17	111	46	61	52	146	73
Crisp Cinnamon Twist	1 serving (13 g)	60	9	2	15	6	9	7	20	10
Double Chocolate Chunk	1 serving (99 g)	430	58	21	111	46	61	52	146	73
Homestyle Oatmeal Raisin	1 serving (102 g)	390	65	15	101	42	55	47	133	66
Petite	1 serving (75 cal)	40	5	2	10	4	6	5	14	7
White Chocolate Macadamia Nut	1 serving (99 g)	470	54	27	121	50	67	57	160	80
Biscotti (any flavor)	1 serving (28 g)	110	15	5	28	12	16	13	37	19
Apricot Granola Bar	1 serving (110 g)	470	56	25	121	50	67	57	160	80
Caramel Brownie	1 serving (126 g)	580	60	36	149	62	82	71	197	99
Chocolate Peanut Butter Stack	1 serving (142 g)	670	67	42	173	71	95	82	228	114
Espresso Brownie	1 serving (82 g)	370	43	21	95	39	52	45	126	63
Espresso Fudge Brownie	1 serving (94 g)	430	48	25	111	46	61	52	146	73
Lemon Bar	1 serving (89 g)	310	44	14	80	33	44	38	105	53
Pecan Diamond	1 serving (86 g)	490	38	37	126	52	70	60	167	83

FOOD	AMOUNT	CAL	CARBS	FAT	WALK	RUN	BIKE	SWIM	YOGA	DANCE
Seven Layer Bar	1 serving (133 g)	600	63	37	155	64	85	73	204	102

Sugar-Free Cookies

■ Murray's

FOOD	AMOUNT	CAL	CARBS	FAT	WALK	RUN	BIKE	SWIM	YOGA	DANCE
Shortbread	8 cookies	120	22	6	31	13	17	15	41	20
Peanut Butter	3 cookies	150	17	9	39	16	21	18	51	26
Oatmeal	3 cookies	150	21	7	39	16	21	18	51	26
Double Fudge	3 cookies	140	23	7	36	15	20	17	48	24
Vanilla Wafer	9 cookies	130	24	5	34	14	18	16	44	22
Lemon Sandwich	3 cookies	130	19	7	34	14	18	16	44	22
Creme Sandwich	3 cookies	130	19	6	34	14	18	16	44	22
Chocolate Chip	3 cookies	140	21	8	36	15	20	17	48	24

■ Pepperidge Farm

FOOD	AMOUNT	CAL	CARBS	FAT	WALK	RUN	BIKE	SWIM	YOGA	DANCE
Sugar Free Milano	3 cookies	170	21	9	44	18	24	21	58	29
Sugar Free Chocolate Chip	3 cookies	170	22	9	44	18	24	21	58	29
Sugar Free Mint Milano	3 cookies	170	21	9	44	18	24	21	58	29

■ Archway, Sugar-Free

FOOD	AMOUNT	CAL	CARBS	FAT	WALK	RUN	BIKE	SWIM	YOGA	DANCE
Oatmeal	1 cookie	100	16	5	26	11	14	12	34	17
Peanut Butter	1 cookie	100	14	6	26	11	14	12	34	17
Rocky Road with Walnuts	1 cookie	100	17	5	26	11	14	12	34	17
Chocolate Chip	1 cookie	100	16	5	26	11	14	12	34	17
Shortbread	1 cookie	107	16	5	28	11	15	13	36	18

■ Archway, Fat Free

FOOD	AMOUNT	CAL	CARBS	FAT	WALK	RUN	BIKE	SWIM	YOGA	DANCE
Archway Fat Free Cinnamon Honey Hearts	1 cookie	106	25	0	27	11	15	13	36	18
Archway Fat Free Devil's Food	1 cookie	60	15	0	15	6	9	7	20	10
Archway Fat Free Lemon Nuggets	1 cookie	115	27	0	30	12	16	14	39	20
Archway Fat Free Oatmeal Raisin	1 cookie	110	25	0	28	12	16	13	37	19
Archway Fat Free Oatmeal Raspberry	1 cookie	109	25	1	28	12	15	13	37	19
Archway Fat Free Sugar Cookies	1 cookie	71	17	0	18	8	10	9	24	12

Portion-Controlled Cookies

■ South Beach Diet

FOOD	AMOUNT	CAL	CARBS	FAT	WALK	RUN	BIKE	SWIM	YOGA	DANCE
South Beach Diet Peanut Butter	1 pack (2 cookies)	100	15	5	26	11	14	12	34	17

FOOD	AMOUNT	CAL	CARBS	FAT	WALK	RUN	BIKE	SWIM	YOGA	DANCE
South Beach Diet Oatmeal Chocolate Chip	1 pack (2 cookies)	100	16	5	26	11	14	12	34	17
South Beach Diet Snack Crackers	1 pack	100	16	4	26	11	14	12	34	17
■ **Nabisco 100 Calorie Packs**										
Cheese Nips Thin Crisps	1 package	100	15	3	26	11	14	12	34	17
Chips Ahoy Thin Crisps	1 package	100	18	3	26	11	14	12	34	17
Honey Maid Cinnamon Thin Crisps	1 package	100	19	2	26	11	14	12	34	17
Oreo Thin Crisps	1 package	100	20	2	26	11	14	12	34	17
Wheat Thin Mini Thin Crisps	1 package	100	16	3	26	11	14	12	34	17
Sandwich Cookies										
■ **General**										
Chocolate cookie with crème filling	1 cookie	47	7	2	12	5	7	6	16	8
Chocolate-coated sandwich	1 cookie	82	11	4	21	9	12	10	28	14
Chocolate sandwich with extra filling	1 cookie	65	9	3	17	7	9	8	22	11
Vanilla sandwich	1 cookie (1 ¾" diameter)	48	7	2	12	5	7	6	16	8
Peanut butter sandwich	1 cookie	67	9	3	17	7	10	8	23	11
■ **Pepperidge Farm Milano**										
Milano	3 cookies	180	21	10	46	19	26	22	61	31
Orange Milano	2 cookies	130	16	7	34	14	18	16	44	22
French Vanilla Milano	2 cookies	130	16	7	34	14	18	16	44	22
Raspberry Milano	2 cookies	130	16	7	34	14	18	16	44	22
Milk Chocolate Milano	3 cookies	170	21	9	44	18	24	21	58	29
Double Chocolate Milano	2 cookies	140	17	8	36	15	20	17	48	24
Mint Milano	2 cookies	130	16	7	34	14	18	16	44	22
Mini Milano	6 cookies	160	18	8	41	17	23	19	54	27
■ **Oreo**										
Oreo	3 cookies	160	25	7	41	17	23	19	54	27
Double Stuf Oreo	2 cookies	140	20	7	36	15	20	17	48	24
Reduced Fat Oreo	3 cookies	150	26	5	39	16	21	18	51	26
Oreo Mint 'n Crème	2 cookies	140	20	7	36	15	20	17	48	24
Mint Chocolate Covered Mint Oreo	1 cookie	90	12	5	23	10	13	11	31	15

FOOD	AMOUNT	CAL	CARBS	FAT	WALK	RUN	BIKE	SWIM	YOGA	DANCE
White Fudge Covered Oreo	1 cookie	110	14	6	28	12	16	13	37	19
Fudge Mint Covered Oreo	1 cookie	90	12	5	23	10	13	11	31	15
Chocolate Cream Golden Uh-Oh Oreo	3 cookies	170	24	7	44	18	24	21	58	29
Bite Size Mini Oreos	9 cookies	140	21	6	36	15	20	17	48	24
Oreo Crunchies Cookie Crumb Topping	1 serving	52	8	2	13	6	7	6	18	9
■ **Keebler**										
E.L Fudge Double Stuffed Sandwich	2 cookies	180	23	9	46	19	26	22	61	31
Vienna Fingers Creme Filled Sandwich	2 cookies	150	22	7	39	16	21	18	51	26
Reduced Fat Vienna Fingers Creme Filled Sandwich	2 cookies	140	24	5	36	15	20	17	48	24
■ **Gamesa**										
Emperador Chocolate Crème Sandwich	2 cookies	120	19	4	31	13	17	15	41	20
Emperador Limon Crème Sandwich	6 cookies	270	45	8	70	29	38	33	92	46
Emperador Fresa Crème Sandwich	2 cookies	120	19	4	31	13	17	15	41	20
Emperador Vanilla Crème Sandwich	2 cookies	120	19	4	31	13	17	15	41	20
■ **Miscellaneous Sandwich Cookies**										
Famous Amos Chocolate Crème Filled Sandwich	3 cookies	160	25	6	41	17	23	19	54	27
Grandma's Fudge Vanilla Sandwich	3 cookies	120	21	4	31	13	17	15	41	20
Grandma's Vanilla Sandwich	5 cookies	210	30	10	54	22	30	26	71	36
Nabisco Cameo Crème Sandwich	2 cookies	140	22	5	36	15	20	17	48	24
Snackwell's Chocolate Sandwich	2 cookies	110	20	3	28	12	16	13	37	19
Snackwell's Crème Sandwich	2 cookies	110	20	3	28	12	16	13	37	19
Chocolate-Dipped Cookies										
■ **Le Petit Ecolier**										
Dark Chocolate	2 biscuits	130	17	6	34	14	18	16	44	22
Hazelnut Chocolate	2 biscuits	130	16	6	34	14	18	16	44	22
Milk Chocolate	2 biscuits	130	17	6	34	14	18	16	44	22

FOOD	AMOUNT	CAL	CARBS	FAT	WALK	RUN	BIKE	SWIM	YOGA	DANCE
Extra Dark Chocolate	2 biscuits	130	15	7	34	14	18	16	44	22
Snack Cakes										
■ Drake's										
Yodels	2 cakes	280	36	14	72	30	40	34	95	48
Coffee Cakes	2 cakes	280	40	12	72	30	40	34	95	48
Devil Dogs	1 cake	170	26	7	44	18	24	21	58	29
Ring Dings	2 cakes	330	43	17	85	35	47	40	112	56
Yankee Doodles	2 cakes	220	33	9	57	23	31	27	75	37
Sunny Doodles	2 cakes	220	33	9	57	23	31	27	75	37
■ Hostess										
Cupcakes	1 cake	180	30	6	46	19	26	22	61	31
Twinkies	1 cake	150	27	5	39	16	21	18	51	26
Ho Hos	3 cakes	380	54	17	98	40	54	46	129	65
Low Fat Hostess Crumb Cake	1 serving	90	19	1	23	10	13	11	31	15
■ Little Debbie										
Marshmallow Pies	1 cookie	180	30	6	46	19	26	22	61	31
Oatmeal Creme Pies	1 cookie	170	26	7	44	18	24	21	58	29
Frosted Fudge Cakes	1 cake	190	26	9	49	20	27	23	65	32
Coffee Cakes	1 cake	200	35	6	52	21	28	24	68	34
Marshmallow Supreme	1 cookie	140	22	5	36	15	20	17	48	24
Devil Squares	2 cakes	270	38	12	70	29	38	33	92	46
Strawberry Shortcake Rolls	1 roll	240	39	9	62	26	34	29	82	41
Boston Crème Rolls	1 roll	270	40	12	70	29	38	33	92	46
Swiss Cake Rolls	2 cakes	270	38	12	70	29	38	33	92	46

Cakes, Pies, and Miscellaneous Baking Needs

Cakes										
■ Angel Food Cake										
Angel food cake	¹⁄₁₂ cake	72	16	0	19	8	10	9	24	12
Angel food cake (prepared from mix)	¹⁄₁₂ cake	128	29	0	33	14	18	16	44	22
■ Butter Cake										
Entenmann's Butter Sunshine Cake	¹⁄₆ cake	320	44	14	82	34	45	39	109	55
Entenmann's All Butter Loaf	¹⁄₈ loaf	220	31	9	57	23	31	27	75	37

FOOD	AMOUNT	CAL	CARBS	FAT	WALK	RUN	BIKE	SWIM	YOGA	DANCE
Cheesecake										
Cheesecake	⅙ cake	257	20	18	66	27	36	31	87	44
No-bake cheesecake	1/12 cake	271	35	13	70	29	38	33	92	46
Weight Watchers New York Style Cheesecake	1 serving	150	21	5	39	16	21	18	51	26
Weight Watchers Triple Chocolate Cheesecake	1 serving	200	32	5	52	21	28	24	68	34
Chocolate Cake										
Homemade Chocolate	1/12 cake	340	51	14	88	36	48	41	116	58
Chocolate cake, with chocolate frosting	⅛ cake	235	35	22	61	25	33	29	80	40
Chocolate Cupcake	1 cupcake	131	29	2	34	14	19	16	45	22
Chocolate Snack, cream filled	1 cake	188	30	7	48	20	27	23	64	32
Entenmann's Iced Devil's Food Cake	⅛ cake	290	38	15	75	31	41	35	99	49
Entenmann's Chocolate Fudge Cake	⅛ cake	270	40	12	70	29	38	33	92	46
Entenmann's Marshmallow Iced Devil's Food Cake	⅛ cake	280	40	14	72	30	40	34	95	48
Entenmann's Fat Free Chocolate	1 slice	130	32	0	34	14	18	16	44	22
Pepperidge Farm Chocolate Fudge Stripe Layer	1 slice	290	38	14	75	31	41	35	99	49
Pepperidge Farm Devil's Food Layer	1 slice	290	40	14	75	31	41	35	99	49
Pepperidge Farm German Chocolate Layer	1 slice	300	37	16	77	32	43	36	102	51
Pillsbury Dark Chocolate Cake Mix (prepared)	1 slice	250	33	12	64	27	35	30	85	43
Pillsbury German Chocolate Cake Mix (prepared)	1 slice	250	34	11	64	27	35	30	85	43
Coffee Cake										
Cinnamon coffee cake, with crumb topping	1/9 cake	263	29	15	68	28	37	32	89	45
Prepared from mix	⅛ cake	178	30	5	46	19	25	22	61	30
Cheese coffee cake	⅙ cake	258	34	12	66	27	37	31	88	44
Fruit-filled coffee cake	⅛ cake	156	26	5	40	17	22	19	53	27
Entenmann's Cheese Filled Crumb Coffee Cake	1/9 cake	200	25	9	52	21	28	24	68	34
Entenmann's Filled Chocolate Chip Crumb Cake	1/9 cake	390	49	21	101	42	55	47	133	66

FOOD	AMOUNT	CAL	CARBS	FAT	WALK	RUN	BIKE	SWIM	YOGA	DANCE
Entenmann's Brownie Crumb Ring	⅛ cake	360	46	19	93	38	51	44	122	61
Entenmann's Fat Free Cinnamon Apple Coffee Cake	1 slice	130	29	0	34	14	18	16	44	22
Hostess Crumb Coffee Cake	1 serving	130	19	5	34	14	18	16	44	22
Little Debbie Apple Streusel Coffee Cake	1 cake	230	39	7	59	24	33	28	78	39
■ Crunch Cake										
Entenmann's Cinnamon Crunch Cake	⅑ cake	320	45	14	82	34	45	39	109	55
Entenmann's Lemon Crunch Cake	⅑ cake	330	49	14	85	35	47	40	112	56
Entenmann's Louisiana Crunch Cake	⅑ cake	330	49	14	85	35	47	40	112	56
■ Gingerbread										
Gingerbread	⅑ cake	263	36	12	68	28	37	32	89	45
Betty Crocker Gingerbread Mix (prepared)	.13 pkg	230	39	6	59	24	33	28	78	39
■ Pound Cake										
Pound	1/12 cake	109	15	5	28	12	15	13	37	19
Butter pound	1/12 cake	109	14	6	28	12	15	13	37	19
Pound cake snack cake	1 cake	276	37	13	71	29	39	34	94	47
Fat-free pound	1 slice (1 oz)	80	17	0	21	9	11	10	27	14
■ Sponge Cake										
Homemade sponge	1/12 cake	187	36	3	48	20	27	23	64	32
Store-bought sponge	1/12 cake	110	23	1	28	12	16	13	37	19
Crème-filled sponge cake snack cake	1 cake	157	27	5	40	17	22	19	53	27
■ White Cake										
White cake	1/12 cake	264	42	9	68	28	37	32	90	45
White cake, with coconut frosting	1/12 cake	399	71	12	103	42	57	49	136	68
Pillsbury White Cake Mix (prepared)	1 slice	280	41	11	72	30	40	34	95	48
■ Yellow Cake										
Homemade yellow	1/12 cake	245	36	10	63	26	35	30	83	42
Yellow cake, with vanilla frosting	⅛ cake	239	37	9	62	25	34	29	81	41

FOOD	AMOUNT	CAL	CARBS	FAT	WALK	RUN	BIKE	SWIM	YOGA	DANCE
Yellow cake, with chocolate frosting	⅛ cake	243	35	11	63	26	34	30	83	41
Entenmann's Fudge Iced Golden Cake	⅛ cake	290	41	13	75	31	41	35	99	49
Entenmann's Light Golden Loaf	⅛ loaf	120	28	0	31	13	17	15	41	20
Pillsbury Yellow Cake Mix (prepared)	1 slice	250	35	11	64	27	35	30	85	43
Pillsbury Light Yellow Cake Mix (prepared)	1 slice	230	43	5	59	24	33	28	78	39
Sweet Rewards Less Fat Cake Mix (prepared)	1 serving	160	37	1	41	17	23	19	54	27
Other Cakes										
Cherry cake, with chocolate frosting	⅛ cake	187	27	9	48	20	27	23	64	32
Fruit cake	1 piece	139	26	4	36	15	20	17	47	24
Entenmann's Banana Cake	⅛ cake	290	40	14	75	31	41	35	99	49
Entenmann's Sour Cream Loaf	⅛ loaf	220	26	12	57	23	31	27	75	37
Pineapple upside-down	⅑ cake	367	58	14	95	39	52	45	125	63
Entenmann's Fat Free Carrot Cake	1 slice	170	40	0	44	18	24	21	58	29
Pepperidge Farm Deluxe Carrot Cake	1 slice	310	39	16	80	33	44	38	105	53
Pillsbury Carrot Cake Mix (prepared)	1 slice	260	35	12	67	28	37	32	88	44
Pie										
Apple Pie										
Homemade apple pie	⅛ pie	411	58	19	106	44	58	50	140	70
Store-bought apple pie	⅙ pie	277	40	12	71	29	39	34	94	47
Fried apple	1 pie	404	55	21	104	43	57	49	137	69
Banquet Frozen Apple Pie	1 serving	292	41	13	75	31	41	36	99	50
Entenmann's Homestyle Apple Pie	⅙ pie	380	57	16	98	40	54	46	129	65
Entenmann's Apple Crumb Pie	⅙ pie	370	63	13	95	39	52	45	126	63
Hostess Apple Pie Snack Cake	1 serving	480	67	22	124	51	68	58	163	82
Mrs. Smith Reduced Fat Frozen Apple Pie	1 slice	250	43	8	64	27	35	30	85	43
Banana Cream Pie										
Banana cream	⅛ pie	387	47	20	100	41	55	47	132	66
No-bake banana cream	⅛ pie	231	29	12	60	25	33	28	79	39

FOOD	AMOUNT	CAL	CARBS	FAT	WALK	RUN	BIKE	SWIM	YOGA	DANCE
Mrs. Smith Frozen Banana Cream Pie	1 slice	280	37	14	72	30	40	34	95	48
■ **Blueberry Pie**										
Homemade blueberry	⅛ pie	360	49	17	93	38	51	44	122	61
Store-bought blueberry	⅛ pie	290	44	13	75	31	41	35	99	49
Hostess Blueberry Pie Snack Cake	1 serving	480	70	21	124	51	68	58	163	82
■ **Cherry Pie**										
Homemade cherry	⅛ pie	486	69	22	125	52	69	59	165	83
Store-bought cherry	⅛ pie	325	50	14	84	35	46	40	111	55
Hostess Cherry Pie Snack Cake	1 serving	470	65	22	121	50	67	57	160	80
Mrs. Smith Reduced Fat Frozen Cherry Pie	1 slice	250	44	8	64	27	35	30	85	43
■ **Chocolate Pie**										
Chocolate cream pie	⅙ pie	344	38	22	89	37	49	42	117	59
Chocolate mousse pie	⅛ pie	247	28	15	64	26	35	30	84	42
Weight Watchers Smart Ones Mississippi Mud Pie	1 pie	160	26	5	41	17	23	19	54	27
■ **Coconut Pie**										
Coconut cream	⅛ pie	143	18	8	37	15	20	17	49	24
No-bake coconut cream	⅛ pie	259	27	17	67	28	37	32	88	44
Coconut custard pie	⅙ pie	270	31	14	70	29	38	33	92	46
Entenmann's Coconut Custard Pie	⅕ pie	390	38	21	101	42	55	47	133	66
■ **Lemon Pie**										
Homemade lemon meringue	⅛ pie	362	50	16	93	39	51	44	123	62
Store-bought lemon meringue	⅙ pie	303	53	10	78	32	43	37	103	52
Fried lemon	1 pie	404	55	21	104	43	57	49	137	69
Hostess Lemon Pie Snack Cake	1 serving	500	66	24	129	53	71	61	170	85
■ **Mince Pie**										
Mince pie	⅛ pie	477	79	18	123	51	68	58	162	81
Mrs. Smith Frozen Mince Pie	1 slice	300	48	11	77	32	43	36	102	51
■ **Peach Pie**										
Peach pie	⅙ pie	261	38	12	67	28	37	32	89	44
Hostess Peach Pie Snack Cake	1 serving	480	68	21	124	51	68	58	163	82
■ **Pecan Pie**										
Homemade pecan	⅛ pie	503	64	27	130	54	71	61	171	86

FOOD	AMOUNT	CAL	CARBS	FAT	WALK	RUN	BIKE	SWIM	YOGA	DANCE
Store-bought pecan	1 oz	452	64	21	116	48	64	55	154	77
Mrs. Smith Frozen Pecan	1 slice	520	73	23	134	55	74	63	177	89
■ **Pumpkin Pie**										
Homemade pumpkin	⅛ pie	316	41	14	81	34	45	38	107	54
Store-bought pumpkin	⅛ pie	229	30	10	59	24	32	28	78	39
Mrs. Smith Frozen Pumpkin	1 slice	270	44	8	70	29	38	33	92	46
■ **Other Pies**										
Boston cream	⅛ pie	232	39	8	60	25	33	28	79	40
Homemade vanilla cream	⅛ pie	350	41	18	90	37	50	43	119	60
Entenmann's Deluxe French Cheese Cake Pie	⅛ pie	390	39	24	101	42	55	47	133	66
Pastry, Pie Shells, and Crusts										
Pie crust	⅛ crust	121	11	8	31	13	17	15	41	21
Frozen pie crust	⅛ crust	82	8	5	21	9	12	10	28	14
Frozen puff pastry	1 shell	259	21	18	67	28	37	32	88	44
Phyllo dough	1 sheet	57	10	1	15	6	8	7	19	10
Homemade graham cracker pie crust	⅛ crust	148	20	7	38	16	21	18	50	25
Chocolate wafer pie crust	⅛ crust	142	15	9	37	15	20	17	48	24
Vanilla wafer pie crust	⅛ crust	117	11	8	30	12	17	14	40	20
Individual graham cracker tart crust	1 tart crust	109	14	5	28	12	15	13	37	19
Egg roll wrapper	7″ square	93	19	0	24	10	13	11	32	16
Wonton wrapper	3-½″ square	23	5	0	6	2	3	3	8	4
Arrowhead Mills Graham Cracker Pie Crust	⅛ crust	100	12	5	26	11	14	12	34	17
Keebler Mini Graham Cracker Crust	1 crust	120	15	6	31	13	17	15	41	20
Keebler Graham Cracker Crust	.13 crust	110	14	5	28	12	16	13	37	19
Keebler Reduced Fat Graham Cracker Crust	.13 crust	90	14	4	23	10	13	11	31	15
Oreo Pie Crust	1 slice	140	18	7	36	15	20	17	48	24
Pillsbury Just Unroll Pie Crust	⅛ crust	120	13	7	31	13	17	15	41	20
Pillsbury Pie Crust Mix	2 tbsp	100	10	6	26	11	14	12	34	17
Mrs. Smith Reduced Fat 9″ Frozen Pie Crust	1 slice	100	13	5	26	11	14	12	34	17

FOOD	AMOUNT	CAL	CARBS	FAT	WALK	RUN	BIKE	SWIM	YOGA	DANCE
Frosting										
Creamy chocolate frosting	2 tbsp	163	26	7	42	17	23	20	55	28
Creamy chocolate frosting (prepared from mix)	1 oz	113	20	4	29	12	16	14	38	19
Coconut frosting	1 oz	121	15	7	31	13	17	15	41	21
Cream cheese frosting	2 tbsp	137	22	5	35	15	19	17	47	23
Creamy vanilla frosting	1 oz	117	19	5	30	12	17	14	40	20
Vanilla frosting (prepared from mix)	1 oz	116	21	4	30	12	16	14	39	20
Glaze frosting	1 oz	101	21	2	26	11	14	12	34	17
White fluffy frosting	1 oz	68	17	0	18	7	10	8	23	12

Jams, Jellies, Fruit Butter, Honey, Molasses, and Pie Filling

Jams and Jellies										
Jam	1 tbsp	56	0	0	14	6	8	7	19	9
Sugar-free jam	1 tbsp	18	8	0	5	2	3	2	6	3
Jelly	1 tbsp	56	15	0	14	6	8	7	19	10
Reduced-sugar jelly	1 tbsp	24	9	0	6	3	3	3	8	4
Orange marmalade	1 tbsp	49	13	0	13	5	7	6	17	8
Apricot jam	1 tbsp	48	13	0	12	5	7	6	16	8
Goodber's Peanut Butter and Jelly Stripes (all flavors)	3 tbsp	240	24	13	62	26	34	29	82	41
Polaner All Fruit Strawberry Spread	1 tbsp	42	10	0	11	4	6	5	14	7
Smucker's Jam (all flavors)	1 tbsp	50	13	0	13	5	7	6	17	9
Smucker's Jelly (all flavors)	1 tbsp	50	13	0	13	5	7	6	17	9
Smucker's Low Sugar Jam (all flavors)	1 tbsp	25	6	0	6	3	4	3	9	4
Smucker's Preserves (all flavors)	1 tbsp	50	13	0	13	5	7	6	17	9
Smucker's Simply Fruit (all flavors)	1 tbsp	40	10	0	10	4	6	5	14	7
Smucker's Squeeze Grape or Strawberry Fruit Spread	1 tbsp	50	13	0	13	5	7	6	17	9
Smucker's Squeeze Reduced Sugar Strawberry Fruit Spread	1 tbsp	20	6	0	5	2	3	2	7	3

FOOD	AMOUNT	CAL	CARBS	FAT	WALK	RUN	BIKE	SWIM	YOGA	DANCE
Smucker's Sugar Free Jam (all flavors)	1 tbsp	10	5	0	3	1	1	1	3	2
Welch's Concord Grape Jelly	1 tbsp	50	13	0	13	5	7	6	17	9
Fruit Butter										
Apple butter	1 tbsp	29	7	0	7	3	4	4	10	5
Smucker's Cider Apple Butter	1 tbsp	45	11	0	12	5	6	5	15	8
Honey										
Honey	1 tbsp	64	17	0	16	7	9	8	22	11
Molasses										
Molasses	1 tbsp	58	15	0	15	6	8	7	20	10
Pie Filling										
Canned apple pie filling	1 can	601	156	0	155	64	85	73	204	102
Canned cherry pie filling	1 can	684	167	1	176	73	97	83	233	117
Reduced-calorie cherry pie filling	1 cup	121	27	0	31	13	17	15	41	21
Blueberry pie filling	1 cup	474	116	1	122	51	67	58	161	81
Solo Poppy Seed Filling	2 tbsp	120	21	3	31	13	17	15	41	20

Pizza

Frozen Pizza

■ **General**

Frozen pepperoni pizza	1 serving	432	42	22	111	46	61	53	147	74
Bagel Bites 3 Cheese Bagel Pizza	4 pieces	200	27	6	52	21	28	24	68	34
Bagel Bites Cheese and Pepperoni Bagel Pizza	4 pieces	210	29	7	54	22	30	26	71	36
Bagel Bites Cheese, Sausage and Pepperoni Bagel Pizza	4 pieces	200	28	6	52	21	28	24	68	34
Celeste Deluxe Pizza with Sausage, Green and Red Peppers and Mushrooms	1 serving	386	33	21	99	41	55	47	131	66
Celeste Pizza for One Cheese Pizza	1 pizza	360	42	14	93	38	51	44	122	61
Celeste Pizza for One Deluxe Pizza	1 pizza	440	42	23	113	47	62	54	150	75
Celeste Pizza for One Zesty 4 Cheese Pizza	1 pizza	440	40	22	113	47	62	54	150	75
DiGiorno 4-Cheese Pizza	1/2 pizza	350	44	12	90	37	50	43	119	60

FOOD	AMOUNT	CAL	CARBS	FAT	WALK	RUN	BIKE	SWIM	YOGA	DANCE
DiGiorno Pepperoni Pizza	⅙ pizza	330	39	13	85	35	47	40	112	56
DiGiorno Supreme Pizza	⅙ pizza	360	41	15	93	38	51	44	122	61
Health Is Wealth Mini Soy Cheese Pizza Bagel	4 pieces	150	28	0	39	16	21	18	51	26
Healthy Choice Cheese French Bread Pizza	1 pizza (6 oz)	360	57	5	93	38	51	44	122	61
Healthy Choice Pepperoni French Bread Pizza	1 pizza (6 oz)	360	56	5	93	38	51	44	122	61
Healthy Choice Supreme French Bread Pizza	1 pizza (6.35 oz)	330	51	5	85	35	47	40	112	56
Healthy Choice Vegetable French Bread Pizza	1 pizza (6 oz)	320	50	5	82	34	45	39	109	55
Jack's Great Combinations Sausage and Pepperoni Pizza	1 serving	348	30	18	90	37	49	42	118	59
Jack's Original Pepperoni Pizza	1 serving	323	30	16	83	34	46	39	110	55
Jeno's Crisp and Tasty Pepperoni Pizza	1 serving	516	46	29	133	55	73	63	176	88
Jeno's Crisp and Tasty Sausage and Pepperoni Pizza	1 serving	491	52	24	127	52	70	60	167	84
Pappalo's Deep Dish Pepperoni Pizza for One	1 serving	525	65	20	135	56	75	64	179	89
Red Baron Pepperoni Pizza	1 serving	442	36	25	114	47	63	54	150	75
Red Baron Premium Singles Deep Dish Pepperoni Pizza	1 serving	480	48	25	124	51	68	58	163	82
Red Baron Special Deluxe 2 Cheese, Sausage, Pepperoni and Onions Pizza	1 serving	337	32	18	87	36	48	41	115	57
Red Baron Supreme Sausage, Mushrooms, and Pepperoni Pizza	1 serving	344	32	18	89	37	49	42	117	59
Stouffer's Deluxe French Bread Pizza with Sausage, Pepperoni and Mushrooms	1 serving	429	44	21	111	46	61	52	146	73
Stouffer's French Bread Pizza with Sausage and Pepperoni	1 serving	448	44	22	115	48	64	55	152	76
Tombstone Brickoven Style Pepperoni Pizza	1 serving	310	39	16	80	33	44	38	105	53
Tombstone Brickoven Style Sausage and Pepperoni Pizza	1 serving	320	30	16	82	34	45	39	109	55
Tombstone Light Veggie Pizza	1 serving	230	31	6	59	24	33	28	78	39
Tombstone Original Extra Cheese Pizza	1 serving	580	74	22	149	62	82	71	197	99

FOOD	AMOUNT	CAL	CARBS	FAT	WALK	RUN	BIKE	SWIM	YOGA	DANCE
Tombstone Original Sausage and Mushroom Pizza	1 serving	290	30	13	75	31	41	35	99	49
Tony's D'primo Deep Dish Sausage Pizza	1 serving	391	41	20	101	42	55	48	133	67
Tony's Pepperoni Pizza with Italian Style Pastry Crust	1 serving	406	36	23	105	43	58	49	138	69
Tony's Sausage and Pepperoni Pizza with Italian Style Pastry Crust	1 serving	434	41	23	112	46	62	53	148	74
Tony's Supreme Sausage, Pepperoni, Mushroom, Green and Red Pepper Pizza	1 serving	400	39	20	103	43	57	49	136	68
Tony's Taco Style Pizza	1 serving	437	43	23	113	47	62	53	149	74
Frozen Pizza Snacks										
Amy's Organic Cheese Pizza Snacks	5 pieces	190	22	7	49	20	27	23	65	32
Health Is Wealth Pizza Munchees	6 munchees	190	32	5	49	20	27	23	65	32
Hot Pockets Pepperoni Pizza	1 piece	360	41	17	93	38	51	44	122	61
Hot Pockets Sausage Pizza	1 piece	380	40	20	98	40	54	46	129	65
Lunchables Extra Cheesey Pizza	1 package	450	63	15	116	48	64	55	153	77
Lunchables Pepperoni Flavored Sausage Pizza	1 package	470	65	17	121	50	67	57	160	80
Totino's Hamburger Pizza Rolls	1 serving	231	26	10	60	25	33	28	79	39
Totino's Pepperoni Party Pizza Crust	1 package	364	35	19	94	39	52	44	124	62
Totino's Pepperoni Pizza Rolls	1 serving	385	39	19	99	41	55	47	131	66
Totino's Sausage and Pepperoni Party Pizza Crust Combos	1 package	385	36	20	99	41	55	47	131	66
Totino's Sausage Pizza Rolls	1 serving	351	40	15	90	37	50	43	119	60
Pizza Dough										
Breadsmith Wheat Pizza Dough	1 oz	65	12	1	17	7	9	8	22	11
Breadsmith White Pizza Dough	1 oz	79	15	1	20	8	11	10	27	13
Little Caesar's										
■ **12″ Round Pizza**										
Cheese Only	⅛ pizza	180	23	6	46	19	26	22	61	31
Pepperoni	⅛ pizza	210	23	8	54	22	30	26	71	36

FOOD	AMOUNT	CAL	CARBS	FAT	WALK	RUN	BIKE	SWIM	YOGA	DANCE
■ 14″ Round Pizza										
Cheese Only	⅒ pizza	200	25	7	52	21	28	24	68	34
Pepperoni	⅒ pizza	230	25	8	59	24	33	28	78	39
Supreme	⅒ pizza	270	31	10	70	29	38	33	92	46
Meatsa	⅒ pizza	280	26	13	72	30	40	34	95	48
Veggie	⅒ pizza	240	32	8	62	26	34	29	82	41
■ 12″ Thin Crust										
Cheese Only	⅛ pizza	140	13	7	36	15	20	17	48	24
Pepperoni	⅛ pizza	170	13	8	44	18	24	21	58	29
■ 14″ Thin Crust										
Cheese Only	⅒ pizza	160	14	7	41	17	23	19	54	27
Pepperoni	⅒ pizza	180	14	9	46	19	26	22	61	31
■ 16″ Round Pizza										
Cheese Only	1/12 pizza	220	27	7	57	23	31	27	75	37
Pepperoni	1/12 pizza	240	27	9	62	26	34	29	82	41
■ 18″ Round Pizza										
Cheese Only	1/14 pizza	230	30	7	59	24	33	28	78	39
Pepperoni	1/14 pizza	260	30	9	67	28	37	32	88	44
■ Medium Deep Dish										
Cheese Only	⅛ pizza	230	27	9	59	24	33	28	78	39
Pepperoni	⅛ pizza	260	27	11	67	28	37	32	88	44
■ Large Deep Dish										
Cheese Only	⅛ pizza	320	37	12	82	34	45	39	109	55
Pepperoni	⅛ pizza	350	38	14	90	37	50	43	119	60
■ Slice										
Cheese Only	⅙ of 14″ pizza	330	42	11	85	35	47	40	112	56
Pepperoni	⅙ of 14″ pizza	390	42	14	101	42	55	47	133	66
■ Additional Toppings for 12″ Cheese Pizza										
Pepperoni	⅛ total topping	25	0	1	7	3	4	3	9	4
Ham	⅛ total topping	6	0	0	1	1	1	1	2	1
Mushroom	⅛ total topping	2	0	0	1	0	0	0	1	0
Beef	⅛ total topping	19	0	1	5	2	3	2	6	3

FOOD	AMOUNT	CAL	CARBS	FAT	WALK	RUN	BIKE	SWIM	YOGA	DANCE
Bacon	⅛ total topping	36	0	3	9	4	5	4	12	6
Italian Sausage	⅛ total topping	19	0	2	5	2	3	2	7	3
Green Pepper	⅛ total topping	2	0	0	0	0	0	0	1	0
Onion	⅛ total topping	2	1	0	1	0	0	0	1	0
Black Olives	⅛ total topping	12	0	2	3	1	2	1	4	2
Pineapple	⅛ total topping	7	2	0	2	1	1	1	2	1
Hot Peppers	⅛ total topping	0	0	0	0	0	0	0	0	0
Tomato	⅛ total topping	2	0	0	0	0	0	0	1	0
Extra Cheese	⅛ total topping	22	0	2	6	2	3	3	7	4

■ Additional Toppings for 14″ Cheese Pizza

FOOD	AMOUNT	CAL	CARBS	FAT	WALK	RUN	BIKE	SWIM	YOGA	DANCE
Pepperoni	¹⁄₁₀ total topping	26	0	2	7	3	4	3	9	4
Ham	¹⁄₁₀ total topping	5	0	0	1	1	1	1	2	1
Mushroom	¹⁄₁₀ total topping	2	0	0	1	0	0	0	1	0
Beef	¹⁄₁₀ total topping	20	0	2	5	2	3	2	7	3
Bacon	¹⁄₁₀ total topping	41	0	4	10	4	6	5	14	7
Italian Sausage	¹⁄₁₀ total topping	22	0	2	6	2	3	3	7	4
Green Pepper	¹⁄₁₀ total topping	2	0	0	0	0	0	0	1	0
Onion	¹⁄₁₀ total topping	3	1	0	1	0	0	0	1	0
Black Olives	¹⁄₁₀ total topping	12	0	2	3	1	2	2	4	2
Pineapple	¹⁄₁₀ total topping	7	2	0	2	1	1	1	2	1
Hot Peppers	¹⁄₁₀ total topping	0	0	0	0	0	0	0	0	0
Tomato	¹⁄₁₀ total topping	2	0	0	1	0	0	0	1	0

FOOD	AMOUNT	CAL	CARBS	FAT	WALK	RUN	BIKE	SWIM	YOGA	DANCE
Extra Cheese	⅒ total topping	26	0	2	7	3	4	3	9	4

Pizza Hut

■ 12″ Medium Pan Pizza

FOOD	AMOUNT	CAL	CARBS	FAT	WALK	RUN	BIKE	SWIM	YOGA	DANCE
Cheese Only	1 slice	270	27	13	70	29	38	33	92	46
Pepperoni	1 slice	280	27	14	72	30	40	34	95	48
Quartered Ham	1 slice	250	27	11	64	27	35	30	85	43
Supreme	1 slice	310	28	16	80	33	44	38	105	53
Super Supreme	1 slice	330	29	17	85	35	47	40	112	56
Chicken Supreme	1 slice	270	28	12	70	29	38	33	92	46
Meat Lovers	1 slice	370	28	22	95	39	52	45	126	63
Veggie Lovers	1 slice	250	28	11	64	27	35	30	85	43
Pepperoni Lovers	1 slice	330	28	18	85	35	47	40	112	56
Sausage Lovers	1 slice	360	28	20	93	38	51	44	122	61

■ 12″ Medium Thin 'N Crispy Pizza

FOOD	AMOUNT	CAL	CARBS	FAT	WALK	RUN	BIKE	SWIM	YOGA	DANCE
Cheese Only	1 slice	200	21	8	52	21	28	24	68	34
Pepperoni	1 slice	210	21	10	54	22	30	26	71	36
Quartered Ham	1 slice	180	21	7	46	19	26	22	61	31
Supreme	1 slice	230	22	11	59	24	33	28	78	39
Super Supreme	1 slice	250	23	13	64	27	35	30	85	43
Chicken Supreme	1 slice	200	22	7	52	21	28	24	68	34
Meat Lovers	1 slice	310	22	18	80	33	44	38	105	53
Veggie Lovers	1 slice	180	23	7	46	19	26	22	61	31
Pepperoni Lovers	1 slice	260	22	14	67	28	37	32	88	44
Sausage Lovers	1 slice	280	22	16	72	30	40	34	95	48

■ 12″ Medium Hand-Tossed Style Pizzas

FOOD	AMOUNT	CAL	CARBS	FAT	WALK	RUN	BIKE	SWIM	YOGA	DANCE
Cheese Only	1 slice	230	28	8	59	24	33	28	78	39
Pepperoni	1 slice	240	27	9	62	26	34	29	82	41
Quartered Ham	1 slice	210	27	6	54	22	30	26	71	36
Supreme	1 slice	260	29	11	67	28	37	32	88	44
Super Supreme	1 slice	280	29	13	72	30	40	34	95	48
Chicken Supreme	1 slice	230	28	7	59	24	33	28	78	39
Meat Lovers	1 slice	330	28	17	85	35	47	40	112	56
Veggie Lovers	1 slice	210	29	6	54	22	30	26	71	36
Pepperoni Lovers	1 slice	290	28	13	75	31	41	35	99	49
Sausage Lovers	1 slice	310	28	16	80	33	44	38	105	53

FOOD	AMOUNT	CAL	CARBS	FAT	WALK	RUN	BIKE	SWIM	YOGA	DANCE
■ 14″ Large Pan Pizzas										
Cheese Only	1 slice	260	25	13	67	28	37	32	88	44
Pepperoni	1 slice	270	25	14	70	29	38	33	92	46
Quartered Ham	1 slice	240	25	11	62	26	34	29	82	41
Supreme	1 slice	290	26	15	75	31	41	35	99	49
Super Supreme	1 slice	310	26	17	80	33	44	38	105	53
Chicken Supreme	1 slice	250	26	11	64	27	35	30	85	43
Meat Lovers	1 slice	350	26	21	90	37	50	43	119	60
Veggie Lovers	1 slice	240	26	11	62	26	34	29	82	41
Pepperoni Lovers	1 slice	320	25	18	82	34	45	39	109	55
Sausage Lovers	1 slice	340	26	20	88	36	48	41	116	58
■ 14″ Large Thin 'N Crispy Pizzas										
Cheese Only	1 slice	190	20	8	49	20	27	23	65	32
Pepperoni	1 slice	200	19	9	52	21	28	24	68	34
Quartered Ham	1 slice	170	19	6	44	18	24	21	58	29
Supreme	1 slice	220	21	11	57	23	31	27	75	37
Super Supreme	1 slice	240	21	12	62	26	34	29	82	41
Chicken Supreme	1 slice	190	21	7	49	20	27	23	65	32
Meat Lovers	1 slice	290	20	17	75	31	41	35	99	49
Veggie Lovers	1 slice	170	21	6	44	18	24	21	58	29
Pepperoni Lovers	1 slice	250	20	13	64	27	35	30	85	43
Sausage Lovers	1 slice	270	21	15	70	29	38	33	92	46
■ 14″ Large Hand-Tossed Style Pizzas										
Cheese Only	1 slice	220	25	8	57	23	31	27	75	37
Pepperoni	1 slice	230	25	9	59	24	33	28	78	39
Quartered Ham	1 slice	200	25	6	52	21	28	24	68	34
Supreme	1 slice	250	26	11	64	27	35	30	85	43
Super Supreme	1 slice	270	27	12	70	29	38	33	92	46
Chicken Supreme	1 slice	210	26	7	54	22	30	26	71	36
Meat Lovers	1 slice	310	26	16	80	33	44	38	105	53
Veggie Lovers	1 slice	190	26	6	49	20	27	23	65	32
Pepperoni Lovers	1 slice	280	26	13	72	30	40	34	95	48
Sausage Lovers	1 slice	290	26	15	75	31	41	35	99	49
■ 14″ Large Stuffed Crust Pizzas										
Cheese Only	1 slice	350	40	13	90	37	50	43	119	60
Pepperoni	1 slice	380	40	16	98	40	54	46	129	65

FOOD	AMOUNT	CAL	CARBS	FAT	WALK	RUN	BIKE	SWIM	YOGA	DANCE
Quartered Ham	1 slice	340	40	12	88	36	48	41	116	58
Supreme	1 slice	410	42	18	106	44	58	50	139	70
Super Supreme	1 slice	430	42	20	111	46	61	52	146	73
Chicken Supreme	1 slice	350	41	12	90	37	50	43	119	60
Meat Lovers	1 slice	500	41	27	129	53	71	61	170	85
Veggie Lovers	1 slice	330	41	11	85	35	47	40	112	56
Pepperoni Lovers	1 slice	440	41	21	113	47	62	54	150	75
Sausage Lovers	1 slice	480	41	25	124	51	68	58	163	82
■ 16″ Full House XL Pizza										
Cheese Only	1 slice	280	30	12	72	30	40	34	95	48
Pepperoni	1 slice	280	30	13	72	30	40	34	95	48
Quartered Ham	1 slice	260	30	10	67	28	37	32	88	44
Supreme	1 slice	310	31	14	80	33	44	38	105	53
Super Supreme	1 slice	330	32	16	85	35	47	40	112	56
Chicken Supreme	1 slice	270	31	10	70	29	38	33	92	46
Meat Lovers	1 slice	370	31	20	95	39	52	45	126	63
Veggie Lovers	1 slice	260	31	10	67	28	37	32	88	44
Pepperoni Lovers	1 slice	340	30	17	88	36	48	41	116	58
Sausage Lovers	1 slice	350	31	19	90	37	50	43	119	60
■ 6″ Personal Pan Pizzas										
Cheese Only	1 whole	620	69	26	160	66	88	75	211	106
Pepperoni	1 whole	640	67	29	165	68	91	78	218	109
Quartered Ham	1 whole	570	67	22	147	61	81	69	194	97
Supreme	1 whole	710	70	34	183	76	101	86	241	121
Super Supreme	1 whole	750	71	37	193	80	106	91	255	128
Chicken Supreme	1 whole	610	70	23	157	65	87	74	207	104
Meat Lovers	1 whole	890	70	49	229	95	126	108	303	152
Veggie Lovers	1 whole	560	70	22	144	60	79	68	190	95
Pepperoni Lovers	1 whole	770	69	39	198	82	109	94	262	131
Sausage Lovers	1 whole	850	71	47	219	91	121	103	289	145
■ 12″ Fit n' Delicious Pizza										
Diced Chicken, Red Onion and Green Pepper	1 slice	170	23	5	44	18	24	21	58	29
Diced Chicken, Mushrooms and Jalapeño	1 slice	170	22	5	44	18	24	21	58	29
Ham, Red Onion and Mushroom	1 slice	160	23	5	41	17	23	19	54	27

FOOD	AMOUNT	CAL	CARBS	FAT	WALK	RUN	BIKE	SWIM	YOGA	DANCE
Ham, Pineapple and Diced Red Tomato	1 slice	160	23	5	41	17	23	19	54	27
Green Pepper, Red Onion and Diced Red Tomato	1 slice	150	23	4	39	16	21	18	51	26
Diced Red Tomato, Mushroom and Jalapeño	1 slice	150	22	4	39	16	21	18	51	26
■ **14″ Fit n' Delicious Pizza**										
Diced Chicken, Red Onion and Green Pepper	1 slice	160	21	5	41	17	23	19	54	27
Diced Chicken, Mushrooms and Jalapeño	1 slice	160	20	5	41	17	23	19	54	27
Ham, Red Onion and Mushroom	1 slice	150	21	5	39	16	21	18	51	26
Ham, Pineapple and Diced Red Tomato	1 slice	150	22	5	39	16	21	18	51	26
Green Pepper, Red Onion and Diced Red Tomato	1 slice	140	22	4	36	15	20	17	48	24
Diced Red Tomato, Mushroom and Jalapeño	1 slice	140	21	4	36	15	20	17	48	24
Papa John's										
■ **Original Crust 14″ Pizza**										
Cheese	1 slice	300	39	11	77	32	43	36	102	51
Pepperoni	1 slice	310	38	13	80	33	44	38	105	53
Sausage	1 slice	330	37	15	85	35	47	40	112	56
Chicken Fajita	1 slice	290	40	9	75	31	41	35	99	49
Steak Fajita	1 slice	300	40	10	77	32	43	36	102	51
The Meats	1 slice	350	38	16	90	37	50	43	119	60
Garden Fresh	1 slice	280	40	9	72	30	40	34	95	48
The Works	1 slice	330	39	11	85	35	47	40	112	56
Spinach Alfredo	1 slice	280	36	11	72	30	40	34	95	48
Grilled Chicken Alfredo	1 slice	310	36	12	80	33	44	38	105	53
Chicken and Bacon	1 slice	340	44	11	88	36	48	41	116	58
Hawaiian BBQ Chicken	1 slice	340	46	11	88	36	48	41	116	58
Grilled Chicken Club	1 slice	320	40	12	82	34	45	39	109	55
Spinach Alfredo Chicken	1 slice	290	37	11	75	31	41	35	99	49
Spicy Italian	1 slice	370	39	11	95	39	52	45	126	63
■ **Original Crust 12″ Pizza**										
Cheese	1 slice	210	27	8	54	22	30	26	71	36
Pepperoni	1 slice	220	27	9	57	23	31	27	75	37

FOOD	AMOUNT	CAL	CARBS	FAT	WALK	RUN	BIKE	SWIM	YOGA	DANCE
Sausage	1 slice	240	26	11	62	26	34	29	82	41
The Meats	1 slice	240	27	11	62	26	34	29	82	41
Garden Fresh	1 slice	200	28	7	52	21	28	24	68	34
The Works	1 slice	230	28	8	59	24	33	28	78	39
Spinach Alfredo	1 slice	200	26	8	52	21	28	24	68	34
Grilled Chicken Alfredo	1 slice	210	26	9	54	22	30	26	71	36
Chicken and Bacon	1 slice	240	32	8	62	26	34	29	82	41
Hawaiian BBQ Chicken	1 slice	240	33	8	62	26	34	29	82	41
Grilled Chicken Club	1 slice	230	28	8	59	24	33	28	78	39
Spinach Alfredo Chicken	1 slice	210	27	8	54	22	30	26	71	36
Spicy Italian	1 slice	260	27	8	67	28	37	32	88	44
■ **Thin Crust Pizza**										
Cheese	1 slice	240	22	13	62	26	34	29	82	41
Pepperoni	1 slice	260	23	15	67	28	37	32	88	44
Sausage	1 slice	280	22	17	72	30	40	34	95	48
The Meats	1 slice	300	23	18	77	32	43	36	102	51
Garden Fresh	1 slice	210	23	11	54	22	30	26	71	36
The Works	1 slice	280	24	14	72	30	40	34	95	48
Spinach Alfredo	1 slice	220	19	13	57	23	31	27	75	37
Grilled Chicken Alfredo	1 slice	240	20	13	62	26	34	29	82	41
Chicken and Bacon	1 slice	290	29	14	75	31	41	35	99	49
Hawaiian BBQ Chicken	1 slice	290	31	14	75	31	41	35	99	49
Grilled Chicken Club	1 slice	270	25	14	70	29	38	33	92	46
Spinach Alfredo Chicken	1 slice	230	21	13	59	24	33	28	78	39
Spicy Italian	1 slice	320	24	14	82	34	45	39	109	55
■ **Pan Crust Pizza**										
Cheese	1 slice	380	39	15	98	40	54	46	129	65
Pepperoni	1 slice	400	38	17	103	43	57	49	136	68
Sausage	1 slice	410	38	19	106	44	58	50	139	70
The Meats	1 slice	420	38	19	108	45	60	51	143	72
Garden Fresh	1 slice	360	40	13	93	38	51	44	122	61
The Works	1 slice	400	39	15	103	43	57	49	136	68
Spinach Alfredo	1 slice	360	36	15	93	38	51	44	122	61
Grilled Chicken Alfredo	1 slice	380	36	16	98	40	54	46	129	65
Chicken and Bacon	1 slice	410	44	16	106	44	58	50	139	70
Hawaiian BBQ Chicken	1 slice	420	46	16	108	45	60	51	143	72

FOOD	AMOUNT	CAL	CARBS	FAT	WALK	RUN	BIKE	SWIM	YOGA	DANCE
Grilled Chicken Club	1 slice	400	39	16	103	43	57	49	136	68
Spinach Alfredo Chicken	1 slice	380	37	16	98	40	54	46	129	65
Spicy Italian	1 slice	450	39	15	116	48	64	55	153	77
■ **Side Items**										
Cheesestick	2 sticks	370	42	16	95	39	52	45	126	63
Breadstick	1 stick	140	26	2	36	15	20	17	48	24
Garlic Parmesan Breadstick	1 stick	170	26	6	44	18	24	21	58	29
Papa's Chicken Strips	2 strips	160	10	8	41	17	23	19	54	27
Papa's Spicy Buffalo Wings	2 wings	160	1	11	41	17	23	19	54	27
Papa's Mild Chipotle Barbecue	2 wings	160	5	10	41	17	23	19	54	27
Papa's Cinnapie	2 slices	200	29	8	52	21	28	24	68	34
Garlic Dipping Sauce	1 cup	150	0	17	39	16	21	18	51	26
Pizza Dipping Sauce	1 cup	20	3	0	5	2	3	2	7	3
Cheese Dipping Sauce	1 cup	70	1	6	18	7	10	9	24	12
Ranch Dipping Sauce	1 cup	110	1	11	28	12	16	13	37	19
Blue Cheese Dipping Sauce	1 cup	170	1	18	44	18	24	21	58	29
Honey Mustard Dipping Sauce	1 cup	150	5	15	39	16	21	18	51	26
BBQ Dipping Sauce	1 cup	40	11	0	10	4	6	5	14	7
Buffalo Dipping Sauce	1 cup	15	2	1	4	2	2	2	5	3
Apple Twist Sweetreat	½ pie	360	54	13	93	38	51	44	122	61
Cinna Swirl Sweetreat	½ pie	400	53	18	103	43	57	49	136	68
Very Berry Sweetreat	½ pie	410	67	12	106	44	58	50	139	70

Fast Food

Breakfast										
■ **Biscuit**										
Egg biscuit	1 biscuit	373	32	33	96	40	53	45	127	64
Egg and bacon biscuit	1 biscuit	458	29	31	118	49	65	56	156	78
Egg and ham biscuit	1 biscuit	461	35	27	119	49	65	56	157	79
Egg and sausage biscuit	1 biscuit	581	41	39	150	62	82	71	198	99
Egg, cheese, and bacon biscuit	1 biscuit	477	33	31	123	51	68	58	162	81
Egg and steak biscuit	1 biscuit	410	21	28	106	44	58	50	139	70
Ham biscuit	1 biscuit	386	44	18	99	41	55	47	131	66
Sausage biscuit	1 biscuit	484	40	32	125	52	69	59	165	82

FOOD	AMOUNT	CAL	CARBS	FAT	WALK	RUN	BIKE	SWIM	YOGA	DANCE
■ **English Muffin**										
English muffin, with butter	1 muffin	189	30	6	49	20	27	23	64	32
English muffin, with cheese and sausage	1 muffin	393	0	24	101	42	56	48	134	67
English muffin, with egg, cheese, and Canadian bacon	1 muffin	289	27	13	74	31	41	35	98	49
English muffin, with egg, cheese, and sausage	1 muffin	487	31	31	126	52	69	59	166	83
■ **French Toast/Pancakes**										
French toast, with butter	2 slices	356	36	19	92	38	50	43	121	61
French toast sticks	5 sticks	513	58	29	132	55	73	62	174	87
Pancakes, with butter and syrup	2 pancakes	520	91	14	134	55	74	63	177	89
■ **Egg**										
Egg and cheese sandwich	1 sandwich	340	26	19	88	36	48	41	116	58
Scrambled egg	2 eggs	199	2	15	51	21	28	24	68	34
■ **Danish**										
Cheese danish	1 danish	353	29	25	91	38	50	43	120	60
Cinnamon danish	1 danish	349	47	17	90	37	50	42	119	59
Fruit-filled danish	1 danish	335	45	16	86	36	48	41	114	57
■ **Croissant**										
Egg and cheese croissant	1 croissant	368	24	25	95	39	52	45	125	63
Egg, cheese, and bacon croissant	1 croissant	413	24	28	106	44	59	50	140	70
Egg, cheese, and ham croissant	1 croissant	474	24	34	122	50	67	58	161	81
Egg, cheese, and sausage croissant	1 croissant	523	25	38	135	56	74	64	178	89
Burgers										
Regular burger	1 sandwich	272	34	10	70	29	39	33	93	46
Regular double burger	1 sandwich	576	39	32	148	61	82	70	196	98
Large burger	1 sandwich	427	37	21	110	45	61	52	145	73
Large double burger	1 sandwich	540	40	27	139	58	77	66	184	92
Large cheeseburger	1 sandwich	563	38	33	145	60	80	68	191	96

FOOD	AMOUNT	CAL	CARBS	FAT	WALK	RUN	BIKE	SWIM	YOGA	DANCE
Large cheeseburger, with ham	1 sandwich	744	38	48	192	79	106	91	253	127
Large double cheeseburger	1 sandwich	704	40	44	181	75	100	86	239	120
Regular cheeseburger	1 sandwich	359	28	20	93	38	51	44	122	61
Regular double cheeseburger	1 sandwich	650	53	35	168	69	92	79	221	111
Chicken										
Chicken fillet sandwich	1 sandwich	515	39	29	133	55	73	63	175	88
Chicken fillet sandwich, with cheese	1 sandwich	632	42	39	163	67	90	77	215	108
Breaded and fried chicken strips	6 pieces	285	16	18	73	30	40	35	97	49
Breaded and fried dark meat	2 pieces (148 g)	431	16	27	111	46	61	52	147	73
Breaded and fried light meat	2 pieces (163 g)	494	20	30	127	53	70	60	168	84
Desserts										
Brownie	1 brownie	243	39	10	63	26	34	30	83	41
Vanilla soft serve ice milk, with cone	1 cone	164	24	6	42	17	23	20	56	28
Caramel sundae	1 sundae	304	49	9	78	32	43	37	103	52
Hot-fudge sundae	1 sundae	284	48	9	73	30	40	35	97	48
Strawberry sundae	1 sundae	268	45	8	69	29	38	33	91	46
Hot Dog										
Plain hot dog	1 dog	242	18	15	62	26	34	29	82	41
Hot dog, with chili	1 dog	296	31	13	76	32	42	36	101	50
Corn dog	1 dog	460	56	19	119	49	65	56	156	78
Mexican										
■ Burritos										
Bean burrito	2 burritos (217 g)	447	71	14	115	48	63	54	152	76
Bean and cheese burrito	2 burritos (186 g)	378	55	12	97	40	54	46	129	64
Bean and chili pepper burrito	2 burritos (204 g)	412	58	15	106	44	58	50	140	70
Bean and meat burrito	2 burritos (231 g)	508	66	18	131	54	72	62	173	87

FOOD	AMOUNT	CAL	CARBS	FAT	WALK	RUN	BIKE	SWIM	YOGA	DANCE
Bean, cheese, and beef burrito	2 burritos (203 g)	331	40	13	85	35	47	40	113	56
Bean, cheese, and chili pepper burrito	2 burritos (336 g)	662	85	23	171	71	94	81	225	113
Beef burrito	2 burritos (220 g)	524	59	21	135	56	74	64	178	89
Beef and chili pepper burrito	2 burritos (201 g)	426	49	17	110	45	60	52	145	73
Beef, cheese, and chili pepper burrito	2 burritos (304 g)	632	64	25	163	67	90	77	215	108
Fruit burrito	1 large burrito	484	73	20	125	52	69	59	165	82
■ Nachos										
Nachos, with cheese	6-8 nachos	346	36	19	89	37	49	42	118	59
Nachos, with cheese and jalapeño peppers	6-8 nachos	608	60	34	157	65	86	74	207	104
Nachos, with cheese, beans, ground beef, and peppers	6-8 nachos	569	56	31	147	61	81	69	194	97
Nachos, with cinnamon and sugar	6-8 nachos	592	63	36	153	63	84	72	201	101
■ Tacos										
Taco	1 large	568	41	32	146	60	81	69	193	97
Tostada, with beans and cheese	1 piece	223	27	10	57	24	32	27	76	38
Tostada, with beans, beef, and cheese	1 piece	333	30	17	86	35	47	41	113	57
Tostada, with beef and cheese	1 piece	315	23	16	81	34	45	38	107	54
■ Chimichanga										
Chimichanga, with beef	1 chimichanga	425	43	20	110	45	60	52	145	72
Chimichanga, with beef and cheese	1 chimichanga	443	39	23	114	47	63	54	151	75
Chimichanga, with beef and red chili peppers	1 chimichanga	424	46	19	109	45	60	52	144	72
Chimichange, with beef, cheese, and red chili peppers	1 chimichanga	364	38	18	94	39	52	44	124	62
■ Enchilada										
Enchilada, with cheese	1 enchilada	310	29	19	80	33	44	38	105	53

FOOD	AMOUNT	CAL	CARBS	FAT	WALK	RUN	BIKE	SWIM	YOGA	DANCE
Enchilada, with cheese and beef	1 enchilada	323	30	18	83	34	46	39	110	55
■ Enchirito										
Enchirito, with beans, cheese, and beef	1 enchirito	344	34	16	89	37	49	42	117	59
■ Frijoles										
Frijoles, with cheese	1 cup	225	29	8	58	24	32	27	77	38
Pizza										
Regular cheese pizza	1 slice	272	34	10	70	29	39	33	93	46
Thick-crust cheese pizza	1 slice	288	33	12	74	31	41	35	98	49
Thin-crust cheese pizza	1 slice	192	17	10	49	20	27	23	65	33
Meat and vegetable–topped pizza	1 slice	332	35	15	86	35	47	40	113	57
Pepperoni pizza	1 slice	298	34	12	77	32	42	36	101	51
Thin-crust pepperoni pizza	1 slice	301	32	13	78	32	43	37	102	51
Salads										
Coleslaw	.75 cup	147	13	11	38	16	21	18	50	25
Vegetable salad, no dressing	1.5 cup	33	7	0	9	4	5	4	11	6
Vegetable salad, with egg and cheese, no dressing	1.5 cup	102	5	6	26	11	14	12	35	17
Vegetable salad, with pasta and seafood, no dressing	1.5 cup	379	32	21	98	40	54	46	129	65
Vegetable salad, with shrimp, no dressing	1.5 cup	106	7	2	27	11	15	13	36	18
Vegetable salad, with turkey, ham, and cheese, no dressing	1.5 cup	267	5	16	69	28	38	32	91	45
Taco salad	1.5 cup	279	24	15	72	30	40	34	95	48
Taco salad, with chili con carne	1.5 cup	290	27	13	75	31	41	35	99	49
Sandwiches										
Plain roast beef sandwich	1 sandwich	346	33	14	89	37	49	42	118	59
Cold-cut sub	1 sub	456	51	19	118	49	65	55	155	78
Roast beef sub	1 sub	410	44	13	106	44	58	50	139	70
Tuna salad sub	1 sub	584	55	28	151	62	83	71	199	99
Ham and cheese sandwich	1 sandwich	352	33	15	91	37	50	43	120	60
Ham, egg, and cheese sandwich	1 sandwich	347	31	16	89	37	49	42	118	59

FOOD	AMOUNT	CAL	CARBS	FAT	WALK	RUN	BIKE	SWIM	YOGA	DANCE
Seafood										
Crab cake	1 cake	160	5	10	41	17	23	19	54	27
Breaded and fried fish fillet	1 fillet	211	15	11	54	22	30	26	72	36
Fish sandwich, with tartar sauce	1 sandwich	431	41	23	111	46	61	52	147	73
Fish sandwich, with tartar sauce and cheese	1 sandwich	523	48	29	135	56	74	64	178	89
Breaded and fried oysters	6 oysters	368	40	18	95	39	52	45	125	63
Breaded and fried clams	.75 cup	451	39	26	116	48	64	55	153	77
Breaded and fried scallops	6 scallops	386	38	19	99	41	55	47	131	66
Breaded and fried shrimp	6-8 shrimp	454	40	25	117	48	64	55	154	77
Shakes										
Chocolate shake	16 fl oz	478	77	14	123	51	68	58	163	81
Strawberry shake	16 fl oz	425	71	11	110	45	60	52	145	72
Vanilla shake	16 fl oz	556	74	25	143	59	79	68	189	95
Sides										
Onion rings	1 serving (8-9 rings)	276	31	16	71	29	39	34	94	47
Fast food hush puppies	5 puppies (78 g)	257	35	12	66	27	36	31	87	44
Corn on the cob, with butter	1 ear	155	32	3	40	17	22	19	53	26
Baked potato, with cheese sauce	1 piece	474	27	29	122	50	67	58	161	81
Baked potato, with cheese sauce and bacon	1 piece	451	44	26	116	48	64	55	153	77
Baked potato, with cheese sauce and broccoli	1 piece	403	47	21	104	43	57	49	137	69
Baked potato, with cheese sauce and chili	1 piece	482	56	22	124	51	68	59	164	82
Baked potato, with sour cream and chives	1 piece	393	50	22	101	42	56	48	134	67
Mashed potatoes	.333 cup	66	13	1	17	7	9	8	22	11
Fries	1 large	539	63	29	139	57	76	66	183	92
Hash browns	.5 cup	151	16	9	39	16	21	18	51	26
Chili con carne	1 cup	256	22	8	66	27	36	31	87	44
Hush puppies	5 pieces	257	35	12	66	27	36	31	87	44
Sushi										
Avocado roll	1 roll	246	33	11	63	26	35	30	84	42

FOOD	AMOUNT	CAL	CARBS	FAT	WALK	RUN	BIKE	SWIM	YOGA	DANCE
Spicy tuna roll	1 roll	290	26	11	75	31	41	35	99	49
Shrimp tempura roll	1 roll	544	75	13	140	58	77	66	185	93
Philadelphia roll	1 roll	319	30	5	82	34	45	39	109	54
Spider roll (fried soft shell crab)	1 roll	317	38	12	82	34	45	39	108	54
California roll	1 roll	266	36	9	69	28	38	32	90	45
Cucumber roll	1 roll	136	30	0	35	14	19	17	46	23
Eel and avocado roll	1 roll	372	31	18	96	40	53	45	127	63
Tuna nigiri	2 pieces over rice	240	27	1	62	26	34	29	82	41
Salmon sashimi	2 pieces, no rice	164	0	6	42	17	23	20	56	28

Arby's

■ Roast Beef Sandwiches and Melts

FOOD	AMOUNT	CAL	CARBS	FAT	WALK	RUN	BIKE	SWIM	YOGA	DANCE
Arby's Melt	1 serving	303	36	12	78	32	43	37	103	52
BBQ Bacon 'n Jack 2for	1 serving	361	42	15	93	38	51	44	123	61
Bacon, Beef and Cheddar	1 serving	521	45	26	134	55	74	63	177	89
Beef and Cheddar	1 serving	445	44	20	115	47	63	54	151	76
French Dip and Swiss	1 serving	473	38	18	122	50	67	58	161	81
French Dip	1 serving	391	37	17	101	42	55	48	133	67
Ham and Swiss Melt	1 serving	275	35	6	71	29	39	33	94	47
Hot Ham and Cheese	1 serving	304	35	7	78	32	43	37	103	52
Jr. Ham and Swiss Melt	1 serving	211	23	5	54	22	30	26	72	36
Junior Roast Beef Sandwich	1 serving	273	34	10	70	29	39	33	93	47
Large Roast Beef	1 serving	547	42	28	141	58	78	67	186	93
Medium Roast Beef	1 serving	416	34	20	107	44	59	51	141	71
Regular Roast Beef	1 serving	320	34	13	82	34	45	39	109	55
Sourdough Ham Melt	1 serving	380	39	14	98	40	54	46	129	65
Sourdough Roast Beef Melt	1 serving	356	40	14	92	38	50	43	121	61
Super Roast Beef	1 serving	398	40	18	103	42	56	48	135	68
Swiss Melt	1 serving	304	37	12	78	32	43	37	103	52

■ Chicken Naturals

FOOD	AMOUNT	CAL	CARBS	FAT	WALK	RUN	BIKE	SWIM	YOGA	DANCE
Crispy Chicken, Bacon and Swiss	1 serving	624	52	29	161	66	89	76	212	106
Grilled Chicken, Bacon and Swiss	1 serving	461	38	16	119	49	65	56	157	79
Crispy Chicken Cordon Bleu Sandwich	1 serving	651	49	31	168	69	92	79	221	111

FOOD	AMOUNT	CAL	CARBS	FAT	WALK	RUN	BIKE	SWIM	YOGA	DANCE
Grilled Chicken Cordon Bleu Sandwich	1 serving	488	35	18	126	52	69	59	166	83
Crispy Chicken Fillet Sandwich	1 serving	577	50	29	149	61	82	70	196	98
Grilled Chicken Fillet Sandwich	1 serving	414	36	16	107	44	59	50	141	71
Chicken Tenders	3 pieces	434	32	21	112	46	62	53	148	74
Chicken Tenders	5 pieces	723	54	35	186	77	103	88	246	123
Grilled SW Chipotle Chicken Sandwich	1 serving	517	37	24	133	55	73	63	176	88
Crispy SW Chipotle Chicken Sandwich	1 serving	680	51	37	175	72	96	83	231	116
■ **Subs**										
French Dip with Au Jus	1 serving	447	48	17	115	48	63	54	152	76
Hot Ham and Swiss	1 serving	497	46	17	128	53	70	60	169	85
Italian	1 serving	621	49	32	160	66	88	76	211	106
Phily Beef and Swiss	1 serving	669	46	35	172	71	95	81	228	114
Roast Beef	1 serving	722	47	41	186	77	102	88	246	123
Turkey	1 serving	632	48	29	163	67	90	77	215	108
■ **Market Fresh Sandwiches and Wraps**										
Chicken Salad with Pecans Sandwich	1 serving	769	78	39	198	82	109	94	262	131
Chicken Salad with Pecans Wrap	1 serving	638	48	38	164	68	90	78	217	109
Corned Beef Reuben Sandwich	1 serving	606	55	33	156	65	86	74	206	103
Roast Beef and Swiss Sandwich	1 serving	777	71	41	200	83	110	95	264	132
Roast Ham and Swiss Sandwich	1 serving	706	74	30	182	75	100	86	240	120
Roast Turkey and Swiss Sandwich	1 serving	725	73	29	187	77	103	88	247	124
Roast Turkey Ranch and Bacon Sandwich	1 serving	834	73	37	215	89	118	101	284	142
Roast Turkey Ranch and Bacon Wrap	1 serving	699	42	36	180	74	99	85	238	119
Roast Turkey Reuben Sandwich	1 serving	611	55	30	157	65	87	74	208	104
Southwest Chicken Wrap	1 serving	568	40	30	146	60	81	69	193	97
Ultimate BLT Sandwich	1 serving	779	76	45	201	83	110	95	265	133
Ultimate BLT Wrap	1 serving	648	46	44	167	69	92	79	220	110

FOOD	AMOUNT	CAL	CARBS	FAT	WALK	RUN	BIKE	SWIM	YOGA	DANCE
■ Market Fresh Salads										
Martha's Vineyard (plain)	1 salad	276	24	8	71	29	39	34	94	47
Santa Fe (plain)	1 salad	500	41	23	129	53	71	61	170	85
Santa Fe Salad with Grilled Chicken	1 salad	306	20	11	79	33	43	37	104	52
Chicken Club Salad (plain)	1 salad	503	31	26	130	54	71	61	171	86
■ Dressings and Salad Add-Ons										
Sliced Almonds	1 serving	81	2	8	21	9	11	10	28	14
Seasoned Tortilla Strips	1 serving	71	9	3	18	8	10	9	24	12
Raspberry Vinaigrette	2.26 oz	194	18	14	50	21	28	24	66	33
Santa Fe Ranch Dressing	2.26 oz	296	4	31	76	32	42	36	101	50
Buttermilk Ranch Dressing	2.26 oz	325	4	34	84	35	46	40	111	55
Light Buttermilk Ranch Dressing	2.26 oz	112	13	6	29	12	16	14	38	19
■ Premium Potatoes										
Curly Fries	small	338	39	20	87	36	48	41	115	58
Curly Fries	medium	406	47	24	105	43	58	49	138	69
Curly Fries	large	631	73	37	163	67	90	77	215	107
Cheddar Cheese Sauce	side order	30	2	2	8	3	4	4	10	5
Homestyle Fries	small	302	44	20	78	32	43	37	103	51
Homestyle Fries	medium	377	55	25	97	40	53	46	128	64
Homestyle Fries	large	566	82	37	146	60	80	69	193	96
Potato Cakes	2 cakes	246	26	18	63	26	35	30	84	42
■ Sidekickers										
Jalapeño Bites	regular	305	29	21	79	32	43	37	104	52
Jalapeño Bites	large	611	58	43	157	65	87	74	208	104
Mozzarella Sticks	regular	426	38	28	110	45	60	52	145	73
Mozzarella Sticks	large	852	76	56	220	91	121	104	290	145
Onion Petals	regular	331	35	23	85	35	47	40	113	56
Onion Petals	large	828	88	57	213	88	117	101	282	141
■ Breakfast										
Bacon 'n Egg Croissant	1 serving	337	23	22	87	36	48	41	115	57
Bacon Biscuit	1 serving	340	28	21	88	36	48	41	116	58
Bacon, Egg and Cheese Biscuit	1 serving	461	30	28	119	49	65	56	157	79
Bacon, Egg and Cheese Croissant	1 serving	378	23	23	97	40	54	46	129	64

FOOD	AMOUNT	CAL	CARBS	FAT	WALK	RUN	BIKE	SWIM	YOGA	DANCE
Bacon, Egg and Cheese Sourdough	1 serving	437	41	16	113	47	62	53	149	74
Bacon, Egg and Cheese Wrap	1 serving	515	50	29	133	55	73	63	175	88
Biscuit (plain)	1 serving	273	28	15	70	29	39	33	93	47
Blueberry Muffin	1 serving	320	49	12	82	34	45	39	109	55
Breakfast Syrup	1 serving	78	20	0	20	8	11	9	27	13
Chicken Biscuit	1 serving	418	39	22	108	45	59	51	142	71
Croissant	1 serving	190	21	10	49	20	27	23	65	32
Egg and Cheese Sourdough	1 serving	392	41	12	101	42	56	48	133	67
French Toastix	1 serving	312	44	13	80	33	44	38	106	53
Ham 'n Cheese Croissant	1 serving	274	22	12	71	29	39	33	93	47
Ham Biscuit	1 serving	316	29	16	81	34	45	38	107	54
Ham, Egg and Cheese Biscuit	1 serving	437	31	23	113	47	62	53	149	74
Ham, Egg and Cheese Croissant	1 serving	434	25	24	112	46	62	53	148	74
Ham, Egg and Cheese Sourdough	1 serving	678	43	35	175	72	96	82	231	116
Ham, Egg and Cheese Wrap	1 serving	568	52	30	146	60	81	69	193	97
Sausage 'n Egg Croissant	1 serving	433	23	32	112	46	61	53	147	74
Sausage Biscuit	1 serving	436	28	31	112	46	62	53	148	74
Sausage Gravy Biscuit	1 serving	961	107	68	248	102	136	117	327	164
Sausage Patty	1 serving	210	0	20	54	22	30	26	71	36
Sausage, Egg and Cheese Croissant	1 serving	474	23	33	122	50	67	58	161	81
Sausage, Egg and Cheese Wrap	1 serving	688	51	45	177	73	98	84	234	117
Sausage, Egg and Cheese Biscuit	1 serving	557	30	38	144	59	79	68	189	95
Sausage, Egg and Cheese Sourdough	1 serving	514	40	28	132	55	73	63	175	88
■ **Desserts**										
Apple Turnover (no icing)	1 turnover	250	35	10	64	27	35	30	85	43
Apple Turnover (with icing)	1 turnover	377	64	15	97	40	53	46	128	64
Cherry Turnover (no icing)	1 turnover	250	35	10	64	27	35	30	85	43
Cherry Turnover (with icing)	1 turnover	377	64	16	97	40	53	46	128	64
Gourmet Chocolate Cookie	1 cookie	202	26	10	52	22	29	25	69	34
■ **Sauces/Condiments**										
Arby's Sauce Packet	1 packet	15	4	0	4	2	2	2	5	3
BBQ Dipping Sauce	1 oz	40	10	0	10	4	6	5	14	7

FOOD	AMOUNT	CAL	CARBS	FAT	WALK	RUN	BIKE	SWIM	YOGA	DANCE
Buffalo Dipping Sauce	1 serving	20	3	1	5	2	3	2	7	3
Bronco Berry Sauce	2 oz	120	30	0	31	13	17	15	41	20
Honey Mustard Dipping Sauce	1 oz	130	5	12	34	14	18	16	44	22
Horsey Sauce Packet	1 packet	60	3	5	15	6	9	7	20	10
Ketchup Packet	1 packet	20	4	0	5	2	3	2	7	3
Light Mayonnaise Packet	1 packet	45	1	5	12	5	6	5	15	8
Marinara Sauce	1 serving	30	4	2	8	3	4	4	10	5
Mayonnaise Packet	1 packet	100	0	11	26	11	14	12	34	17
Red Ranch Sauce	1 serving	70	5	6	18	7	10	9	24	12
Tangy Southwest Sauce	2 oz	330	5	35	85	35	47	40	112	56
Three Pepper Sauce Packet	1 packet	20	3	1	5	2	3	2	7	3
■ Shakes										
Chocolate Shake	regular	510	83	13	131	54	72	62	173	87
Chocolate Shake	large	660	110	17	170	70	94	80	224	112
Jamocha Shake	regular	500	81	13	129	53	71	61	170	85
Jamocha Shake	large	650	107	17	168	69	92	79	221	111
Strawberry Shake	regular	500	81	13	129	53	71	61	170	85
Strawberry Shake	large	650	107	17	168	69	92	79	221	111
Vanilla Shake	regular	500	82	13	129	53	71	61	170	85
Vanilla Shake	large	650	107	17	168	69	92	79	221	111
Au Bon Pain										
■ Breakfast Sandwiches										
Arugula and Tomato Frittata	1 serving	290	27	13	75	31	41	35	99	49
Cholesterol and Fat Free Eggs	1 serving	25	1	0	6	3	4	3	9	4
Cinnamon Raisin French Toast	1 serving	830	137	20	214	88	118	101	282	141
Egg on a Bagel	1 serving	400	63	5	103	43	57	49	136	68
Egg on a Bagel with Bacon	1 serving	480	63	12	124	51	68	58	163	82
Egg on a Bagel with Cheese	1 serving	480	63	11	124	51	68	58	163	82
Egg on a Bagel with Cheese and Bacon	1 serving	560	63	18	144	60	79	68	190	95
Eggs BLT Sandwich	1 serving	790	61	41	204	84	112	96	269	135
Ham and Cheddar Frittata	1 serving	320	25	14	82	34	45	39	109	55
Scrambled Egg, Bacon and Salsa Wrap	1 serving	491	41	25	127	52	70	60	167	84
■ Other Sandwiches										
Asian Chicken Salad	1 sandwich	430	50	16	111	46	61	52	146	73

FOOD	AMOUNT	CAL	CARBS	FAT	WALK	RUN	BIKE	SWIM	YOGA	DANCE
Barbecue Pulled Pork	1 sandwich	610	83	18	157	65	87	74	207	104
Chicken Mozzarella	1 sandwich	740	73	24	191	79	105	90	252	126
Chicken Tarragon with Field Greens	1 sandwich	800	71	42	206	85	113	97	272	136
Chili Dijon Chicken Breast, Wisconsin Aged Cheddar	1 sandwich	530	52	17	137	56	75	64	180	90
Hickory Smoked Turkey Club, Aged Wisconsin Cheddar, Bacon	1 sandwich	710	59	32	183	76	101	86	241	121
Mozzarella, Tomato and Pesto	1 sandwich	820	67	43	211	87	116	100	279	140
Roasted Portabello and Goat Cheese	1 sandwich	560	63	27	144	60	79	68	190	95
Spicy Tuna on Multigrain	1 sandwich	690	72	33	178	73	98	84	235	118
Steak and Gorgonzola on Onion Roll	1 sandwich	780	76	39	201	83	111	95	265	133
Turkey, Guacamole, Swiss on Baguette	1 sandwich	760	77	28	196	81	108	92	259	129

■ Wraps

FOOD	AMOUNT	CAL	CARBS	FAT	WALK	RUN	BIKE	SWIM	YOGA	DANCE
Chicken Caesar Wrap	1 wrap	591	63	24	152	63	84	72	201	101
Chicken Salsa Wrap	1 wrap	440	68	8	113	47	62	54	150	75
Chopped Cobb Wrap	1 wrap	561	65	20	145	60	80	68	191	96
Egg Salad Wrap	1 wrap	650	83	25	168	69	92	79	221	111
Fields and Feta Wrap	1 wrap	551	90	26	142	59	78	67	187	94
Mediterranean	1 wrap	571	80	22	147	61	81	69	194	97
Southwest Tuna	1 wrap	541	68	25	139	58	77	66	184	92

■ Baked Sandwiches

FOOD	AMOUNT	CAL	CARBS	FAT	WALK	RUN	BIKE	SWIM	YOGA	DANCE
Grilled Chicken, Blue Cheese, Caramelized Onion	1 sandwich	672	64	29	173	72	95	82	229	114
Grilled Chicken, Melted Gouda, Caramelized Onion, Chipotle Mayonnaise	1 sandwich	660	68	25	170	70	94	80	224	112
Mozzarella, Tomato, Basil Pesto, Caramelized Onion	1 sandwich	638	66	30	164	68	90	78	217	109
Roasted Turkey Cranberry, Wensleydale Cheese, Roasted Almond	1 sandwich	554	80	12	143	59	79	67	188	94

FOOD	AMOUNT	CAL	CARBS	FAT	WALK	RUN	BIKE	SWIM	YOGA	DANCE
Steak, Melted Swiss, Caramelized Onions, Portobello Mushrooms, and Jalapeño Mayonnaise	1 sandwich	690	68	28	178	73	98	84	235	118
Tuna, Aged Shelburne Farms Cheddar, Roasted Red Peppers	1 sandwich	553	62	18	143	59	78	67	188	94

■ Salads

FOOD	AMOUNT	CAL	CARBS	FAT	WALK	RUN	BIKE	SWIM	YOGA	DANCE
Asian Chicken Side Salad	1 salad	220	14	11	57	23	31	27	75	37
Caesar Salad	1 salad	240	23	11	62	26	34	29	82	41
Chef's Salad	1 salad	270	8	15	70	29	38	33	92	46
Chicken Caesar Salad	1 salad	530	40	22	137	56	75	64	180	90
Chicken Pesto Salad	1 salad	420	14	30	108	45	60	51	143	72
Large Garden Salad	1 salad	110	19	2	28	12	16	13	37	19
Small Garden Salad	1 salad	50	10	1	13	5	7	6	17	9
Gorgonzola and Walnut Salad	1 salad	340	10	28	88	36	48	41	116	58
Mediterranean Chicken Salad	1 salad	290	14	16	75	31	41	35	99	49
Steak Salad with Cranberries and Mandarin Oranges	1 salad	290	46	7	75	31	41	35	99	49
Thai Chicken	1 salad	140	14	3	36	15	20	17	48	24
Tuna Garden Salad	1 salad	400	25	24	103	43	57	49	136	68
Tuna Nicoise Salad	1 salad	300	19	15	77	32	43	36	102	51
Turkey Medallion Cobb Salad	1 salad	370	27	18	95	39	52	45	126	63
Watermelon and Goat Cheese Salad	1 salad	250	31	10	64	27	35	30	85	43

■ Dressings

FOOD	AMOUNT	CAL	CARBS	FAT	WALK	RUN	BIKE	SWIM	YOGA	DANCE
Balsamic Vinaigrette	2.5 oz	150	9	12	39	16	21	18	51	26
Blue Cheese	2.5 oz	370	3	39	95	39	52	45	126	63
Caesar	2.5 oz	390	6	38	101	42	55	47	133	66
Fat Free Raspberry Vinaigrette	2.5 oz	80	19	0	21	9	11	10	27	14
Lite Honey Mustard	2.5 oz	240	26	15	62	26	34	29	82	41
Lite Olive Oil Vinaigrette	2.5 oz	150	7	14	39	16	21	18	51	26
Lite Ranch	2.5 oz	200	5	16	52	21	28	24	68	34

■ Soups

FOOD	AMOUNT	CAL	CARBS	FAT	WALK	RUN	BIKE	SWIM	YOGA	DANCE
Chicken Chili with Beans	1 cup	180	26	4	46	19	26	22	61	31
Black Bean Soup	1 cup	100	29	1	26	11	14	12	34	17
Clam Chowder	1 cup	220	20	13	57	23	31	27	75	37
Mediterranean Seafood Stew	1 cup	140	12	4	36	15	20	17	48	24

FOOD	AMOUNT	CAL	CARBS	FAT	WALK	RUN	BIKE	SWIM	YOGA	DANCE
Low Fat Garden Vegetable Soup	1 cup	50	9	1	13	5	7	6	17	9
Low Fat French Onion Soup	1 cup	80	12	3	21	9	11	10	27	14
Italian Wedding Soup	1 cup	100	12	4	26	11	14	12	34	17
Low Fat Chicken Noodle Soup	1 cup	100	14	2	26	11	14	12	34	17
Potato Leek Soup	1 cup	190	19	12	49	20	27	23	65	32
Potato Cheese Soup	1 cup	160	16	9	41	17	23	19	54	27
Baked Stuffed Potato Soup	1 cup	230	21	14	59	24	33	28	78	39
Broccoli Cheese Soup	1 cup	210	14	14	54	22	30	26	71	36
Chicken Florentine	1 cup	160	18	8	41	17	23	19	54	27
Chicken Noodle Soup	1 cup	100	14	2	26	11	14	12	34	17
Chicken Vegetable Stew	1 cup	200	18	11	52	21	28	24	68	34
Corn and Green Chili Bisque	1 cup	170	19	9	44	18	24	21	58	29
Corn Chili	1 cup	230	28	13	59	24	33	28	78	39
Curried Rice and Lentil	1 cup	100	20	1	26	11	14	12	34	17
French Moroccan Tomato Lentil	1 cup	120	21	2	31	13	17	15	41	20
French Onion Soup	1 cup	80	12	3	21	9	11	10	27	14
Garden Vegetable	1 cup	50	9	1	13	5	7	6	17	9
Harvest Pumpkin Soup	1 cup	140	15	7	36	15	20	17	48	24
Jamaican Black Bean	1 cup	120	30	1	31	13	17	15	41	20
Macaroni and Cheese Soup	1 cup	290	21	17	75	31	41	35	99	49
Mediterranean Pepper	1 cup	70	12	2	18	7	10	9	24	12
Old Fashioned Tomato	1 cup	130	19	5	34	14	18	16	44	22
Old Fashioned Tomato Rice	1 cup	80	16	1	21	9	11	10	27	14
Pasta e Fagioli	1 cup	160	24	6	41	17	23	19	54	27
Red Beans, Italian Sausage and Rice	1 cup	130	26	4	34	14	18	16	44	22
Red Lentil and Mango	1 cup	150	25	3	39	16	21	18	51	26
Southern Black-Eyed Pea	1 cup	120	21	1	31	13	17	15	41	20
Southwest Tortilla Soup	1 cup	130	16	7	34	14	18	16	44	22
Southwest Vegetable	1 cup	70	11	2	18	7	10	9	24	12
Split Pea with Ham	1 cup	140	28	1	36	15	20	17	48	24
Tomato Basil Bisque	1 cup	140	20	5	36	15	20	17	48	24
Tomato Florentine	1 cup	80	12	2	21	9	11	10	27	14
Turkey Chili with Beans	1 cup	200	27	4	52	21	28	24	68	34
Turkey Cranberry Stew	1 cup	240	20	10	62	26	34	29	82	41

FOOD	AMOUNT	CAL	CARBS	FAT	WALK	RUN	BIKE	SWIM	YOGA	DANCE
Tuscan Vegetable	1 cup	110	16	4	28	12	16	13	37	19
Vegetable Beef Barley	1 cup	90	14	2	23	10	13	11	31	15
Vegetarian Chili	1 cup	120	29	2	31	13	17	15	41	20
Vegetarian Lentil	1 cup	90	21	1	23	10	13	11	31	15
Vegetarian Minestrone	1 cup	80	14	1	21	9	11	10	27	14
Wild Mushroom Bisque	1 cup	130	16	6	34	14	18	16	44	22

■ Yogurt, Candy, and Fruit

FOOD	AMOUNT	CAL	CARBS	FAT	WALK	RUN	BIKE	SWIM	YOGA	DANCE
Assorted Nuts	4 oz	730	24	64	188	78	104	89	248	124
Chocolate Covered Espresso Beans	1.4 oz	180	22	12	46	19	26	22	61	31
Fruit Cup	small	70	16	0	18	7	10	9	24	12
Fruit Cup	large	140	32	1	36	15	20	17	48	24
Fruit Sours	4 oz	400	105	0	103	43	57	49	136	68
Granola	8 oz	1120	68	64	289	119	159	136	381	191
Kookaburra Black Licorice	1.4 oz	130	31	1	34	14	18	16	44	22
Kookaburra Red Licorice	1.4 oz	140	31	1	36	15	20	17	48	24
Maple Roasted Cashews	4 oz	650	45	49	168	69	92	79	221	111
Summit Blend	4 oz	500	63	27	129	53	71	61	170	85
Tamari Roast	4 oz	770	41	61	198	82	109	94	262	131
Plain, Low Fat Yogurt	small	190	36	2	49	20	27	23	65	32
Strawberry Yogurt with Fruit	large	380	75	5	98	40	54	46	129	65
Strawberry Yogurt with Granola and Fruit	small	310	56	6	80	33	44	38	105	53
Strawberry Yogurt with Granola and Fruit	large	620	112	13	160	66	88	75	211	106
Blueberry Yogurt with Fruit	large	380	75	5	98	40	54	46	129	65
Blueberry Yogurt with Granola and Fruit	small	310	56	6	80	33	44	38	105	53
Blueberry Yogurt with Granola and Fruit	large	620	112	13	160	66	88	75	211	106
Vanilla Yogurt with Fruit	large	370	64	4	95	39	52	45	126	63
Vanilla Yogurt with Granola and Fruit	small	310	56	6	80	33	44	38	105	53
Vanilla Yogurt with Granola and Fruit	large	620	112	13	160	66	88	75	211	106

Burger King

■ Whoppers

FOOD	AMOUNT	CAL	CARBS	FAT	WALK	RUN	BIKE	SWIM	YOGA	DANCE
Original	1 serving	670	51	39	173	71	95	82	228	114

FOOD	AMOUNT	CAL	CARBS	FAT	WALK	RUN	BIKE	SWIM	YOGA	DANCE
Original, No Mayo	1 serving	510	51	22	131	54	72	62	173	87
Original, Low Carb	1 serving	280	3	20	72	30	40	34	95	48
Original, with Cheese	1 serving	760	52	47	196	81	108	92	259	129
Original, with Cheese (no mayo)	1 serving	600	52	30	155	64	85	73	204	102
Original, with Cheese (low carb)	1 serving	370	5	28	95	39	52	45	126	63
Original Double Whopper	1 serving	900	51	57	232	96	128	109	306	153
Original Double Whopper (no mayo)	1 serving	740	51	39	191	79	105	90	252	126
Original Double Whopper (low carb)	1 serving	540	3	40	139	58	77	66	184	92
Original Double Whopper, with Cheese	1 serving	990	52	64	255	105	140	120	337	169
Original Double Whopper, with Cheese (no mayo)	1 serving	830	52	47	214	88	118	101	282	141
Original Double Whopper, with Cheese (low carb)	1 serving	630	5	47	162	67	89	77	214	107
Original Triple Whopper	1 serving	1130	51	74	291	120	160	137	384	193
Original Triple Whopper (no mayo)	1 serving	980	51	57	253	104	139	119	333	167
Original Triple Whopper, with Cheese	1 serving	1230	52	82	317	131	174	150	418	210
Original Triple Whopper, with Cheese (no mayo)	1 serving	1070	52	65	276	114	152	130	364	182
Original Whopper Jr.	1 serving	370	31	21	95	39	52	45	126	63
Original Whopper Jr. (no mayo)	1 serving	290	31	12	75	31	41	35	99	49
Original Whopper Jr. (low carb)	1 serving	140	1	10	36	15	20	17	48	24
Original Whopper Jr. with Cheese	1 serving	410	32	24	106	44	58	50	139	70
Original Whopper Jr. with Cheese (no mayo)	1 serving	330	31	16	85	35	47	40	112	56
Original Whopper Jr. with Cheese (low carb)	1 serving	190	2	14	49	20	27	23	65	32
Bacon	1 strip	15	0	1	4	2	2	2	5	3
■ **Fire Grilled Burgers**										
Hamburger	1 burger	290	30	12	75	31	41	35	99	49
Cheeseburger	1 burger	330	31	16	85	35	47	40	112	56
Double Hamburger	1 burger	410	30	21	106	44	58	50	139	70
Double Cheeseburger	1 burger	500	31	29	129	53	71	61	170	85
Bacon Cheeseburger	1 burger	370	31	19	95	39	52	45	126	63

FOOD	AMOUNT	CAL	CARBS	FAT	WALK	RUN	BIKE	SWIM	YOGA	DANCE
Bacon Double Cheeseburger	1 burger	540	32	32	139	58	77	66	184	92
Angus Steakburger	1 burger	560	59	22	144	60	79	68	190	95
Low Carb Angus Steakburger	1 burger	260	2	18	67	28	37	32	88	44
Angus Bacon and Cheese	1 burger	710	61	33	183	76	101	86	241	121
Low Carb Angus Bacon and Cheese	1 burger	410	4	29	106	44	58	50	139	70
■ **Chicken, Fish, and Veggie**										
TenderGrill Chicken Sandwich, with honey mustard	1 sandwich	450	53	10	116	48	64	55	153	77
TenderGrill Chicken Sandwich, with mayo	1 sandwich	510	49	19	131	54	72	62	173	87
TenderGrill Chicken Sandwich (no sauce)	1 sandwich	400	49	7	103	43	57	49	136	68
Chicken Whopper Sandwich	1 sandwich	570	48	25	147	61	81	69	194	97
Chicken Whopper Sandwich (no mayo)	1 sandwich	410	48	7	106	44	58	50	139	70
Chicken Whopper Sandwich (low carb)	1 sandwich	160	3	4	41	17	23	19	54	27
Original Chicken Sandwich	1 sandwich	560	52	28	144	60	79	68	190	95
Original Chicken Sandwich (no mayo)	1 sandwich	460	52	17	119	49	65	56	156	78
Tendercrisp Chicken Sandwich	1 sandwich	780	73	43	201	83	111	95	265	133
Spicy Tendercrisp Chicken Sandwich	1 sandwich	720	74	36	186	77	102	88	245	123
Spicy Tendercrisp Chicken Sandwich (no sauce or mayo)	1 sandwich	570	73	21	147	61	81	69	194	97
Chicken Tenders	4 pieces	170	10	9	44	18	24	21	58	29
Chicken Tenders	5 pieces	210	12	12	54	22	30	26	71	36
Chicken Tenders	6 pieces	250	15	14	64	27	35	30	85	43
Chicken Tenders	8 pieces	340	20	19	88	36	48	41	116	58
Chicken Fries	6 pieces	260	18	15	67	28	37	32	88	44
Chicken Fries	9 pieces	390	26	23	101	42	55	47	133	66
BK Fish Filet Sandwich	1 sandwich	630	67	30	162	67	89	77	214	107
BK Fish Filet Sandwich, without tartar sauce	1 sandwich	470	65	13	121	50	67	57	160	80
Spicy BK Fish Filet Sandwich	1 sandwich	620	67	29	160	66	88	75	211	106

FOOD	AMOUNT	CAL	CARBS	FAT	WALK	RUN	BIKE	SWIM	YOGA	DANCE
BK Veggie Burger	1 sandwich	420	46	16	108	45	60	51	143	72
BK Veggie Burger, with Cheese	1 sandwich	470	47	20	121	50	67	57	160	80
BK Veggie Burger (no mayo)	1 sandwich	340	46	8	88	36	48	41	116	58
■ **French Fries**										
Small French Fries	1 order	230	29	11	59	24	33	28	78	39
Medium French Fries	1 order	360	46	18	93	38	51	44	122	61
Large French Fries	1 order	500	63	25	129	53	71	61	170	85
King French Fries	1 order	600	76	30	155	64	85	73	204	102
Small Onion Rings	1 order	180	22	9	46	19	26	22	61	31
Medium Onion Rings	1 order	320	40	16	82	34	45	39	109	55
Large Onion Rings	1 order	480	60	23	124	51	68	58	163	82
King Onion Rings	1 order	550	70	27	142	59	78	67	187	94
Mott's Strawberry Flavored Applesauce	1 serving	90	23	0	23	10	13	11	31	15
■ **Dipping Sauces, Dressings, Jams, and Syrup**										
Barbecue Dipping Sauce	1 oz	40	9	0	10	4	6	5	14	7
Honey Flavored Dipping Sauce	1 oz	90	23	0	23	10	13	11	31	15
Honey Mustard Dipping Sauce	1 oz	90	9	6	23	10	13	11	31	15
Sweet and Sour Dipping Sauce	1 oz	45	10	0	12	5	6	5	15	8
Ranch Dipping Sauce	1 oz	140	1	15	36	15	20	17	48	24
Zesty Onion Ring Dipping Sauce	1 oz	150	3	15	39	16	21	18	51	26
Buffalo Dipping Sauce	1 oz	80	2	8	21	9	11	10	27	14
Ketchup	1 packet	10	3	0	3	1	1	1	3	2
■ **Salad Dressings and Toppings**										
Ken's Border Ranch	2 oz	110	7	8	28	12	16	13	37	19
Ken's Light Italian	2 oz	120	5	11	31	13	17	15	41	20
Ken's Ranch	2 oz	190	2	20	49	20	27	23	65	32
Ken's Creamy Caesar	2 oz	210	4	21	54	22	30	26	71	36
Ken's Honey Mustard	2 oz	270	15	23	70	29	38	33	92	46
Garlic Parmesan Toast	1 serving	70	9	3	18	7	10	9	24	12
■ **Jams and syrup**										
Grape Jam	1 serving	30	7	0	8	3	4	4	10	5
Strawberry Jam	1 serving	30	7	0	8	3	4	4	10	5

FOOD	AMOUNT	CAL	CARBS	FAT	WALK	RUN	BIKE	SWIM	YOGA	DANCE
Breakfast Syrup	1 oz	80	21	0	21	9	11	10	27	14
■ **Salads**										
Side Garden Salad	1 salad	15	3	0	4	2	2	2	5	3
TenderGrill Chicken Garden	1 salad	230	11	8	59	24	33	28	78	39
TenderGrill Chicken Caesar	1 salad	220	7	7	57	23	31	27	75	37
Tendercrisp Chicken Garden	1 salad	410	34	21	106	44	58	50	139	70
Tendercrisp Chicken Caesar	1 salad	400	31	21	103	43	57	49	136	68
■ **Desserts**										
Dutch Apple Pie	1 serving	300	45	13	77	32	43	36	102	51
Hershey's Sundae Pie	1 serving	300	31	18	77	32	43	36	102	51
Croissan'wich										
Croissan'wich with Bacon, Egg and Cheese	1 serving	340	26	20	88	36	48	41	116	58
Croissan'wich with Ham, Egg and Cheese	1 serving	340	26	18	88	36	48	41	116	58
Croissan'wich with Sausage, Egg and Cheese	1 serving	470	26	32	121	50	67	57	160	80
Croissan'wich with Sausage and Cheese	1 serving	370	23	25	95	39	52	45	126	63
Croissan'wich with Egg and Cheese	1 serving	300	26	17	77	32	43	36	102	51
Double Croissan'wich with Sausage, Egg and Cheese	1 serving	680	26	51	175	72	96	83	231	116
Double Croissan'wich with Bacon, Egg and Cheese	1 serving	430	27	27	111	46	61	52	146	73
Double Croissan'wich with Ham, Egg and Cheese	1 serving	420	27	23	108	45	60	51	143	72
Double Croissan'wich with Sausage, Bacon, Egg and Cheese	1 serving	560	27	39	144	60	79	68	190	95
Double Croissan'wich with Ham, Bacon, Egg and Cheese	1 serving	430	27	25	111	46	61	52	146	73
Double Croissan'wich with Ham, Sausage, Egg and Cheese	1 serving	550	27	37	142	59	78	67	187	94
■ **Other Breakfast Items**										
French Toast Sticks	5 sticks	390	46	20	101	42	55	47	133	66
Small Hash Brown Rounds	1 serving	230	23	15	59	24	33	28	78	39
Medium Hash Brown Rounds	1 serving	390	38	25	101	42	55	47	133	66

FOOD	AMOUNT	CAL	CARBS	FAT	WALK	RUN	BIKE	SWIM	YOGA	DANCE
■ **Shakes**										
Vanilla	Small	400	57	15	103	43	57	49	136	68
Vanilla	Medium	560	79	21	144	60	79	68	190	95
Vanilla	Large	820	117	30	211	87	116	100	279	140
Vanilla	King	1070	151	39	276	114	152	130	364	182
Chocolate	Small	470	75	14	121	50	67	57	160	80
Chocolate	Medium	690	114	20	178	73	98	84	235	118
Chocolate	Large	950	151	29	245	101	135	116	323	162
Chocolate	King	1260	204	38	325	134	179	153	429	215
Strawberry	Small	460	73	14	119	49	65	56	156	78
Strawberry	Medium	660	111	19	170	70	94	80	224	112
Strawberry	Large	930	148	28	240	99	132	113	316	158
Strawberry	King	1230	200	36	317	131	174	150	418	210
Cousins Subs										
■ **7 ½" Subs**										
BLT	1 7-½" sub	591	47	38	152	63	84	72	201	101
Cheese Steak	1 7-½" sub	503	49	19	130	54	71	61	171	86
Chicken Breast	1 7-½" sub	569	50	27	147	61	81	69	194	97
Chicken Cheddar Deluxe	1 7-½" sub	669	51	39	172	71	95	81	228	114
Club	1 7-½" sub	657	51	35	169	70	93	80	223	112
Double Cheese Steak	1 7-½" sub	747	49	36	193	80	106	91	254	127
Garden Veggie	1 7-½" sub	390	51	12	101	42	55	47	133	66
Gyro	1 7-½" sub	710	61	41	183	76	101	86	241	121
Ham and Provolone	1 7-½" sub	612	50	34	158	65	87	74	208	104
Hot Veggie	1 7-½" sub	472	55	17	122	50	67	57	161	80
Italian Special	1 7-½" sub	817	50	51	211	87	116	99	278	139
Meatball and Provolone	1 7-½" sub	723	54	38	186	77	103	88	246	123

FOOD	AMOUNT	CAL	CARBS	FAT	WALK	RUN	BIKE	SWIM	YOGA	DANCE
Pepperoni Melt	1 7-½" sub	730	50	45	188	78	104	89	248	124
Philly Cheese Steak	1 7-½" sub	531	55	19	137	57	75	65	181	90
Pizza Sub	1 7-½" sub	709	55	39	183	76	101	86	241	121
Roast Beef	1 7-½" sub	607	50	30	156	65	86	74	206	103
Seafood with Crab	1 7-½" sub	642	60	38	165	68	91	78	218	109
Spicy Chicken Sedona	1 7-½" sub	530	54	18	137	56	75	64	180	90
Three Cheese	1 7-½" sub	685	50	44	177	73	97	83	233	117
Tuna	1 7-½" sub	666	49	40	172	71	94	81	227	113
Turkey Breast	1 7-½" sub	537	50	28	138	57	76	65	183	91
■ Better Bunch										
Mini Chicken Breast	1 4" sub	185	25	1	48	20	26	23	63	32
Mini Club	1 4" sub	193	26	3	50	21	27	23	66	33
Mini Garden Veggie	1 4" sub	136	26	1	35	14	19	17	46	23
Mini Ham	1 4" sub	178	26	2	46	19	25	22	61	30
Mini Hot Veggie	1 4" sub	144	27	1	37	15	20	18	49	25
Mini Roast Beef	1 4" sub	205	25	3	53	22	29	25	70	35
Mini Turkey Breast	1 4" sub	177	26	2	46	19	25	22	60	30
Chicken Breast	1 7-½" sub	366	50	2	94	39	52	45	124	62
Club	1 7-½" sub	381	51	5	98	41	54	46	130	65
Garden Veggie	1 7-½" sub	266	50	2	69	28	38	32	90	45
Ham	1 7-½" sub	336	50	4	87	36	48	41	114	57
Hot Veggie	1 7-½" sub	287	55	2	74	31	41	35	98	49
Roast Beef	1 7-½" sub	405	50	6	104	43	57	49	138	69
Turkey Breast	1 7-½" sub	335	50	3	86	36	48	41	114	57

FOOD	AMOUNT	CAL	CARBS	FAT	WALK	RUN	BIKE	SWIM	YOGA	DANCE
■ Mini Subs										
Mini BLT	1 4″ sub	298	24	19	77	32	42	36	101	51
Mini Chicken Breast	1 4″ sub	287	25	13	74	31	41	35	98	49
Mini Chicken Cheddar Deluxe	1 4″ sub	329	26	19	85	35	47	40	112	56
Mini Club	1 4″ sub	337	27	18	87	36	48	41	115	57
Mini Garden Veggie	1 4″ sub	216	26	7	56	23	31	26	73	37
Mini Ham and Provolone	1 4″ sub	316	26	18	81	34	45	38	107	54
Mini Hot Veggie	1 4″ sub	254	28	10	65	27	36	31	86	43
Mini Italian Special	1 4″ sub	403	25	25	104	43	57	49	137	69
Mini Meatball and Provolone	1 4″ sub	361	27	19	93	38	51	44	123	61
Mini Pepperoni Melt	1 4″ sub	348	26	21	90	37	49	42	118	59
Mini Pizza Sub	1 4″ sub	336	28	18	87	36	48	41	114	57
Mini Roast Beef	1 4″ sub	306	25	15	79	33	43	37	104	52
Mini Seafood with Crab	1 4″ sub	323	31	19	83	34	46	39	110	55
Mini Three Cheese	1 4″ sub	363	25	23	94	39	51	44	123	62
Mini Tuna	1 4″ sub	335	25	20	86	36	48	41	114	57
Mini Turkey Breast	1 4″ sub	279	26	14	72	30	40	34	95	48
■ Specials										
Balsamic Garden Turkey	1 7-½″ sub	501	50	18	129	53	71	61	170	85
Chicken Salad	1 7-½″ sub	569	61	26	147	61	81	69	194	97
Sunny Hunny Ham	1 7-½″ sub	530	53	20	137	56	75	64	180	90
■ Breads										
Mini Garlic Herb	1 4″ bread	120	22	1	31	13	17	15	41	20
Mini Italian	1 4″ bread	120	22	1	31	13	17	15	41	20
Mini Parmesan Asiago	1 4″ bread	124	22	1	32	13	18	15	42	21
Mini Wheat	1 4″ bread	120	22	2	31	13	17	15	41	20
Italian	1 7-½″ sub	240	44	2	62	26	34	29	82	41
Parmesan Asiago	1 7-½″ sub	248	45	2	64	26	35	30	84	42
Wheat	1 7-½″ sub	240	44	3	62	26	34	29	82	41

FOOD	AMOUNT	CAL	CARBS	FAT	WALK	RUN	BIKE	SWIM	YOGA	DANCE
Low Carb Wraps	1 serving	188	19	8	48	20	27	23	64	32
■ **Salads**										
Chef Salad	1 serving	332	26	14	86	35	47	40	113	57
Chicken Sedona Salad	1 serving	232	16	5	60	25	33	28	79	40
Garden Salad	1 serving	241	24	11	62	26	34	29	82	41
Garden Salad with Chicken Breast	1 serving	355	26	12	91	38	50	43	121	60
Italian Salad	1 serving	409	25	24	105	44	58	50	139	70
Seafood Salad	1 serving	320	35	11	82	34	45	39	109	55
Side Salad	1 serving	135	14	6	35	14	19	16	46	23
Tuna Salad	1 serving	629	24	46	162	67	89	77	214	107
■ **Soups**										
Beef Steak and Noodle Soup	Large	165	19	4	43	18	23	20	56	28
Beef Steak and Noodle Soup	Regular	105	12	3	27	11	15	13	36	18
Cheddar Cheese Cauliflower Soup	Large	179	21	8	46	19	25	22	61	30
Cheddar Cheese Cauliflower Soup	Regular	114	13	5	29	12	16	14	39	19
Cheddar Cheese Soup	Large	316	29	18	81	34	45	38	107	54
Cheddar Cheese Soup	Regular	201	18	11	52	21	29	24	68	34
Chicken Dumpling Soup	Large	234	26	7	60	25	33	28	80	40
Chicken Dumpling Soup	Regular	149	17	4	38	16	21	18	51	25
Chicken Noodle Soup	Large	179	25	6	46	19	25	22	61	30
Chicken Noodle Soup	Regular	114	16	4	29	12	16	14	39	19
Chicken with Rice Soup	Large	344	21	14	89	37	49	42	117	59
Chicken with Rice Soup	Regular	219	13	9	56	23	31	27	74	37
Chili	Large	344	41	12	89	37	49	42	117	59
Chili	Regular	219	26	8	56	23	31	27	74	37
Cream of Broccoli with Cheese	Large	261	21	11	67	28	37	32	89	44
Cream of Broccoli with Cheese	Regular	166	13	7	43	18	24	20	56	28
Cream of Mushroom	Large	303	21	17	78	32	43	37	103	52
Cream of Mushroom	Regular	193	13	11	50	21	27	23	66	33
Cream of Potato Soup	Large	261	33	12	67	28	37	32	89	44
Cream of Potato Soup	Regular	166	21	8	43	18	24	20	56	28
Eight Bean Soup with Ham	Large	165	29	1	43	18	23	20	56	28
Eight Bean Soup with Ham	Regular	105	18	1	27	11	15	13	36	18

FOOD	AMOUNT	CAL	CARBS	FAT	WALK	RUN	BIKE	SWIM	YOGA	DANCE
Fiesta Tortilla Soup with Chicken	Large	179	18	8	46	19	25	22	61	30
Fiesta Tortilla Soup with Chicken	Regular	114	11	5	29	12	16	14	39	19
New England Clam Chowder	Large	234	39	4	60	25	33	28	80	40
New England Clam Chowder	Regular	149	25	3	38	16	21	18	51	25
Tomato Basil with Raviolini	Large	151	30	1	39	16	21	18	51	26
Tomato Basil with Raviolini	Regular	96	19	1	25	10	14	12	33	16
Vegetable Beef	Large	110	18	3	28	12	16	13	37	19
Vegetable Beef	Regular	70	11	2	18	7	10	9	24	12

Denny's

■ Breakfast

FOOD	AMOUNT	CAL	CARBS	FAT	WALK	RUN	BIKE	SWIM	YOGA	DANCE
Meat Lover's Breakfast	1 serving	1250	109	68	322	133	177	152	425	213
Original Grand Slam	1 serving	770	56	44	198	82	109	94	262	131
All-American Slam with hash browns	1 serving	970	21	76	250	103	138	118	330	165
French Slam	2 pieces	1180	74	75	304	126	167	144	401	201
Grand Slam Slugger with hash browns	1 serving	1050	96	55	271	112	149	128	357	179
Meat Lover's Scramble	1 serving	1310	104	73	338	140	186	159	446	223
Heartland Scramble	1 serving	1210	118	61	312	129	172	147	412	206
Denver Scramble with hash browns	1 serving	1080	106	49	278	115	153	131	367	184
Meat Lover's Bowl	1 serving	1540	121	94	397	164	218	187	524	262
Country Sausage Bowl	1 serving	1680	127	108	433	179	238	204	571	286
Ham and Mushroom Bowl	1 serving	1530	121	96	394	163	217	186	520	261
Lumberjack Slam with hash browns	1 serving	1170	109	57	302	125	166	142	398	199
Ultimate Omelette	1 serving	600	7	49	155	64	85	73	204	102
Veggie-Cheese Omelette	1 serving	480	10	37	124	51	68	58	163	82
Veggie-Cheese Omelette with Egg Beaters	1 serving	346	11	22	89	37	49	42	118	59
Ham and Cheddar Omelette	1 serving	595	5	47	153	63	84	72	202	101
Ham and Cheddar Omelette with Egg Beaters	1 serving	468	5	32	121	50	66	57	159	80
Country Fried Steak and Eggs	1 serving	464	13	34	120	49	66	56	158	79
T-Bone Steak and Eggs	1 serving	991	1	77	255	106	141	121	337	169
Steakhouse Strip and Eggs	1 serving	560	3	37	144	60	79	68	190	95

FOOD	AMOUNT	CAL	CARBS	FAT	WALK	RUN	BIKE	SWIM	YOGA	DANCE
Moons Over My Hammy	1 serving	841	42	51	217	90	119	102	286	143
Belgian Waffle Platter	1 waffle	619	28	45	160	66	88	75	211	105
Fabulous French Toast Platter	3 pieces	1261	110	79	325	134	179	153	429	215
Cherry Fruit Filled Pancakes	1 serving	1070	103	55	276	114	152	130	364	182
Blueberry Fruit Filled Pancakes	1 serving	1076	103	55	277	115	153	131	366	183
Apple Cinnamon Fruit Filled Pancakes	1 serving	1080	106	56	278	115	153	131	367	184
Buttermilk Pancake Platter	3 pieces	660	83	25	170	70	94	80	224	112
Buttermilk Pancake	3 pieces	420	82	5	108	45	60	51	143	72
Country-Fried Potatoes	1 serving	394	23	20	102	42	56	48	134	67
Hashed Browns	1 serving	197	20	12	51	21	28	24	67	34
Hashed Browns with Cheddar Cheese	1 serving	280	21	19	72	30	40	34	95	48
Hashed Browns with Onions, Cheese, Gravy	1 serving	493	54	25	127	53	70	60	168	84
Grits	1 serving	80	18	0	21	9	11	10	27	14
One Egg	1 serving	120	1	10	31	13	17	15	41	20
Two Eggs and More Breakfast	1 serving	678	20	55	175	72	96	82	231	116
Egg Beaters Egg Substitute	1 serving	56	2	0	14	6	8	7	19	10
Ham, Grilled Slice, Homey Smoked	1 serving	85	6	3	22	9	12	10	29	14
Bacon	4 strips	162	1	18	42	17	23	20	55	28
Sausage	4 links	354	0	32	91	38	50	43	120	60
Sausage Patties	2 patties	295	1	28	76	31	42	36	100	50
Toast (dry)	1 slice	90	17	1	23	10	13	11	31	15
English Muffin (dry)	1 serving	150	27	2	39	16	21	18	51	26
Bagel (dry)	1 bagel	310	65	1	80	33	44	38	105	53
Biscuit	1 serving	192	22	10	49	20	27	23	65	33
Quaker Oatmeal	1 serving	100	18	2	26	11	14	12	34	17
Kellogg's Dry Cereal	1 serving	100	23	0	26	11	14	12	34	17
Musselman's Applesauce	1 serving	60	15	0	15	6	9	7	20	10
Banana	1 whole	110	29	0	28	12	16	13	37	19
Grapefruit	½ fruit	60	16	0	15	6	9	7	20	10
Grapes	1 serving	55	15	1	14	6	8	7	19	9
Maple-Flavored Syrup	3 tbsp	143	36	0	37	15	20	17	49	24
Sugar-Free Maple-Flavored Syrup	3 tbsp	23	9	0	6	2	3	3	8	4

FOOD	AMOUNT	CAL	CARBS	FAT	WALK	RUN	BIKE	SWIM	YOGA	DANCE
Whipped Margarine	1 serving	87	0	10	22	9	12	11	30	15
Cream Cheese	1 serving	100	1	10	26	11	14	12	34	17
Whipped Cream	1 dollop	23	2	2	6	2	3	3	8	4
Blueberry Topping	3 oz	106	26	0	27	11	15	13	36	18
Cinnamon Apple Filling	1 serving	90	19	2	23	10	13	11	31	15
Cherry Topping	3 oz	86	21	0	22	9	12	10	29	15
■ Carb-Watch Items										
Two Egg & Three Meat Breakfast	1 serving	653	10	44	168	70	93	79	222	111
Ultimate Carb-Watch Omelette	1 serving	662	11	53	171	71	94	81	225	113
Carb-Watch Ham & Cheddar Omelette	1 serving	610	8	47	157	65	87	74	207	104
Carb-Watch Mushroom Swiss Burger	1 serving	625	13	45	161	67	89	76	213	106
Carb-Watch Bacon-Cheddar Burger	1 serving	514	13	36	132	55	73	63	175	88
Carb-Watch T-Bone	1 serving	791	8	57	204	84	112	96	269	135
Carb-Watch Steakhouse Strip	1 serving	304	13	8	78	32	43	37	103	52
Carb-Watch Grilled Chicken Dinner	1 serving	314	8	8	81	33	45	38	107	53
Carb-Watch Grilled Tilapia	1 serving	300	11	11	77	32	43	36	102	51
■ Desserts										
Apple Pie	1 serving	470	68	21	121	50	67	57	160	80
Coconut Cream Pie	1 serving	701	100	32	181	75	99	85	238	119
French Silk Pie	1 serving	737	58	56	190	78	105	90	251	126
Apple Crisp a la Mode	1 serving	723	133	21	186	77	103	88	246	123
Chocolate Peanut Butter Pie	1 serving	653	64	39	168	70	93	79	222	111
Cheesecake	1 serving	580	51	38	149	62	82	71	197	99
Carrot Cake	1 serving	799	99	45	206	85	113	97	272	136
Hershey's Chocolate Cake	1 serving	631	79	33	163	67	90	77	215	107
Hot Fudge Brownie a la Mode	1 serving	997	147	42	257	106	141	121	339	170
Hot Fudge Brownie (kids)	1 serving	344	49	16	89	37	49	42	117	59
Banana Split	1 serving	894	121	43	230	95	127	109	304	152
Double Scoop/Sundae	1 serving	375	29	27	97	40	53	46	128	64
Single Scoop/Sundae (Delicious Dip)	1 serving	188	14	14	48	20	27	23	64	32
Milkshake (vanilla/chocolate)	1 serving	560	76	26	144	60	79	68	190	95

FOOD	AMOUNT	CAL	CARBS	FAT	WALK	RUN	BIKE	SWIM	YOGA	DANCE
Malted Milkshake (vanilla/chocolate)	1 serving	583	82	26	150	62	83	71	198	99
Floats (Root Beer or Cola)	1 serving	280	47	10	72	30	40	34	95	48
Oreo Blender Blaster	1 serving	895	112	46	231	95	127	109	304	152
Oreo Blender Blaster (kids)	1 serving	580	72	29	149	62	82	71	197	99

■ Toppings

FOOD	AMOUNT	CAL	CARBS	FAT	WALK	RUN	BIKE	SWIM	YOGA	DANCE
Chocolate Topping	2 oz	133	34	1	34	14	19	16	45	23
Fudge Topping	2 oz	201	30	10	52	21	29	24	68	34

■ Fit Fare

FOOD	AMOUNT	CAL	CARBS	FAT	WALK	RUN	BIKE	SWIM	YOGA	DANCE
Slim Slam (without topping)	1 serving	490	63	11	126	52	70	60	167	83
Skinny Moons	1 serving	560	73	12	144	60	79	68	190	95
Veggie EB Veggie Omelette with English Muffin	1 serving	330	37	8	85	35	47	40	112	56
Boca Burger with Small Fruit Bowl	1 serving	508	78	11	131	54	72	62	173	87
Turkey Breast Salad (no dressing)	1 serving	230	13	10	59	24	33	28	78	39
Grilled Chicken Breast Salad	1 serving	310	13	13	80	33	44	38	105	53
Side Garden Salad (no dressing)	1 serving	113	6	7	29	12	16	14	38	19
Vegetable Beef Soup	1 serving	79	11	1	20	8	11	10	27	13
Chicken Noodle	1 serving	110	16	6	28	12	16	13	37	19
Grilled Chicken Breast Dinner	1 serving	190	12	3	49	20	27	23	65	32
Tilapia, Rice, Green Beans and Tomato Slices	1 serving	410	44	11	106	44	58	50	139	70
Baked Potato (plain with skin)	1 serving	220	51	0	57	23	31	27	75	37
Mashed Potatoes	1 serving	168	23	7	43	18	24	20	57	29
Corn	1 serving	110	23	2	28	12	16	13	37	19
Green Beans	1 serving	40	8	1	10	4	6	5	14	7

■ Sandwiches/Salads/Soups

FOOD	AMOUNT	CAL	CARBS	FAT	WALK	RUN	BIKE	SWIM	YOGA	DANCE
Club Sandwich	1 serving	602	45	38	155	64	85	73	205	103
Super Bird Sandwich	1 serving	479	32	29	123	51	68	58	163	82
Grilled Chicken Sandwich (no dressing)	1 serving	476	56	14	123	51	68	58	162	81
Bacon, Lettuce, & Tomato	1 serving	610	50	38	157	65	87	74	207	104
BBQ Chicken Sandwich	1 serving	1089	86	62	281	116	154	132	370	186
Classic Burger	1 serving	694	56	35	179	74	98	84	236	118
Classic Burger with Cheese	1 serving	852	57	48	220	91	121	104	290	145

FOOD	AMOUNT	CAL	CARBS	FAT	WALK	RUN	BIKE	SWIM	YOGA	DANCE
Chicken Ranch Melt	1 serving	838	57	47	216	89	119	102	285	143
Philly Melt	1 serving	874	58	50	225	93	124	106	297	149
Italian Chicken Melt	1 serving	1134	68	62	292	121	161	138	386	193
Boca Burger	1 serving	452	64	11	116	48	64	55	154	77
Mushroom Swiss Burger	1 serving	880	63	49	227	94	125	107	299	150
Spicy Buffalo Chicken Melt	1 serving	880	70	47	227	94	125	107	299	150
Vegetable Beef	1 cup	79	11	1	20	8	11	10	27	13
Chicken Noodle	1 cup	110	16	6	28	12	16	13	37	19
Broccoli & Cheddar	1 cup	190	4	14	49	20	27	23	65	32
Fish Sandwich	1 serving	589	30	30	152	63	84	72	200	100
Clam Chowder	1 serving	624	55	42	161	66	89	76	212	106
Taco Salad	1 serving	505	57	22	130	54	72	61	172	86
Chef's Salad	1 serving	365	14	16	94	39	52	44	124	62
Grilled Chicken Breast Salad	1 serving	259	10	11	67	28	37	32	88	44
Turkey Breast Salad (no dressing)	1 serving	248	12	8	64	26	35	30	84	42
Fried Chicken Strip Salad	1 serving	438	26	26	113	47	62	53	149	75
Coleslaw	1 serving	274	14	24	71	29	39	33	93	47
Side Caesar (with dressing)	1 serving	362	20	26	93	39	51	44	123	62
Side Garden Salad (no dressing)	1 serving	113	6	7	29	12	16	14	38	19
French Fries (unsalted)	1 serving	423	57	20	109	45	60	51	144	72
Seasoned Fries	1 serving	261	35	12	67	28	37	32	89	44
Onion Rings	1 serving	381	38	23	98	41	54	46	130	65
■ **Seniors**										
Senior Omelette	1 serving	429	8	20	111	46	61	52	146	73
Senior Scram, Egg & Cheddar	1 serving	735	33	51	189	78	104	89	250	125
Senior Starter	1 serving	544	23	42	140	58	77	66	185	93
Senior French Toast Slam	1 serving	591	37	43	152	63	84	72	201	101
Senior Belgian Waffle Slam	1 serving	700	29	51	180	75	99	85	238	119
Senior Biscuits & Gravy	1 serving	791	40	55	204	84	112	96	269	135
Senior Grilled Tilapia	1 serving	248	0	10	64	26	35	30	84	42
Senior Lemon Pepper Tilapia	1 serving	509	6	41	131	54	72	62	173	87
Senior Fried Shrimp Dinner	1 serving	149	14	6	38	16	21	18	51	25
Senior Turkey & Stuffing	1 serving	360	57	9	93	38	51	44	122	61
Senior Grilled Chicken Breast	1 serving	200	15	5	52	21	28	24	68	34

FOOD	AMOUNT	CAL	CARBS	FAT	WALK	RUN	BIKE	SWIM	YOGA	DANCE
Senior Country Fried Steak	1 serving	341	18	23	88	36	48	41	116	58
Senior Chicken Strip Dinner	1 serving	285	31	10	73	30	40	35	97	49
Senior Club	1 serving	540	34	31	139	58	77	66	184	92
Senior Bacon Cheddar Burger	1 serving	433	27	25	112	46	61	53	147	74
Grilled Cheese Sandwich	1 serving	510	40	30	131	54	72	62	173	87
Senior Fish and Chips	1 serving	756	64	47	195	81	107	92	257	129
■ **Kid's D-Zone**										
Smiley Alien Pancakes (with meat)	1 serving	463	63	22	119	49	66	56	157	79
Smiley Alien Pancakes (without meat)	1 serving	344	62	9	89	37	49	42	117	59
Junior Grand Slam	1 serving	397	33	25	102	42	56	48	135	68
French-toastix	1 serving	627	71	71	162	67	89	76	213	107
Jr. Dippers with Marinara & Fries	1 serving	860	80	43	222	92	122	105	293	147
Jr. Dippers with Applesauce & Marinara	1 serving	566	50	27	146	60	80	69	193	96
Burgerlicious	1 serving	296	24	17	76	32	42	36	101	50
Cosmic Cheeseburger	1 serving	341	24	20	88	36	48	41	116	58
Flying Saucer Pizza	1 serving	331	48	14	85	35	47	40	113	56
Galactic Grilled Cheese	1 serving	334	28	20	86	36	47	41	114	57
Moons and Stars Chicken Nuggets	1 serving	190	9	13	49	20	27	23	65	32
Macaroni & Cheese	1 serving	353	48	13	91	38	50	43	120	60
Thanksgiving Jr.	1 serving	290	49	14	75	31	41	35	99	49
Thanksgiving Jr. with Red Grapes	1 serving	350	64	14	90	37	50	43	119	60
Moon Crater Mashed with Brown Gravy	1 serving	145	20	6	37	15	21	18	49	25
Cucumber Craverz	1 serving	164	3	16	42	17	23	20	56	28
Astronaut Applesauce	1 serving	84	19	0	22	9	12	10	29	14
Goldfish Galaxy	1 serving	284	0	3	73	30	40	35	97	48
Deep-Sea Salad with Ranch	1 serving	240	13	20	62	26	34	29	82	41
Anti-Gravity Grapes	1 serving	60	15	0	15	6	9	7	20	10
Neutron Brownie	1 serving	344	49	16	89	37	49	42	117	59
Delicious Dip Sundae	1 serving	413	59	19	106	44	59	50	140	70
■ **Appetizers and Entrees**										
Sampler	1 serving	1405	124	80	362	150	199	171	478	239
Buffalo Wings	9 wings	974	11	72	251	104	138	118	331	166

FOOD	AMOUNT	CAL	CARBS	FAT	WALK	RUN	BIKE	SWIM	YOGA	DANCE
Mozzarella Sticks	8 sticks	710	49	41	183	76	101	86	241	121
Smothered Cheese Fries	1 serving	767	69	48	198	82	109	93	261	131
Buffalo Chicken Strips	5 strips	734	43	42	189	78	104	89	250	125
Chicken Strips	5 strips	720	56	33	186	77	102	88	245	123
Nacho	1 serving	1278	117	64	329	136	181	155	435	218
Mini Burgers with Onion Rings	1 serving	2044	179	122	527	218	290	249	695	348
T-Bone Steak Dinner	1 serving	860	0	65	222	92	122	105	293	147
Steakhouse Strip Dinner	1 serving	410	3	27	106	44	58	50	139	70
Country-Fried Steak	1 serving	644	30	46	166	69	91	78	219	110
Steakhouse Strip & Shrimp	1 serving	517	7	33	133	55	73	63	176	88
Blackened Steakhouse Strip	1 serving	775	7	66	200	83	110	94	264	132
Fried Shrimp Dinner	1 serving	258	19	11	66	27	37	31	88	44
Roast Turkey and Stuffing (including gravy)	1 serving	435	62	10	112	46	62	53	148	74
Grilled Tilapia Dinner	1 serving	470	33	18	121	50	67	57	160	80
Lemon Pepper Tilapia	1 serving	773	38	47	199	82	110	94	263	132
Grilled Chicken Dinner	1 serving	200	15	5	52	21	28	24	68	34
Hickory Grilled Chicken	1 serving	766	18	48	197	82	109	93	261	130
Fish & Chips	1 serving	958	83	54	247	102	136	117	326	163
Baked Potato, plain with skin	1 serving	220	51	0	57	23	31	27	75	37
Mashed Potatoes	1 serving	168	23	7	43	18	24	20	57	29
Vegetable Rice Pilaf	1 serving	173	33	3	45	18	25	21	59	29
Bread Stuffing (plain)	1 serving	100	19	1	26	11	14	12	34	17
Dunkin' Donuts										
■ Sandwiches										
Steak and Cheddar Egg Sandwich	1 sandwich	600	41	40	155	64	85	73	204	102
Sausage Egg Cheese Croissant Sandwich	1 sandwich	690	40	51	178	73	98	84	235	118
Bacon Egg Cheese Bagel Sandwich	1 sandwich	540	69	18	139	58	77	66	184	92
Bacon Egg Cheese Croissant Sandwich	1 sandwich	520	40	33	134	55	74	63	177	89
Bacon Egg Cheese English Muffin Sandwich	1 sandwich	360	36	16	93	38	51	44	122	61
Egg Cheese Bagel Sandwich	1 sandwich	470	65	15	121	50	67	57	160	80

FOOD	AMOUNT	CAL	CARBS	FAT	WALK	RUN	BIKE	SWIM	YOGA	DANCE
Egg Cheese Biscuit Sandwich	1 sandwich	410	32	25	106	44	58	50	139	70
Egg Cheese Croissant Sandwich	1 sandwich	480	40	31	124	51	68	58	163	82
Egg Cheese English Muffin Sandwich	1 sandwich	280	34	9	72	30	40	34	95	48
Ham Egg Cheese Bagel Sandwich	1 sandwich	510	65	16	131	54	72	62	173	87
Ham Egg Cheese Croissant Sandwich	1 sandwich	520	40	32	134	55	74	63	177	89
Ham Egg Cheese English Muffin Sandwich	1 sandwich	310	34	10	80	33	44	38	105	53
Sausage Egg Cheese Bagel Sandwich	1 sandwich	660	63	35	170	70	94	80	224	112
Sausage Egg Cheese English Muffin Sandwich	1 sandwich	530	37	32	137	56	75	64	180	90
Sausage Egg Cheese Biscuit Sandwich	1 sandwich	610	32	43	157	65	87	74	207	104
Supreme Omelet on a Croissant	1 sandwich	590	42	38	152	63	84	72	201	101
Southwestern Chicken Panini	1 panini	420	57	10	108	45	60	51	143	72
Meatball Panini	1 panini	480	56	19	124	51	68	58	163	82
Steak Panini	1 panini	450	56	12	116	48	64	55	153	77

Einstein Bros.

■ Breakfast Menu

FOOD	AMOUNT	CAL	CARBS	FAT	WALK	RUN	BIKE	SWIM	YOGA	DANCE
Yogurt Parfait	1 cup	220	44	1	57	23	31	27	75	37
Spinach and Bacon Panini	1 sandwich	930	72	49	240	99	132	113	316	158
Lox and Bagel	1 sandwich	660	79	27	170	70	94	80	224	112

■ Frittata Sandwiches

FOOD	AMOUNT	CAL	CARBS	FAT	WALK	RUN	BIKE	SWIM	YOGA	DANCE
Plain with Cheddar	1 sandwich	590	74	20	152	63	84	72	201	101
Smoked Bacon and Cheddar	1 sandwich	680	75	26	175	72	96	83	231	116
Black Forest Ham and Swiss	1 sandwich	660	76	21	170	70	94	80	224	112
Turkey Sausage and Cheddar	1 sandwich	660	74	23	170	70	94	80	224	112
Santa Fe	1 sandwich	720	78	28	186	77	102	88	245	123

FOOD	AMOUNT	CAL	CARBS	FAT	WALK	RUN	BIKE	SWIM	YOGA	DANCE
■ Hot Grilled Panini										
Italian Chicken Panini	1 sandwich	690	68	27	178	73	98	84	235	118
Ham and Cheese	1 sandwich	620	68	22	160	66	88	75	211	106
Cali Club	1 sandwich	750	68	34	193	80	106	91	255	128
■ Sandwiches										
Roasted Turkey on Artisan Wheat	1 sandwich	590	50	28	152	63	84	72	201	101
Black Forest Ham on Challah Roll	1 sandwich	570	61	23	147	61	81	69	194	97
Albacore Tuna Salad on Artisan Wheat	1 sandwich	400	49	9	103	43	57	49	136	68
Turkey on Asiago Bagel	1 sandwich	600	81	18	155	64	85	73	204	102
Veg Out on Sesame Bagel	1 sandwich	500	82	13	129	53	71	61	170	85
Einstein Club on Grilled Rustic White	1 sandwich	670	54	29	173	71	95	82	228	114
Club Mex on Challah	1 sandwich	730	60	38	188	78	104	89	248	124
Cobbie on Challah	1 sandwich	620	59	29	160	66	88	75	211	106
Hummus and Feta on Ciabatta	1 sandwich	450	77	10	116	48	64	55	153	77
■ Salads										
Chicken Caesar	1 salad	740	25	54	191	79	105	90	252	126
Bros Bistro	1 salad	810	37	69	209	86	115	99	276	138
Chicken Chipotle	1 salad	630	38	40	162	67	89	77	214	107
■ Soups										
Broccoli Sharp Cheddar	1 bowl	540	31	35	139	58	77	66	184	92
Chicken Noodle	1 bowl	510	39	21	131	54	72	62	173	87
Chicken and Wild Rice	1 bowl	440	67	9	113	47	62	54	150	75
Low Fat Vegetarian Minestrone	1 bowl	360	62	10	93	38	51	44	122	61
New England Clam Chowder	1 bowl	370	25	25	95	39	52	45	126	63
Turkey Chili	1 bowl	330	34	11	85	35	47	40	112	56
Caribbean Crab Chowder	1 bowl	520	30	38	134	55	74	63	177	89

FOOD	AMOUNT	CAL	CARBS	FAT	WALK	RUN	BIKE	SWIM	YOGA	DANCE
■ **Desserts**										
Apple Cinnamon Coffee Cake	1 serving	660	106	25	170	70	94	80	224	112
Banana Nut Muffin	1 muffin	640	81	32	165	68	91	78	218	109
Blueberry Coffee Cake	1 serving	610	97	25	157	65	87	74	207	104
Blueberry Muffin	1 muffin	540	80	22	139	58	77	66	184	92
Chocolate Chip Coffee Cake	1 serving	730	108	31	188	78	104	89	248	124
Cinnamon Twist	1 twist	370	41	21	95	39	52	45	126	63
Cinnamon Walnut Strudel	1 serving	550	63	31	142	59	78	67	187	94
Heavenly Chocolate Chip Cookie	1 cookie	389	52	19	100	41	55	47	132	66
Honey Roasted Peanut Butter Cookie	1 cookie	389	43	20	100	41	55	47	132	66
Lemon Pound Cake	1 slice	510	62	28	131	54	72	62	173	87
Marble Pound Cake	1 slice	370	47	20	95	39	52	45	126	63
Oatmeal Raisin Cookie	1 cookie	319	54	10	82	34	45	39	109	54
■ **Beverages**										
SpontaneiTEA	1 drink	50	12	0	13	5	7	6	17	9
Mel's Cool Cap	1 large	290	32	16	75	31	41	35	99	49
Blackberry Lemonade	1 drink	310	76	0	80	33	44	38	105	53
Jimmy Dean Rollergrill Program										
8:1 All Meat Hot Dog	1 serving	160	2	16	41	17	23	19	54	27
Cheddarwurst	1 serving	300	3	27	77	32	43	36	102	51
Bratwurst	1 serving	270	1	23	70	29	38	33	92	46
Pepperjack Cheese Smoked Sausage	1 serving	290	4	26	75	31	41	35	99	49
Pork Sausage	1 serving	370	1	36	95	39	52	45	126	63
Black Pepper Smoked Sausage	1 serving	250	1	23	64	27	35	30	85	43
5:1 All Meat Hot Dog	1 serving	280	2	25	72	30	40	34	95	48
Jalapeño Mesquite	1 serving	290	5	26	75	31	41	35	99	49
Mesquite Smoked	1 serving	290	2	25	75	31	41	35	99	49
Polish Smoked	1 serving	290	2	26	75	31	41	35	99	49
4:1 All Beef Hot Dog	1 serving	360	4	32	93	38	51	44	122	61
5:1 All Beef Hot Dog	1 serving	290	5	26	75	31	41	35	99	49
■ **Desserts**										
Cream Cheese Danish	1 danish	450	63	19	116	48	64	55	153	77
Cherry Danish	1 danish	371	69	8	96	40	53	45	126	63

FOOD	AMOUNT	CAL	CARBS	FAT	WALK	RUN	BIKE	SWIM	YOGA	DANCE
Cinnamon Roll	1 roll	453	84	10	117	48	64	55	154	77
Bear Claw	1 claw	412	76	9	106	44	58	50	140	70
Glazed Old Fashioned Donut	1 donut	484	62	22	125	52	69	59	165	82
Concha Sweet Bread	1 serving	480	67	18	124	51	68	58	163	82
Raspberry Cheese Turnover	1 turnover	570	63	28	147	61	81	69	194	97
Apple Turnover	1 turnover	560	63	26	144	60	79	68	190	95
Cream Cheese Turnover	1 turnover	575	63	29	148	61	82	70	196	98
Blueberry Cheese Turnover	1 turnover	575	63	28	148	61	82	70	196	98
Almond Bear Claw	1 claw	575	63	28	148	61	82	70	196	98
Blueberry Muffin	1 muffin	555	72	28	143	59	79	68	189	95
Banana Walnut Muffin	1 muffin	605	72	30	156	64	86	74	206	103
Lemon Poppyseed Muffin	1 muffin	610	72	29	157	65	87	74	207	104
Cream Cheese Muffin	1 muffin	645	72	36	166	69	91	78	219	110
Double Chocolate Chip Muffin	1 muffin	620	72	29	160	66	88	75	211	106
Honey Bran Muffin	1 muffin	620	72	29	160	66	88	75	211	106
Banana Nut Pound Cake	1 serving	445	50	20	115	47	63	54	151	76
Marble Pound Cake	1 serving	450	50	21	116	48	64	55	153	77
Pink Iced Cookie	1 cookie	452	60	24	116	48	64	55	154	77
Diet Pepsi Slurpee	12 fl oz	5	3	0	1	1	1	1	2	1
Crystal Light Slurpee	12 fl oz	50	11	0	13	5	7	6	17	9
Peppermint Pattie Cocoa	8 fl oz	180	36	3	46	19	26	22	61	31

Little Caesar's

■ Sides

FOOD	AMOUNT	CAL	CARBS	FAT	WALK	RUN	BIKE	SWIM	YOGA	DANCE
Crazy Bread	1 stick	90	15	3	23	10	13	11	31	15
Crazy Sauce	1 serving	45	9	0	12	5	6	5	15	8
Baby Pan! Pan!	1 piece	360	34	16	93	38	51	44	122	61
Italian Cheese Bread	1 piece	130	13	6	34	14	18	16	44	22
Chicken Wings	1 wing	70	0	5	18	7	10	9	24	12
Cinnamon Crazy Bread	2 sticks	100	19	2	26	11	14	12	34	17

■ Deli Sandwiches

FOOD	AMOUNT	CAL	CARBS	FAT	WALK	RUN	BIKE	SWIM	YOGA	DANCE
Italian	1 sandwich	800	66	45	206	85	113	97	272	136
Veggie	1 sandwich	600	67	28	155	64	85	73	204	102
Ham & Cheese	1 sandwich	640	66	29	165	68	91	78	218	109

FOOD	AMOUNT	CAL	CARBS	FAT	WALK	RUN	BIKE	SWIM	YOGA	DANCE
■ Individual Size Salads										
Tossed	1 salad	100	15	3	26	11	14	12	34	17
Antipasto	1 salad	140	6	8	36	15	20	17	48	24
Greek	1 salad	120	11	7	31	13	17	15	41	20
Caesar	1 salad	90	12	3	23	10	13	11	31	15
■ Salad Dressings										
Italian	1.5 oz	220	2	23	57	23	31	27	75	37
Ranch	1.5 oz	230	2	24	59	24	33	28	78	39
Fat Free Italian	1.5 oz	25	5	0	6	3	4	3	9	4
Greek	1.5 oz	270	0	29	70	29	38	33	92	46
Caesar	1.5 oz	230	1	25	59	24	33	28	78	39
Long John Silver's										
■ Fish										
Battered Fish	1 piece	260	17	16	67	28	37	32	88	44
Baked Cod	1 piece	120	1	5	31	13	17	15	41	20
Fish Sandwich	1 piece	470	48	23	121	50	67	57	160	80
Ultimate Fish Sandwich	1 piece	530	49	28	137	56	75	64	180	90
Shrimp and Seafood Salad	1 salad	260	22	12	67	28	37	32	88	44
Battered Shrimp	1 piece	45	3	3	12	5	6	5	15	8
Buttered Lobster Bites (snack box)	4 oz	250	27	9	64	27	35	30	85	43
Popcorn Shrimp (snack box)	4 oz	270	23	16	70	29	38	33	92	46
Breaded Clams	3 oz	240	22	13	62	26	34	29	82	41
■ Sauces and Dressings										
Lite Italian Dressing	1 pouch	20	3	1	5	2	3	2	7	3
Garden Ranch Dressing	1 pouch	230	2	24	59	24	33	28	78	39
Thousand Island Dressing	1 pouch	220	7	21	57	23	31	27	75	37
Cocktail Sauce	1 oz	25	6	0	6	3	4	3	9	4
Tartar Sauce	1 oz	100	4	9	26	11	14	12	34	17
■ Sides										
Regular Fries	3 oz	230	34	10	59	24	33	28	78	39
Large Fries	5 oz	390	56	17	101	42	55	47	133	66
Hush Puppies	1 pup	60	9	3	15	6	9	7	20	10
Lobster Stuffed Crab Cake	1 cake	170	16	9	44	18	24	21	58	29
Slaw	4 oz	200	15	15	52	21	28	24	68	34
Corn Cobbette	1 cobbette	90	14	3	23	10	13	11	31	15

FOOD	AMOUNT	CAL	CARBS	FAT	WALK	RUN	BIKE	SWIM	YOGA	DANCE
Cheesesticks	3 sticks	140	12	8	36	15	20	17	48	24
Rice	4 oz	180	34	4	46	19	26	22	61	31
Crumblies	1 oz	170	14	12	44	18	24	21	58	29
Clam Chowder	1 bowl	220	23	10	57	23	31	27	75	37
■ **Desserts**										
Chocolate Cream Pie	1 serving	310	24	22	80	33	44	38	105	53
Pineapple Cream Pie	1 serving	290	39	13	75	31	41	35	99	49
Pecan Pie	1 serving	370	55	15	95	39	52	45	126	63
McDonald's										
■ **Sandwiches**										
Hamburger	1 burger	260	33	9	67	28	37	32	88	44
Cheeseburger	1 burger	310	35	12	80	33	44	38	105	53
Double Cheeseburger	1 burger	460	37	23	119	49	65	56	156	78
Quarter Pounder	1 burger	420	40	18	108	45	60	51	143	72
Quarter Pounder with Cheese	1 burger	510	43	25	131	54	72	62	173	87
Double Quarter Pounder with Cheese	1 burger	730	46	40	188	78	104	89	248	124
Big Mac	1 burger	560	47	30	144	60	79	68	190	95
Big N' Tasty	1 burger	470	41	23	121	50	67	57	160	80
Big N' Tasty with Cheese	1 burger	520	43	26	134	55	74	63	177	89
Fillet-o-Fish	1 sandwich	400	42	18	103	43	57	49	136	68
McChicken	1 sandwich	370	41	16	95	39	52	45	126	63
Spicy Chicken Sandwich	1 sandwich	510	64	17	131	54	72	62	173	87
Grilled Chicken Sandwich	1 sandwich	420	52	9	108	45	60	51	143	72
Crispy Chicken Sandwich	1 sandwich	500	63	16	129	53	71	61	170	85
Grilled Chicken Club Sandwich	1 sandwich	590	54	22	152	63	84	72	201	101
Crispy Chicken Club Sandwich	1 sandwich	680	64	29	175	72	96	83	231	116
Grilled Chicken Ranch BLT Sandwich	1 sandwich	490	54	13	126	52	70	60	167	83
Crispy Chicken Ranch BLT Sandwich	1 sandwich	580	64	20	149	62	82	71	197	99

FOOD	AMOUNT	CAL	CARBS	FAT	WALK	RUN	BIKE	SWIM	YOGA	DANCE
■ French Fries										
Small	2.6 oz	250	30	13	64	27	35	30	85	43
Medium	4 oz	380	47	20	98	40	54	46	129	65
Large	6 oz	570	70	30	147	61	81	69	194	97
■ McNuggets and Breast Strips										
4 Piece McNuggets	2.3 oz	170	10	10	44	18	24	21	58	29
6 Piece McNuggets	3.4 oz	250	15	15	64	27	35	30	85	43
10 Piece McNuggets	5.6 oz	420	26	24	108	45	60	51	143	72
20 Piece McNuggets	11.3 oz	840	51	49	216	89	119	102	286	143
3 Piece Chicken Breast Strips	4.7 oz	380	28	20	98	40	54	46	129	65
5 Piece Chicken Breast Strips	7.8 oz	630	46	33	162	67	89	77	214	107
10 Piece Chicken Breast Strips	15.6 oz	1270	92	66	327	135	180	155	432	216
■ Sauces, Dressings, and Jams										
Barbecue Sauce	1 package	45	11	0	12	5	6	5	15	8
Honey	1 package	50	12	0	13	5	7	6	17	9
Hot Mustard Sauce	1 package	50	9	2	13	5	7	6	17	9
Sweet and Sour Sauce	1 package	50	11	0	13	5	7	6	17	9
Spicy Buffalo Sauce	1.5 oz	60	1	6	15	6	9	7	20	10
Creamy Ranch Sauce	1.5 oz	200	3	21	52	21	28	24	68	34
Tangy Honey Mustard Sauce	1.5 oz	70	13	2	18	7	10	9	24	12
Southwestern Chipotle Barbecue Sauce	1.5 oz	70	16	0	18	7	10	9	24	12
■ Jam										
Grape Jam	.5 oz	35	9	0	9	4	5	4	12	6
Strawberry Preserves	.5 oz	35	9	0	9	4	5	4	12	6
■ Dressings										
Newman's Own Cobb	2 oz	120	9	9	31	13	17	15	41	20
Newman's Own Creamy Caesar	2 oz	190	4	18	49	20	27	23	65	32
Newman's Own Low Fat Balsamic Vinaigrette	1.5 oz	40	4	3	10	4	6	5	14	7
Newman's Own Low Fat Family Recipe Italian	1.5 oz	50	7	3	13	5	7	6	17	9
Newman's Own Ranch	2 oz	170	9	15	44	18	24	21	58	29
■ Salads										
Bacon Ranch Salad with Grilled Chicken	1 salad	280	12	9	72	30	40	34	95	48

FOOD	AMOUNT	CAL	CARBS	FAT	WALK	RUN	BIKE	SWIM	YOGA	DANCE
Bacon Ranch Salad with Crispy Chicken	1 salad	340	23	16	88	36	48	41	116	58
Bacon Ranch Salad (no chicken)	1 salad	140	10	7	36	15	20	17	48	24
Caesar Salad with Grilled Chicken	1 salad	220	12	6	57	23	31	27	75	37
Caesar Salad with Crispy Chicken	1 salad	300	22	13	77	32	43	36	102	51
Caesar Salad (no chicken)	1 salad	90	9	4	23	10	13	11	31	15
California Cobb with Grilled Chicken	1 salad	280	12	11	72	30	40	34	95	48
California Cobb with Crispy Chicken	1 salad	360	22	18	93	38	51	44	122	61
California Cobb (no chicken)	1 salad	160	9	9	41	17	23	19	54	27
Fruit and Walnut Salad	1 salad	310	44	13	80	33	44	38	105	53
Side Salad	1 salad	20	4	0	5	2	3	2	7	3
Butter Garlic Croutons	.5 oz	60	10	1	15	6	9	7	20	10
■ **Breakfast**										
Egg McMuffin	1 serving	300	30	12	77	32	43	36	102	51
Sausage McMuffin	1 serving	380	31	22	98	40	54	46	129	65
Sausage McMuffin with Egg	1 serving	450	31	27	116	48	64	55	153	77
English Muffin	1 serving	170	27	5	44	18	24	21	58	29
Bacon, Egg and Cheese Biscuit	1 serving	440	36	24	113	47	62	54	150	75
Sausage Biscuit with Egg	1 serving	500	36	31	129	53	71	61	170	85
Sausage Biscuit	1 serving	410	34	26	106	44	58	50	139	70
Biscuit	1 serving	240	31	11	62	26	34	29	82	41
Bacon, Egg and Cheese McGriddles	1 serving	450	46	21	116	48	64	55	153	77
Sausage, Egg and Cheese McGriddles	1 serving	560	47	32	144	60	79	68	190	95
Sausage McGriddles	1 serving	420	44	22	108	45	60	51	143	72
Big Breakfast	1 serving	730	53	46	188	78	104	89	248	124
Deluxe Breakfast	1 serving	1220	136	61	314	130	173	148	415	208
Sausage Burrito	1 serving	300	26	16	77	32	43	36	102	51
Hot Cakes and Sausage	1 serving	770	104	33	198	82	109	94	262	131
Hot Cakes (with 2 pats margarine and syrup)	1 serving	600	102	17	155	64	85	73	204	102
Sausage Patty	1 serving	170	2	15	44	18	24	21	58	29

FOOD	AMOUNT	CAL	CARBS	FAT	WALK	RUN	BIKE	SWIM	YOGA	DANCE
Scrambled Eggs	2 eggs	190	5	12	49	20	27	23	65	32
Hash Browns	1 serving	140	15	8	36	15	20	17	48	24
Warm Cinnamon Rolls	1 serving	420	57	18	108	45	60	51	143	72
Deluxe Warm Cinnamon Rolls	1 serving	590	86	24	152	63	84	72	201	101
■ Desserts and Shakes										
Fruit 'n Yogurt Parfait	1 serving	160	31	2	41	17	23	19	54	27
Fruit 'n Yogurt Parfait, No Granola	1 serving	130	25	2	34	14	18	16	44	22
Apple Dippers with Low Fat Caramel Dip	1 serving	100	24	1	26	11	14	12	34	17
Apple Dippers	1 package	35	8	0	9	4	5	4	12	6
Low Fat Caramel Dip	1 serving	70	15	1	18	7	10	9	24	12
Vanilla, Reduced Fat Ice Cream Cone	1 cone	150	24	4	39	16	21	18	51	26
Kiddie Cone	1 cone	45	8	1	12	5	6	5	15	8
Strawberry Sundae	1 serving	280	51	6	72	30	40	34	95	48
Hot Caramel Sundae	1 serving	340	62	7	88	36	48	41	116	58
Hot Fudge Sundae	1 serving	330	55	9	85	35	47	40	112	56
McFlurry with M&M's Candies	12 oz	620	96	20	160	66	88	75	211	106
McFlurry with Oreos	12 oz	560	88	16	144	60	79	68	190	95
Chocolate Triple Thick Shake	12 oz	440	76	10	113	47	62	54	150	75
Chocolate Triple Thick Shake	16 oz	580	102	14	149	62	82	71	197	99
Chocolate Triple Thick Shake	21 oz	770	134	18	198	82	109	94	262	131
Chocolate Triple Thick Shake	32 oz	1160	203	27	299	124	165	141	395	198
Strawberry Triple Thick Shake	12 oz	420	73	10	108	45	60	51	143	72
Strawberry Triple Thick Shake	16 oz	560	97	13	144	60	79	68	190	95
Strawberry Triple Thick Shake	21 oz	740	128	18	191	79	105	90	252	126
Strawberry Triple Thick Shake	32 oz	1110	194	26	286	118	157	135	378	189
Vanilla Triple Thick Shake	12 oz	420	72	10	108	45	60	51	143	72
Vanilla Triple Thick Shake	16 oz	550	96	13	142	59	78	67	187	94
Vanilla Triple Thick Shake	21 oz	740	128	18	191	79	105	90	252	126
Vanilla Triple Thick Shake	32 oz	1110	193	26	286	118	157	135	378	189
Baked Apple Pie	1 serving	250	34	11	64	27	35	30	85	43
McDonaldland Chocolate Chip Cookie	2 oz	270	39	11	70	29	38	33	92	46
McDonaldland Cookies	2 oz	250	42	8	64	27	35	30	85	43
Chocolate Chip Cookie	1 cookie	160	22	7	41	17	23	19	54	27

FOOD	AMOUNT	CAL	CARBS	FAT	WALK	RUN	BIKE	SWIM	YOGA	DANCE
Oatmeal Raisin Cookie	1 cookie	140	22	5	36	15	20	17	48	24
Sugar Cookie	1 cookie	150	22	6	39	16	21	18	51	26

P.F. Chang's

■ Appetizers

FOOD	AMOUNT	CAL	CARBS	FAT	WALK	RUN	BIKE	SWIM	YOGA	DANCE
Chang's Chicken in Soothing Lettuce Wraps	1 serving	630	92	8	162	67	89	77	214	107
Chang's Spare Ribs	1 serving	1410	47	109	363	150	200	172	480	240
Chang's Vegetarian Lettuce Wraps	1 serving	370	71	4	95	39	52	45	126	63
Crab Wontons	1 serving	520	51	26	134	55	74	63	177	89
Harvest Spring Rolls	1 serving	640	106	17	165	68	91	78	218	109
Northern Style Spare Ribs	1 serving	1090	6	95	281	116	155	133	371	186
Peking Dumplings (pan-fried)	1 serving	420	31	22	108	45	60	51	143	72
Peking Dumplings (steamed)	1 serving	400	31	20	103	43	57	49	136	68
Salt & Pepper Calamari	1 serving	590	35	37	152	63	84	72	201	101
Seared Ahi Tuna	1 serving	220	18	5	57	23	31	27	75	37
Shanghai Street Dumplings	1 serving	860	90	46	222	92	122	105	293	147
Shrimp Dumplings (pan-fried)	1 serving	360	26	17	93	38	51	44	122	61
Shrimp Dumplings (steamed)	1 serving	320	26	12	82	34	45	39	109	55
Vegetable Dumplings (pan-fried)	1 serving	340	47	12	88	36	48	41	116	58
Vegetable Dumplings (steamed)	1 serving	300	47	8	77	32	43	36	102	51

■ Salads and Soups

FOOD	AMOUNT	CAL	CARBS	FAT	WALK	RUN	BIKE	SWIM	YOGA	DANCE
Wild Alaskan Sockeye Salmon Salad	1 serving	470	18	30	121	50	67	57	160	80
Hot and Sour Soup	1 cup	56	2	4	14	6	8	7	19	10
Oriental Chicken Salad	1 serving	940	49	56	242	100	133	114	320	160
Peanut Chicken Salad	1 serving	1080	47	69	278	115	153	131	367	184
Pin Rice Noodle Soup	1 serving	270	55	2	70	29	38	33	92	46
Warm Duck Spinach Salad	1 serving	940	44	66	242	100	133	114	320	160
Wonton Soup	1 cup	52	4	3	13	6	7	6	18	9

■ Traditions

FOOD	AMOUNT	CAL	CARBS	FAT	WALK	RUN	BIKE	SWIM	YOGA	DANCE
Almond Cashew Chicken	1 lunch portion	740	51	30	191	79	105	90	252	126
Almond Cashew Chicken	1 dinner portion	850	57	33	219	91	121	103	289	145

FOOD	AMOUNT	CAL	CARBS	FAT	WALK	RUN	BIKE	SWIM	YOGA	DANCE
Beef with Broccoli	1 lunch portion	760	23	49	196	81	108	92	259	129
Beef with Broccoli	1 dinner portion	910	24	59	235	97	129	111	310	155
Crispy Honey Chicken	1 lunch portion	860	84	36	222	92	122	105	293	147
Crispy Honey Chicken	1 dinner portion	960	90	37	247	102	136	117	327	164
Lo Mein Beef	1 lunch portion	850	90	34	219	91	121	103	289	145
Lo Mein Beef	1 dinner portion	990	90	42	255	105	140	120	337	169
Lo Mein Chicken	1 lunch portion	720	92	20	186	77	102	88	245	123
Lo Mein Chicken	1 dinner portion	810	93	25	209	86	115	99	276	138
Lo Mein Combo	1 lunch portion	900	94	35	232	96	128	109	306	153
Lo Mein Combo	1 dinner portion	960	94	37	247	102	136	117	327	164
Lo Mein Pork	1 lunch portion	740	91	25	191	79	105	90	252	126
Lo Mein Pork	1 dinner portion	840	92	31	216	89	119	102	286	143
Lo Mein Shrimp	1 lunch portion	700	92	20	180	75	99	85	238	119
Lo Mein Shrimp	1 dinner portion	790	94	24	204	84	112	96	269	135
Lo Mein Vegetable	1 lunch portion	550	93	12	142	59	78	67	187	94
Lo Mein Vegetable	1 dinner portion	560	95	12	144	60	79	68	190	95
Moo Goo Gai Pan	1 serving	610	32	25	157	65	87	74	207	104
Shrimp with Lobster Sauce	1 lunch portion	490	21	24	126	52	70	60	167	83
Shrimp with Lobster Sauce	1 dinner portion	560	22	27	144	60	79	68	190	95

■ Vegetarian plates

FOOD	AMOUNT	CAL	CARBS	FAT	WALK	RUN	BIKE	SWIM	YOGA	DANCE
Buddha's Feast (steamed)	1 serving	200	44	2	52	21	28	24	68	34
Buddha's Feast (stir-fried)	1 serving	370	64	7	95	39	52	45	126	63
Coconut Curry Vegetables	1 serving	950	79	63	245	101	135	116	323	162

FOOD	AMOUNT	CAL	CARBS	FAT	WALK	RUN	BIKE	SWIM	YOGA	DANCE
Garlic Snap Peas	1 serving	220	20	7	57	23	31	27	75	37
Ma Po Tofu	1 serving	760	40	52	196	81	108	92	259	129
Shanghai Cucumbers	1 serving	120	8	6	31	13	17	15	41	20
Sichuan Style Asparagus	1 serving	170	29	4	44	18	24	21	58	29
Sichuan Style Long Beans	1 serving	190	36	4	49	20	27	23	65	32
Stir Fried Spicy Eggplant	1 serving	510	60	29	131	54	72	62	173	87
Spinach Stir Fried with Garlic	1 serving	110	15	4	28	12	16	13	37	19
■ Chicken and Duck										
Cantonese Roasted Duck	1 serving	1160	109	59	299	124	165	141	395	198
Chang's Spicy Chicken	1 serving	990	70	51	255	105	140	120	337	169
Chicken with Black Bean Sauce	1 serving	640	31	22	165	68	91	78	218	109
Ginger Chicken and Broccoli	1 serving	620	43	21	160	66	88	75	211	106
Kung Pao Chicken	1 regular serving	1230	51	78	317	131	174	150	418	210
Kung Pao Chicken	training table	930	38	50	240	99	132	113	316	158
Mango Chicken	1 serving	730	68	19	188	78	104	89	248	124
Mu Shu Chicken	1 serving	750	55	31	193	80	106	91	255	128
Orange Peel Chicken	1 serving	1090	73	60	281	116	155	133	371	186
Philip's Better Lemon Chicken	1 serving	810	94	21	209	86	115	99	276	138
Spicy Ground Chicken and Eggplant	1 serving	890	70	43	229	95	126	108	303	152
Sweet and Sour Chicken	1 serving	800	89	31	206	85	113	97	272	136
■ Seafood										
Wild Alaskan Sockeye Salmon Lemon Pepper	1 serving	670	32	36	173	71	95	82	228	114
Alaskan Sockeye Salmon Steamed with Ginger	1 serving	740	49	36	191	79	105	90	252	126
Cantonese Scallops	1 serving	370	20	13	95	39	52	45	126	63
Cantonese Shrimp	1 serving	380	17	15	98	40	54	46	129	65
Crispy Honey Shrimp	1 serving	860	85	37	222	92	122	105	293	147
Hot Fish (Catfish)	1 serving	960	86	42	247	102	136	117	327	164
Kung Pao Scallops	1 serving	1180	56	76	304	126	167	144	401	201
Kung Pao Shrimp	1 serving	1230	52	79	317	131	174	150	418	210
Lemon Pepper Shrimp	1 serving	520	31	25	134	55	74	63	177	89
Lemon Scallops	1 serving	720	96	18	186	77	102	88	245	123
Oolong Marinated Seabass	1 serving	740	39	30	191	79	105	90	252	126

FOOD	AMOUNT	CAL	CARBS	FAT	WALK	RUN	BIKE	SWIM	YOGA	DANCE
Orange Peel Shrimp	1 serving	1070	74	60	276	114	152	130	364	182
Sichuan from the Sea Calamari	1 serving	720	88	21	186	77	102	88	245	123
Sichuan from the Sea Scallops	1 serving	630	66	19	162	67	89	77	214	107
Sichuan from the Sea Shrimp	1 serving	630	52	21	162	67	89	77	214	107
Spicy Salt and Pepper Prawns	1 serving	770	28	50	198	82	109	94	262	131
■ **Meat**										
Beef a la Sichuan	1 serving	990	55	55	255	105	140	120	337	169
Mongolian Beef	1 serving	1080	18	72	278	115	153	131	367	184
Mu Shu Pork	1 serving	780	53	38	201	83	111	95	265	133
Orange Peel Beef	1 serving	1330	69	82	343	142	189	162	452	227
Sichuan Style Pork	1 serving	910	43	47	235	97	129	111	310	155
Sweet and Sour Pork	1 serving	910	89	43	235	97	129	111	310	155
Wok Seared Lamb	1 serving	1270	22	95	327	135	180	155	432	216
■ **Noodles, Meins, and Rice**										
Cantonese Chow Fun Beef	1 serving	1080	101	48	278	115	153	131	367	184
Cantonese Chow Fun Chicken	1 serving	930	105	34	240	99	132	113	316	158
Chow Mein Beef	1 serving	770	90	24	198	82	109	94	262	131
Chow Mein Chicken	1 serving	670	92	16	173	71	95	82	228	114
Chow Mein Combo	1 serving	1130	150	28	291	120	160	137	384	193
Chow Mein Pork	1 serving	800	92	27	206	85	113	97	272	136
Chow Mein Shrimp	1 serving	750	94	20	193	80	106	91	255	128
Chow Mein Vegetable	1 serving	520	95	7	134	55	74	63	177	89
Dan-Dan Noodles	1 serving	1070	128	30	276	114	152	130	364	182
Double Pan-Fried Noodles Beef	1 serving	1240	111	61	320	132	176	151	422	211
Double Pan-Fried Noodles Chicken	1 serving	1140	113	53	294	121	162	139	388	194
Double Pan-Fried Noodles Combo	1 serving	1390	116	70	358	148	197	169	473	237
Double Pan-Fried Noodles Pork	1 serving	1170	113	57	302	125	166	142	398	199
Double Pan-Fried Noodles Shrimp	1 serving	1130	114	53	291	120	160	137	384	193
Double Pan-Fried Noodles Vegetable	1 serving	980	114	44	253	104	139	119	333	167
Garlic Noodles	1 serving	610	107	12	157	65	87	74	207	104
P.F. Chang's Fried Rice Beef	1 serving	1080	144	28	278	115	153	131	367	184
P.F. Chang's Fried Rice Chicken	1 serving	960	145	17	247	102	136	117	327	164

FOOD	AMOUNT	CAL	CARBS	FAT	WALK	RUN	BIKE	SWIM	YOGA	DANCE
P.F. Chang's Fried Rice Combo	1 serving	1130	150	28	291	120	160	137	384	193
P.F. Chang's Fried Rice Pork	1 serving	990	145	22	255	105	140	120	337	169
P.F. Chang's Fried Rice Shrimp	1 serving	950	146	17	245	101	135	116	323	162
P.F. Chang's Fried Rice Vegetable	1 serving	820	147	12	211	87	116	100	279	140
Sichuan Chicken Chow Fun	1 serving	690	97	19	178	73	98	84	235	118
Singapore Street Noodles	1 serving	600	67	24	155	64	85	73	204	102
Vegetable Chow Fun	1 serving	440	100	2	113	47	62	54	150	75
Brown Rice	1 serving	350	73	3	90	37	50	43	119	60
White Rice	1 serving	410	88	1	106	44	58	50	139	70
■ **Dessert**										
Banana Spring Rolls	1 serving	1860	235	97	479	198	264	226	633	317
New York Style Cheesecake	1 serving	870	72	58	224	93	123	106	296	148
Great Wall of Chocolate	1 serving	1883	325	71	485	201	267	229	640	321
Panera Bread										
■ **Baked Soufflés**										
Spinach and Artichoke	6.25 oz	480	35	30	124	51	68	58	163	82
Spinach and Bacon	6.25 oz	510	34	34	131	54	72	62	173	87
■ **Soup**										
Baked Potato Soup	1 cup	230	21	14	59	24	33	28	78	39
Boston Clam Chowder	1 cup	200	19	11	52	21	28	24	68	34
Broccoli Cheddar Soup	1 cup	230	13	16	59	24	33	28	78	39
Cream of Chicken and Wild Rice Soup	1 cup	200	19	12	52	21	28	24	68	34
French Onion Soup (no cheese or croutons)	1 cup	80	12	3	21	9	11	10	27	14
French Onion Soup with Cheese and Croutons	1 cup	200	21	10	52	21	28	24	68	34
Low-Fat Chicken Noodle Soup	1 cup	100	15	2	26	11	14	12	34	17
Low-Fat Vegetarian Black Bean Soup	1 cup	160	31	1	41	17	23	19	54	27
Low-Fat Vegetarian Garden Vegetable Soup	1 cup	90	17	1	23	10	13	11	31	15
Low-Fat Vegetarian Moroccan Tomato Lentil Soup	1 cup	120	22	2	31	13	17	15	41	20
Portobello and Roasted Garlic Bisque	1 cup	220	15	16	57	23	31	27	75	37
Vegetarian Roasted Tomato and Pepper Bisque	1 cup	260	19	20	67	28	37	32	88	44

FOOD	AMOUNT	CAL	CARBS	FAT	WALK	RUN	BIKE	SWIM	YOGA	DANCE
■ **Sandwiches**										
Asiago Roast Beef	1 sandwich	670	55	27	173	71	95	82	228	114
Bacon Turkey Bravo	1 sandwich	740	82	25	191	79	105	90	252	126
Chicken Salad Sandwich on Artisan Sesame Semolina	1 sandwich	740	80	27	191	79	105	90	252	126
Chicken Salad Sandwich on Nine Grain	1 sandwich	660	59	30	170	70	94	80	224	112
Chicken Bacon Dijon Panini on Artisan Country	1 sandwich	810	88	29	209	86	115	99	276	138
Chicken Bacon Dijon Panini on French	1 sandwich	690	60	29	178	73	98	84	235	118
Chicken Caesar Sandwich on Artisan Three Cheese	1 sandwich	750	71	32	193	80	106	91	255	128
Chicken Caesar Sandwich on Asiago Cheese Focaccia	1 sandwich	920	78	46	237	98	130	112	313	157
Frontega Chicken Panini	1 sandwich	890	75	43	229	95	126	108	303	152
Garden Veggie Sandwich	1 sandwich	640	90	25	165	68	91	78	218	109
Italian Combo Sandwich	1 sandwich	1110	91	56	286	118	157	135	378	189
Peanut Butter and Jelly on Artisan French	1 sandwich	590	93	15	152	63	84	72	201	101
Peanut Butter and Jelly on French	1 sandwich	460	66	15	119	49	65	56	156	78
PepperBlue Steak Sandwich	1 sandwich	850	89	39	219	91	121	103	289	145
Portobello and Mozzarella Panini	1 sandwich	750	78	37	193	80	106	91	255	128
Sierra Turkey Sandwich	1 sandwich	950	75	54	245	101	135	116	323	162
Smoked Ham and Swiss on Artisan Stone-Milled Rye	1 sandwich	760	73	31	196	81	108	92	259	129
Smoked Ham and Swiss on Rye	1 sandwich	690	52	35	178	73	98	84	235	118
Smoked Turkey Breast on Artisan Country	1 sandwich	590	77	15	152	63	84	72	201	101
Smoked Turkey Breast on Sourdough	1 sandwich	430	44	14	111	46	61	52	146	73

FOOD	AMOUNT	CAL	CARBS	FAT	WALK	RUN	BIKE	SWIM	YOGA	DANCE
Smokehouse Turkey Panini on Artisan Three Cheese	1 sandwich	680	73	23	175	72	96	83	231	116
Smokehouse Turkey Panini on Asiago Focaccia	1 sandwich	840	77	37	216	89	119	102	286	143
Tuna Salad on Artisan Multigrain	1 sandwich	810	75	42	209	86	115	99	276	138
Tuna Salad on Honey Wheat	1 sandwich	720	51	44	186	77	102	88	245	123
Turkey Artichoke Panini	1 sandwich	840	83	37	216	89	119	102	286	143
Tuscan Chicken Sandwich	1 sandwich	720	77	27	186	77	102	88	245	123

■ **Hand-Tossed Salads**

FOOD	AMOUNT	CAL	CARBS	FAT	WALK	RUN	BIKE	SWIM	YOGA	DANCE
Asian Sesame Chicken Salad	1 salad	430	33	19	111	46	61	52	146	73
Bistro Steak Salad	1 salad	630	16	57	162	67	89	77	214	107
Caesar Salad	1 salad	440	25	32	113	47	62	54	150	75
Classic Café Salad	1 salad	400	18	37	103	43	57	49	136	68
Fandango Salad	1 salad	390	26	27	101	42	55	47	133	66
Fresh Fruit Cup	10 oz	150	37	0	39	16	21	18	51	26
Grilled Chicken Caesar Salad	1 salad	560	26	34	144	60	79	68	190	95
Greek Salad	1 salad	520	17	48	134	55	74	63	177	89

■ **Dressings**

FOOD	AMOUNT	CAL	CARBS	FAT	WALK	RUN	BIKE	SWIM	YOGA	DANCE
Balsamic Vinaigrette	2 oz	350	8	36	90	37	50	43	119	60
Caesar Dressing	2 oz	200	3	21	52	21	28	24	68	34
Fat-Free Poppyseed Dressing	2 oz	25	6	0	6	3	4	3	9	4
Fat-Free Raspberry Dressing	2 oz	50	9	1	13	5	7	6	17	9
Greek Dressing	2 oz	290	2	32	75	31	41	35	99	49
Reduced-Sugar Asian Sesame Vinaigrette	2 oz	110	8	8	28	12	16	13	37	19

Pizza Hut

■ **Appetizers**

FOOD	AMOUNT	CAL	CARBS	FAT	WALK	RUN	BIKE	SWIM	YOGA	DANCE
Hot Wings	2 pieces	110	1	6	28	12	16	13	37	19
Mild Wings	2 pieces	110	<1	7	28	12	16	13	37	19
Wing Ranch Dipping Sauce	1.5 oz	210	4	22	54	22	30	26	71	36
Wing Blue Cheese Dipping Sauce	1.5 oz	230	2	24	59	24	33	28	78	39
Breadsticks	1 breadstick	150	20	6	39	16	21	18	51	26

FOOD	AMOUNT	CAL	CARBS	FAT	WALK	RUN	BIKE	SWIM	YOGA	DANCE
Cheese Breadsticks	1 breadstick	200	21	10	52	21	28	24	68	34
■ **Dressings and Dipping Sauces**										
Breadstick Dipping Sauce	3 oz	45	9	0	12	5	6	5	15	8
Ranch Dressing	2 tbsp	100	2	10	26	11	14	12	34	17
Thousand Island Dressing	2 tbsp	110	6	9	28	12	16	13	37	19
French Dressing	2 tbsp	140	11	11	36	15	20	17	48	24
Italian Dressing	2 tbsp	140	2	15	36	15	20	17	48	24
Caesar Dressing	2 tbsp	150	1	16	39	16	21	18	51	26
Lite Ranch Dressing	2 tbsp	70	0	7	18	7	10	9	24	12
Lite Italian Dressing	2 tbsp	60	5	5	15	6	9	7	20	10
■ **Desserts**										
Cinnamon Sticks	2 pieces	170	27	5	44	18	24	21	58	29
White Icing Dipping Cup	2 oz	190	46	0	49	20	27	23	65	32
Apple Dessert Pizza	1 slice	260	53	4	67	28	37	32	88	44
Cherry Dessert Pizza	1 slice	240	47	4	62	26	34	29	82	41
Quiznos										
Small Turkey Lite	1 sub	334	52	6	86	36	47	41	114	57
Small Honey Bourbon Chicken	1 sub	359	45	6	93	38	51	44	122	61
Small Sierra Smoked Turkey with Raspberry Chipotle Sauce	1 sub	350	53	6	90	37	50	43	119	60
Red Lobster										
■ **Fantastic Fresh Fish**										
Tilapia (lunch portion)	1 lunch portion	186	0	6	48	20	26	23	63	32
Tilapia (dinner portion)	1 dinner portion	346	0	10	89	37	49	42	118	59
Tilapia in a Bag (lunch portion)	1 lunch portion	297	15	9	77	32	42	36	101	51
Tilapia in a Bag (dinner portion)	1 dinner portion	563	30	16	145	60	80	68	191	96
Rainbow Trout (lunch portion)	1 lunch portion	273	2	14	70	29	39	33	93	47
Rainbow Trout (dinner portion)	1 dinner portion	512	6	25	132	55	73	62	174	87
Atlantic Salmon (lunch portion)	1 lunch portion	258	0	12	66	27	37	31	88	44
Atlantic Salmon (dinner portion)	1 dinner portion	578	0	33	149	62	82	70	197	98

FOOD	AMOUNT	CAL	CARBS	FAT	WALK	RUN	BIKE	SWIM	YOGA	DANCE
■ Signature Shellfish										
Jumbo Shrimp Cocktail Appetizer	1 serving	138	1	2	36	15	20	17	47	24
Jumbo Shrimp Cocktail Dinner	1 serving	228	2	4	59	24	32	28	78	39
Live Maine Lobster	1 serving	145	2	1	37	15	21	18	49	25
Rock Lobster Tail	1 serving	258	0	3	66	27	37	31	88	44
Snow Crab Legs	1 serving	262	0	5	68	28	37	32	89	45
King Crab Legs	1 serving	490	0	9	126	52	70	60	167	83
Grilled Jumbo Shrimp Dinner	1 serving	142	1	3	37	15	20	17	48	24
Lobster Chops	1 serving	321	0	9	83	34	46	39	109	55
■ Sauce										
Large Cocktail Sauce	1 serving	87	17	2	22	9	12	11	30	15
Melted Butter	1 serving	189	0	21	49	20	27	23	64	32
■ Sides/Accompaniments										
Garden Salad	1 serving	52	9	2	13	6	7	6	18	9
Red Wine Vinaigrette	1 serving	50	5	3	13	5	7	6	17	9
Petite Shrimp Topping	1 serving	30	1	1	8	3	4	4	10	5
Cheddar Bay Biscuits	1 serving	160	17	9	41	17	23	19	54	27
Baked Potato with Pico de Gallo	1 serving	185	37	2	48	20	26	23	63	32
Wild Rice Pilaf	1 serving	204	36	5	53	22	29	25	69	35
Seasonal Vegetables with Butter	1 serving	143	9	11	37	15	20	17	49	24
Seasoned Fresh Broccoli	1 serving	56	10	0	14	6	8	7	19	10
7-Eleven										
Black Forest Ham & Mozzarella Cheese on Cracked Wheat Bread	1 sandwich	610	29	59	157	65	87	74	207	104
Mediterranean Style Turkey Sandwich	1 sandwich	400	43	14	103	43	57	49	136	68
Ham & Cheese Round	1 sandwich	290	36	8	75	31	41	35	99	49
Barbecue Deluxe	1 sandwich	310	53	5	80	33	44	38	105	53
100% Beef Cheeseburger	1 sandwich	390	33	21	101	42	55	47	133	66
Chuckwagon	1 sandwich	360	39	16	93	38	51	44	122	61
Chicken & Swiss	1 sandwich	380	30	22	98	40	54	46	129	65

FOOD	AMOUNT	CAL	CARBS	FAT	WALK	RUN	BIKE	SWIM	YOGA	DANCE
Double Charbroil Del.	1 sandwich	500	41	26	129	53	71	61	170	85
1/4 lb. Cheeseburger	1 sandwich	610	44	36	157	65	87	74	207	104
Twin Chili Dogs	1 sandwich	630	55	36	162	67	89	77	214	107
Egg Salad	1 sandwich	330	42	15	85	35	47	40	112	56
Deli Style Stacker®	1 sandwich	250	28	8	64	27	35	30	85	43
Chicken Salad	1 sandwich	340	43	15	88	36	48	41	116	58
Ham & Cheese Wedge	1 sandwich	220	28	7	57	23	31	27	75	37
Turkey Club	1 sandwich	250	29	7	64	27	35	30	85	43
Tuna Salad	1 sandwich	330	43	14	85	35	47	40	112	56
Turkey & Cheese Wedge	1 sandwich	240	30	7	62	26	34	29	82	41
Ham & Swiss on Rye	1 sandwich	280	29	9	72	30	40	34	95	48
Mega Muffaletta	1 sandwich	390	36	19	101	42	55	47	133	66
Mega Small Turkey & Cheese	1 sandwich	340	37	9	88	36	48	41	116	58
Mega Ham & Cheese	1 sandwich	330	39	11	85	35	47	40	112	56
Mega Turkey & Cheese	1 sandwich	310	40	10	80	33	44	38	105	53
Mega Turkey Club	1 sandwich	320	40	10	82	34	45	39	109	55
Ham & Cheese Sub	1 sandwich	460	49	23	119	49	65	56	156	78
Ham & Cheese Sub Selects	1 sandwich	400	44	13	103	43	57	49	136	68
Italian Sub Selects	1 sandwich	450	42	21	116	48	64	55	153	77
Twin Sausage & Biscuit	1 sandwich	350	25	24	90	37	50	43	119	60
Sausage & Cheese on a Biscuit	1 sandwich	410	27	29	106	44	58	50	139	70

FOOD	AMOUNT	CAL	CARBS	FAT	WALK	RUN	BIKE	SWIM	YOGA	DANCE
Sausage, Egg & Cheese on a Biscuit	1 sandwich	380	28	26	98	40	54	46	129	65
H&C Hot Pockets	1 sandwich	540	74	18	139	58	77	66	184	92
Pepp. Hot Pockets	1 sandwich	590	76	22	152	63	84	72	201	101
Hot Pockets Brand RollerStix Philly Steak & Cheese	1 piece	230	23	12	59	24	33	28	78	39
Ham, Egg & Cheese Croissant	1 sandwich	390	34	22	101	42	55	47	133	66
San Luis 5 oz. Red Hot Beef	1 burrito	340	39	17	88	36	48	41	116	58
San Luis 5 oz. Bean & Cheese	1 burrito	310	44	10	80	33	44	38	105	53
San Luis10 oz. Bean & Cheese	1 burrito	620	88	19	160	66	88	75	211	106
San Luis 10 oz. Green Chili Beef & Bean	1 burrito	720	83	33	186	77	102	88	245	123
San Luis 10 oz. Red Hot Beef	1 burrito	690	78	34	178	73	98	84	235	118
De/posada Cheese Chimichanga	1 chimichanga	300	39	12	77	32	43	36	102	51
De/posada Beef Chimichanga	1 chimichanga	360	37	18	93	38	51	44	122	61
De/posada Beef & Jack Cheese	1 burrito	300	36	11	77	32	43	36	102	51
The Bomb Beef Spicy Red Hot	.5 burrito	500	60	21	129	53	71	61	170	85
The Bomb Beef & Green Chili	.5 burrito	470	57	21	121	50	67	57	160	80
Egg, Sausage, Cheese HBW Cheese	1 burrito	520	51	25	134	55	74	63	177	89
Egg, Bacon, Cheese HBW Burrito	1 burrito	550	51	27	142	59	78	67	187	94
Beef, Steak & Jalapeño HBW Burrito	1 burrito	390	61	8	101	42	55	47	133	66
Sausage & Biscuit	1 sandwich	240	14	17	62	26	34	29	82	41
Sausage, Egg & Cheese Biscuit	1 sandwich	430	29	27	111	46	61	52	146	73
Ham, Egg & Cheese English Muffin	1 sandwich	260	30	8	67	28	37	32	88	44
Sausage, Egg & Cheese English Muffin	1 sandwich	370	29	20	95	39	52	45	126	63
Char-Broil & Cheese	1 sandwich	350	36	15	90	37	50	43	119	60

FOOD	AMOUNT	CAL	CARBS	FAT	WALK	RUN	BIKE	SWIM	YOGA	DANCE
Chicken & Swiss	1 sandwich	380	30	22	98	40	54	46	129	65
100% Beef Cheeseburger	1 sandwich	390	33	21	101	42	55	47	133	66
Hot Jalapeño Biscuit	1 sandwich	350	21	24	90	37	50	43	119	60
HEC Croissant	1 sandwich	340	28	20	88	36	48	41	116	58
SEC Pancake	1 sandwich	420	37	25	108	45	60	51	143	72
Scrambled Egg, Bacon, Cheese Burrito	1 burrito	320	31	16	82	34	45	39	109	55
Scrambled Egg, Sausage, Cheese Burrito	1 burrito	280	31	13	72	30	40	34	95	48
Deep-Fried Red Hot Beef & Bean	1 burrito	390	36	24	101	42	55	47	133	66
Deep-Fried Green Chili Beef & Bean	1 burrito	380	36	22	98	40	54	46	129	65
Green Chili Beef & Bean	1 burrito	340	39	17	88	36	48	41	116	58
Red Chili Beef & Bean	1 burrito	390	36	24	101	42	55	47	133	66
Ready Pac Chef Salad	1 container	350	9	25	90	37	50	43	119	60
Ready Pac Chicken Caesar Salad	1.33 cups	230	4	21	59	24	33	28	78	39

Subway

■ Breakfast Sandwiches

FOOD	AMOUNT	CAL	CARBS	FAT	WALK	RUN	BIKE	SWIM	YOGA	DANCE
Cheese and Egg on Deli Roll	1 sandwich	270	35	9	70	29	38	33	92	46
Chipotle Steak and Cheese on Deli Roll	1 sandwich	470	38	25	121	50	67	57	160	80
Double Bacon and Cheese on Deli Roll	1 sandwich	460	37	23	119	49	65	56	156	78
Honey Mustard Ham and Egg on Deli Roll	1 sandwich	270	43	5	70	29	38	33	92	46
Western with Cheese on Deli Roll	1 sandwich	360	38	14	93	38	51	44	122	61

■ Sandwiches with 6 Grams of Fat or Less

FOOD	AMOUNT	CAL	CARBS	FAT	WALK	RUN	BIKE	SWIM	YOGA	DANCE
6" Ham	1 sandwich	290	47	5	75	31	41	35	99	49
6" Oven Roasted Chicken Breast	1 sandwich	330	47	5	85	35	47	40	112	56

FOOD	AMOUNT	CAL	CARBS	FAT	WALK	RUN	BIKE	SWIM	YOGA	DANCE
6″ Roast Beef	1 sandwich	290	45	5	75	31	41	35	99	49
6″ Subway Club	1 sandwich	320	47	6	82	34	45	39	109	55
6″ Sweet Onion Teriyaki	1 sandwich	370	59	5	95	39	52	45	126	63
6″ Turkey Breast	1 sandwich	280	46	5	72	30	40	34	95	48
6″ Turkey Breast and Ham	1 sandwich	290	47	5	75	31	41	35	99	49
6″ Veggie Delite	1 sandwich	230	44	3	59	24	33	28	78	39
■ Cold Sandwiches										
6″ Cold Cut Combo	1 sandwich	410	47	17	106	44	58	50	139	70
6″ Tuna	1 sandwich	530	45	31	137	56	75	64	180	90
■ Deli Sandwiches										
Ham Deli	1 sandwich	210	36	4	54	22	30	26	71	36
Roast Beef Deli	1 sandwich	220	35	5	57	23	31	27	75	37
Tuna Deli	1 sandwich	350	35	18	90	37	50	43	119	60
Turkey Breast Deli	1 sandwich	210	36	4	54	22	30	26	71	36
■ Toasted Sandwiches										
6″ Cheese Steak	1 sandwich	360	47	10	93	38	51	44	122	61
6″ Chicken and Bacon Ranch	1 sandwich	530	47	25	137	56	75	64	180	90
6″ Chicken Parmesan	1 sandwich	510	64	18	131	54	72	62	173	87
6″ Chipotle Southwest Cheese Steak	1 sandwich	450	48	20	116	48	64	55	153	77
6″ Italian BMT	1 sandwich	450	47	21	116	48	64	55	153	77
6″ Meatball Marinara	1 sandwich	560	63	24	144	60	79	68	190	95
6″ Spicy Italian	1 sandwich	480	46	25	124	51	68	58	163	82

FOOD	AMOUNT	CAL	CARBS	FAT	WALK	RUN	BIKE	SWIM	YOGA	DANCE
6" Subway Melt	1 sandwich	380	48	12	98	40	54	46	129	65
■ Salads—6 Grams of Fat or Less										
Grilled Chicken Breast and Baby Spinach	1 salad	140	11	3	36	15	20	17	48	24
Grilled Chicken Breast Strips	1 salad	140	12	3	36	15	20	17	48	24
Ham	1 salad	120	15	3	31	13	17	15	41	20
Roast Beef	1 salad	130	13	4	34	14	18	16	44	22
Subway Club	1 salad	160	15	4	41	17	23	19	54	27
Turkey Breast	1 salad	120	14	3	31	13	17	15	41	20
Turkey Breast and Ham	1 salad	130	15	3	34	14	18	16	44	22
Veggie Delite	1 salad	60	12	1	15	6	9	7	20	10
■ Other Salads										
BMT	1 salad	290	15	19	75	31	41	35	99	49
Cold Cut Combo	1 salad	250	14	15	64	27	35	30	85	43
■ Dressings										
Atkins Sweet As Honey Mustard	2 oz	200	1	22	52	21	28	24	68	34
Fat Free Italian	2 oz	35	7	0	9	4	5	4	12	6
Ranch	2 oz	200	1	22	52	21	28	24	68	34
■ Breads										
6" Hearty Italian	1 serving	210	41	3	54	22	30	26	71	36
6" Honey Oat	1 serving	250	48	4	64	27	35	30	85	43
6" Italian White	1 serving	190	38	3	49	20	27	23	65	32
6" Italian Herbs and Cheese	1 serving	240	40	6	62	26	34	29	82	41
6" Monterey Cheddar	1 serving	240	39	6	62	26	34	29	82	41
6" Parmesan Oregano	1 serving	210	40	4	54	22	30	26	71	36
6" Roasted Garlic	1 serving	230	45	3	59	24	33	28	78	39
6" Sourdough	1 serving	210	41	3	54	22	30	26	71	36
6" Wheat	1 serving	200	40	3	52	21	28	24	68	34
Atkins Friendly Wrap	1 serving	120	13	5	31	13	17	15	41	20
Deli Style Roll	1 serving	170	32	3	44	18	24	21	58	29
■ Condiments/Toppings										
Bacon	2 strips	45	0	4	12	5	6	5	15	8
Cheddar Cheese	2 triangles	60	0	5	15	6	9	7	20	10
Chipotle Southwest	1.5 tbsp	100	1	10	26	11	14	12	34	17
Fat Free Honey Mustard	1.5 tbsp	30	7	0	8	3	4	4	10	5

FOOD	AMOUNT	CAL	CARBS	FAT	WALK	RUN	BIKE	SWIM	YOGA	DANCE
Fat Free Sweet Onion	1.5 tbsp	40	9	0	10	4	6	5	14	7
Light Mayo	1 tbsp	50	1	5	13	5	7	6	17	9
Mayonnaise	1 tbsp	110	0	12	28	12	16	13	37	19
Mustard (Yellow and Deli Brown)	2 tsp	5	1	0	1	1	1	1	2	1
Olive Oil Blend	1 tsp	45	0	5	12	5	6	5	15	8
Pepperjack Cheese	2 triangles	50	0	4	13	5	7	6	17	9
Processed American Cheese	2 triangles	40	1	4	10	4	6	5	14	7
Provolone Cheese	2 half circles	50	0	4	13	5	7	6	17	9
Ranch	amount on wrap	70	0	8	18	7	10	9	24	12
Shredded Monterey Blend	1 serving	50	1	5	13	5	7	6	17	9
Swiss Cheese Triangles	2 triangles	50	0	5	13	5	7	6	17	9
Vinegar	1 tsp	0	0	0	0	0	0	0	0	0

■ Soup

FOOD	AMOUNT	CAL	CARBS	FAT	WALK	RUN	BIKE	SWIM	YOGA	DANCE
Brown and Wild Rice with Chicken	1 cup	190	17	11	49	20	27	23	65	32
Cheese with Ham and Bacon	1 cup	240	17	15	62	26	34	29	82	41
Chicken and Dumpling	1 cup	130	16	5	34	14	18	16	44	22
Chili Con Carne	1 cup	240	23	10	62	26	34	29	82	41
Cream of Broccoli	1 cup	130	15	6	34	14	18	16	44	22
Cream of Potato with Bacon	1 cup	200	21	11	52	21	28	24	68	34
Golden Broccoli and Cheese	1 cup	180	16	11	46	19	26	22	61	31
Minestrone	1 cup	90	7	4	23	10	13	11	31	15
New England Clam Chowder	1 cup	110	16	4	28	12	16	13	37	19
Roasted Chicken Noodle	1 cup	60	7	2	15	6	9	7	20	10
Spanish Style Chicken with Rice	1 cup	90	13	2	23	10	13	11	31	15
Tomato Garden Vegetable with Rotini	1 cup	100	20	1	26	11	14	12	34	17
Vegetable Beef	1 cup	90	15	1	23	10	13	11	31	15

■ Carb Conscious

FOOD	AMOUNT	CAL	CARBS	FAT	WALK	RUN	BIKE	SWIM	YOGA	DANCE
Tuna Salad	1 salad	360	12	29	93	38	51	44	122	61
Chicken and Bacon Ranch Wrap	1 wrap	440	18	27	113	47	62	54	150	75
Tuna Wrap	1 wrap	440	16	32	113	47	62	54	150	75
Turkey and Bacon Melt	1 wrap	380	20	24	98	40	54	46	129	65
Turkey Breast Wrap	1 wrap	190	18	6	49	20	27	23	65	32

FOOD	AMOUNT	CAL	CARBS	FAT	WALK	RUN	BIKE	SWIM	YOGA	DANCE
■ **Desserts**										
Berry Lishus	1 small	110	28	0	28	12	16	13	37	19
Berry Lishus with Banana	1 small	140	35	0	36	15	20	17	48	24
Chocolate Chip	1 cookie	210	30	10	54	22	30	26	71	36
Chocolate Chunk	1 cookie	220	30	10	57	23	31	27	75	37
Double Chocolate	1 cookie	210	30	10	54	22	30	26	71	36
M&M's	1 cookie	210	30	10	54	22	30	26	71	36
Oatmeal Raisin	1 cookie	200	30	8	52	21	28	24	68	34
Peach Pizazz	1 small	100	26	0	26	11	14	12	34	17
Peanut Butter	1 cookie	220	26	12	57	23	31	27	75	37
Pineapple Delight	1 small	130	33	0	34	14	18	16	44	22
Pineapple Delight with Banana	1 small	160	40	0	41	17	23	19	54	27
Sugar	1 cookie	230	28	12	59	24	33	28	78	39
Sunrise Refresher	1 small	120	29	0	31	13	17	15	41	20
White Macadamia Nut	1 cookie	220	28	11	57	23	31	27	75	37
Taco Bell										
■ **Big Bell Value Menu**										
Grande Soft Taco	1 serving	450	44	21	116	48	64	55	153	77
Double Decker Taco	1 serving	340	39	14	88	36	48	41	116	58
Spicy Chicken Soft Taco	1 serving	180	21	7	46	19	26	22	61	31
Spicy Chicken Burrito	1 serving	420	51	19	108	45	60	51	143	72
1/2 lb Bean Burrito Especial	1 serving	600	82	21	155	64	85	73	204	102
1/2 lb Beef Combo Burrito	1 serving	470	52	19	121	50	67	57	160	80
1/2 lb Beef and Potato Burrito	1 serving	540	66	25	139	58	77	66	184	92
Cheesy Fiesta Potatoes	1 serving	290	28	18	75	31	41	35	99	49
Caramel Apple Empanada	1 serving	290	37	15	75	31	41	35	99	49
■ **Tacos**										
Taco	1 serving	170	13	10	44	18	24	21	58	29
Taco Supreme	1 serving	220	14	14	57	23	31	27	75	37
Double Decker Taco Supreme	1 serving	380	41	18	98	40	54	46	129	65
Soft Taco, Beef	1 serving	210	21	10	54	22	30	26	71	36
Soft Taco Supreme, Beef	1 serving	260	23	14	67	28	37	32	88	44
Ranchero Chicken Soft Taco	1 serving	270	21	14	70	29	38	33	92	46
Grilled Steak Soft Taco	1 serving	280	21	17	72	30	40	34	95	48
■ **Gorditas**										
Gordita Supreme, Beef	1 serving	310	30	16	80	33	44	38	105	53

FOOD	AMOUNT	CAL	CARBS	FAT	WALK	RUN	BIKE	SWIM	YOGA	DANCE
Gordita Supreme, Chicken	1 serving	290	28	12	75	31	41	35	99	49
Gordita Supreme, Steak	1 serving	290	28	13	75	31	41	35	99	49
Gordita Baja, Beef	1 serving	350	31	19	90	37	50	43	119	60
Gordita Baja, Chicken	1 serving	320	29	15	82	34	45	39	109	55
Gordita Baja, Steak	1 serving	320	29	16	82	34	45	39	109	55
Gordita Nacho Cheese, Beef	1 serving	300	32	13	77	32	43	36	102	51
Gordita Nacho Cheese, Chicken	1 serving	270	30	10	70	29	38	33	92	46
Gordita Nacho Cheese, Steak	1 serving	270	30	11	70	29	38	33	92	46
■ **Chalupas**										
Chalupa Supreme, Beef	1 serving	400	31	24	103	43	57	49	136	68
Chalupa Supreme, Chicken	1 serving	370	29	21	95	39	52	45	126	63
Chalupa Supreme, Steak	1 serving	370	29	22	95	39	52	45	126	63
Chalupa Baja, Beef	1 serving	430	32	28	111	46	61	52	146	73
Chalupa Baja, Chicken	1 serving	400	30	24	103	43	57	49	136	68
Chalupa Baja, Steak	1 serving	410	30	25	106	44	58	50	139	70
Chalupa Nacho Cheese, Beef	1 serving	380	33	22	98	40	54	46	129	65
Chalupa Nacho Cheese, Chicken	1 serving	350	31	18	90	37	50	43	119	60
Chalupa Nacho Cheese, Steak	1 serving	360	31	20	93	38	51	44	122	61
■ **Burritos**										
Bean Burrito	1 serving	370	55	10	95	39	52	45	126	63
7-Layer Burrito	1 serving	530	68	21	137	56	75	64	180	90
Chili Cheese Burrito	1 serving	390	40	18	101	42	55	47	133	66
Burrito Supreme, Beef	1 serving	440	52	18	113	47	62	54	150	75
Burrito Supreme, Chicken	1 serving	410	50	14	106	44	58	50	139	70
Burrito Supreme, Steak	1 serving	420	50	16	108	45	60	51	143	72
Fiesta Burrito, Beef	1 serving	390	51	14	101	42	55	47	133	66
Fiesta Burrito, Chicken	1 serving	370	49	11	95	39	52	45	126	63
Fiesta Burrito, Steak	1 serving	370	49	12	95	39	52	45	126	63
Grilled Stuft Burrito, Beef	1 serving	720	80	32	186	77	102	88	245	123
Grilled Stuft Burrito, Chicken	1 serving	670	77	25	173	71	95	82	228	114
Grilled Stuft Burrito, Steak	1 serving	680	77	27	175	72	96	83	231	116
■ **Specialties**										
Tostada	1 serving	250	29	10	64	27	35	30	85	43
Crunchwrap Supreme	1 serving	560	70	24	144	60	79	68	190	95
Mexican Pizza	1 serving	540	47	31	139	58	77	66	184	92

FOOD	AMOUNT	CAL	CARBS	FAT	WALK	RUN	BIKE	SWIM	YOGA	DANCE
Enchirito, Beef	1 serving	380	35	18	98	40	54	46	129	65
Enchirito, Chicken	1 serving	350	33	14	90	37	50	43	119	60
Enchirito, Steak	1 serving	360	33	16	93	38	51	44	122	61
Meximelt	1 serving	290	23	16	75	31	41	35	99	49
Fiesta Taco Salad	1 serving	860	82	46	222	92	122	105	293	147
Fiesta Taco Salad (without shell)	1 serving	490	43	25	126	52	70	60	167	83
Fiesta Taco Salad (without shell or red strips)	1 serving	420	34	21	108	45	60	51	143	72
Express Taco Salad	1 serving	630	58	34	162	67	89	77	214	107
Express Taco Salad (without chips)	1 serving	410	32	21	106	44	58	50	139	70
Cheese Quesadilla	1 serving	490	39	28	126	52	70	60	167	83
Chicken Quesadilla	1 serving	540	40	30	139	58	77	66	184	92
Steak Quesadilla	1 serving	540	40	31	139	58	77	66	184	92
Zesty Chicken Border Bowl	1 serving	730	69	40	188	78	104	89	248	124
Zesty Chicken Border Bowl (no dressing)	1 serving	490	64	16	126	52	70	60	167	83
Southwest Steak Border Bowl	1 serving	690	79	28	178	73	98	84	235	118
■ Nachos and Sides										
Nachos	1 serving	320	32	20	82	34	45	39	109	55
Nachos Supreme	1 serving	460	42	26	119	49	65	56	156	78
Nachos Bellgrande	1 serving	790	79	44	204	84	112	96	269	135
Pintos 'n Cheese	1 serving	180	20	7	46	19	26	22	61	31
Mexican Rice	1 serving	200	26	9	52	21	28	24	68	34
Cinnamon Twists	1 serving	160	27	5	41	17	23	19	54	27
Wendy's										
■ Salads										
Mandarin Chicken Salad	1 salad (348 g)	170	18	2	44	18	24	21	58	29
Mandarin Chicken Salad with Crispy Noodles, Roasted Almonds and Oriental Sesame Dressing	1 salad (447 g)	450	53	26	116	48	64	55	153	77
Spring Mix Salad	1 salad (313 g)	180	13	11	46	19	26	22	61	31
Spring Mix Salad with Home-style Garlic Croutons and House Vinaigrette Dressing	1 salad (391 g)	440	30	32	113	47	62	54	150	75

FOOD	AMOUNT	CAL	CARBS	FAT	WALK	RUN	BIKE	SWIM	YOGA	DANCE
Chicken BLT Salad	1 salad (374 g)	340	12	18	88	36	48	41	116	58
Chicken BLT Salad with Homestyle Garlic Croutons and Honey Mustard Dressing	1 salad (452 g)	690	32	47	178	73	98	84	235	118
Taco Supremo Salad	1 salad (494 g)	380	33	17	98	40	54	46	129	65
Taco Supremo Salad with Salsa, Reduced Fat Sour Cream, and Taco Chips	1 salad (650 g)	670	70	30	173	71	95	82	228	114
Homestyle Chicken Strips Salad	1 salad (417 g)	450	35	22	116	48	64	55	153	77
Homestyle Chicken Strips Salad with Creamy Ranch Dressing	1 salad (481 g)	680	40	45	175	72	96	83	231	116
Side Salad	1 salad (166 g)	35	8	0	9	4	5	4	12	6
Caesar Side Salad	1 salad (99 g)	70	3	5	18	7	10	9	24	12
Caesar Side Salad with Homestyle Garlic Croutons and Caesar Dressing	1 salad (141 g)	260	13	20	67	28	37	32	88	44
Oriental Sesame Dressing	1 packet	190	21	11	49	20	27	23	65	32
House Vinaigrette Dressing	1 packet	190	8	18	49	20	27	23	65	32
Honey Mustard Dressing	1 packet	280	11	26	72	30	40	34	95	48
Creamy Ranch Dressing	1 packet	230	5	23	59	24	33	28	78	39
Fat Free French Dressing	1 packet	80	19	0	21	9	11	10	27	14
Reduced Fat Creamy Ranch	1 packet	100	6	8	26	11	14	12	34	17
Low Fat Honey Mustard	1 packet	110	21	3	28	12	16	13	37	19
Salsa	85 g	30	6	0	8	3	4	4	10	5
Caesar Dressing	1 packet	120	1	13	31	13	17	15	41	20
Reduced Fat Sour Cream	1 packet	50	2	4	13	5	7	6	17	9
Homestyle Garlic Croutons	1 packet	70	9	3	18	7	10	9	24	12
Roasted Almonds	1 packet	130	4	11	34	14	18	16	44	22
Crispy Noodles	1 packet	60	10	2	15	6	9	7	20	10
Taco Chips	1 bag	210	29	9	54	22	30	26	71	36
■ **Frosty**										
Junior Frosty	1 drink (113 g)	160	28	4	41	17	23	19	54	27

FOOD	AMOUNT	CAL	CARBS	FAT	WALK	RUN	BIKE	SWIM	YOGA	DANCE
Small Frosty	1 drink (227 g)	330	56	8	85	35	47	40	112	56
Medium Frosty	1 drink (298 g)	430	74	11	111	46	61	52	146	73
Fix 'n Mix Frosty	1 drink (117 g)	170	29	4	44	18	24	21	58	29
Oreo Cookie Crumbles	1 packet (21 g)	100	15	5	26	11	14	12	34	17
Butterfinger Candy Crumbles	1 packet (28 g)	130	20	5	34	14	18	16	44	22
M&M's Candy Crumbles	1 packet (28 g)	140	20	6	36	15	20	17	48	24
■ **Sides**										
Mandarin Orange Cup	5 oz	80	19	0	21	9	11	10	27	14
Low-Fat Strawberry Flavored Yogurt	1 container (194 g)	200	37	2	52	21	28	24	68	34
Low-Fat Strawberry Flavored Yogurt with Granola Topping	1 container + 1 packet	310	52	7	80	33	44	38	105	53
Plain Baked Potato	10 oz	270	61	0	70	29	38	33	92	46
Sour Cream and Chives Baked Potato	1 potato (311 g)	320	63	4	82	34	45	39	109	55
Broccoli and Cheese Baked Potato	1 potato (397 g)	340	69	4	88	36	48	41	116	58
Bacon and Cheese Baked Potato	1 potato (366 g)	460	69	13	119	49	65	56	156	78
Small Chili	8 oz	220	23	6	57	23	31	27	75	37
Large Chili	12 oz	330	35	9	85	35	47	40	112	56
Kids' Meal French Fries	3.2 oz	280	37	14	72	30	40	34	95	48
Medium French Fries	5 oz	440	58	21	113	47	62	54	150	75
Biggie French Fries	5.6 oz	490	64	24	126	52	70	60	167	83
Great Biggie French Fries	6.7 oz	590	77	28	152	63	84	72	201	101
■ **Chicken Strips/Nuggets**										
Homestyle Chicken Strips	3 strips	410	33	18	106	44	58	50	139	70
4-Piece Chicken Nuggets	4 nuggets	180	10	11	46	19	26	22	61	31
5-Piece Chicken Nuggets	5 nuggets	220	13	14	57	23	31	27	75	37
Deli Honey Mustard Sauce	1 packet	170	6	16	44	18	24	21	58	29
Spicy Southwest Chipotle Sauce	1 packet	150	5	15	39	16	21	18	51	26

FOOD	AMOUNT	CAL	CARBS	FAT	WALK	RUN	BIKE	SWIM	YOGA	DANCE
Heartland Ranch Sauce	1 packet	200	1	22	52	21	28	24	68	34
Barbecue Sauce	1 packet	45	10	0	12	5	6	5	15	8
Sweet and Sour Sauce	1 packet	50	13	0	13	5	7	6	17	9
Honey Mustard Nugget Sauce	1 packet	130	6	12	34	14	18	16	44	22
■ **Burgers**										
Jr. Hamburger	117 g	280	34	9	72	30	40	34	95	48
Jr. Cheeseburger	129 g	320	34	13	82	34	45	39	109	55
Jr. Cheeseburger Deluxe	179 g	360	37	16	93	38	51	44	122	61
Jr. Bacon Cheeseburger	165 g	380	34	18	98	40	54	46	129	65
Hamburger, Kids' Meal	110 g	270	33	9	70	29	38	33	92	46
Cheeseburger, Kids' Meal	122 g	320	34	13	82	34	45	39	109	55
Classic Single with Everything	218 g	420	37	19	108	45	60	51	143	72
Big Bacon Classic	282 g	580	46	29	149	62	82	71	197	99
■ **Chicken Sandwiches**										
Ultimate Chicken Grill Sandwich	225 g	360	44	7	93	38	51	44	122	61
Spicy Chicken Fillet Sandwich	224 g	510	57	18	131	54	72	62	173	87
Homestyle Chicken Fillet Sandwich	230 g	540	57	22	139	58	77	66	184	92

Deli

Sausage and Wurst										
Beerwurst pork and beef salami	2 oz	155	2	13	40	17	22	19	53	26
Beerwurst pork salami	1 slice (23 g)	55	0	4	14	6	8	7	19	9
Berliner pork sausage	1 slice (23 g)	53	1	4	14	6	8	6	18	9
Blood sausage	1 slice (25 g)	95	0	9	24	10	13	11	32	16
Pork and beef chorizo	1 link	273	1	23	70	29	39	33	93	47
Pork bratwurst	1 link	283	2	25	73	30	40	34	96	48
Veal bratwurst	1 link	286	0	27	74	30	41	35	97	49
Chicken bratwurst	1 link	148	0	9	38	16	21	18	50	25
Light smoked beef, pork, and turkey bratwurst	1 serving (2.66 oz)	123	1	9	32	13	17	15	42	21
Braunschweiger sausage	1 slice (1 oz)	92	1	8	24	10	13	11	31	16

FOOD	AMOUNT	CAL	CARBS	FAT	WALK	RUN	BIKE	SWIM	YOGA	DANCE
Meatless sausage	1 link	64	0	5	16	7	9	8	22	11
Beef sausage	1 oz	113	0	11	29	12	16	14	38	19
Smoked beef sausage	1 oz	88	1	8	23	9	12	11	30	15
Reduced-fat turkey sausage	1 oz	56	3	3	14	6	8	7	19	10
Louis Rich smoked turkey sausage	1 oz	45	1	3	12	5	6	5	15	8
Pork sausage	1 link (24 g)	81	0	7	21	9	11	10	28	14
Italian pork sausage	1 link (83 g)	286	4	23	74	30	41	35	97	49
Kielbasa	1 oz	88	1	8	23	9	12	11	30	15
Knackwurst	1 link (72 g)	221	2	20	57	24	31	27	75	38
Liverwurst	1 oz	92	1	8	24	10	13	11	31	16
Polish sausage	1 oz	92	0	8	24	10	13	11	31	16
Pork and beef sausage	1 link (13 g)	51	0	5	13	5	7	6	18	9
Smoked pork sausage	1 link (68 g)	265	1	22	68	28	38	32	90	45
Smoked pork and beef sausage	1 link (68 g)	218	2	20	56	23	31	26	74	37
Thuringer or cervelat	2 oz	203	2	17	52	22	29	25	69	35
Oscar Mayer Thuringer Cervelat Beef Summer Sausage	2 slices (46 g)	142	1	12	37	15	20	17	48	24
Oscar Mayer Thuringer Cervelat Summer Sausage	2 slices (46 g)	140	0	12	36	15	20	17	48	24
Canned Vienna sausage	1 sausage (16 g)	37	0	3	9	4	5	4	13	6
Oscar Mayer Braunschweiger Sausage	1 slice (1 oz)	93	1	8	24	10	13	11	32	16
Oscar Mayer Pork Sausage Links	2 links (48 g)	165	0	15	42	18	23	20	56	28
Smoked pork and beef sausage with cheddar cheese	1 oz	83	1	7	21	9	12	10	28	14
Turkey breakfast sausage links	2 links (56 g)	132	1	10	34	14	19	16	45	22
Swisswurst	1 oz	86	0	8	22	9	12	10	29	15
Yachtwurst	2 oz	150	1	13	39	16	21	18	51	26
Turkey and pork sausage	1 patty, cooked	77	0	6	20	8	11	9	26	13

FOOD	AMOUNT	CAL	CARBS	FAT	WALK	RUN	BIKE	SWIM	YOGA	DANCE
Spread										
Liverwurst spread	.25 cup	168	3	14	43	18	24	20	57	29
Chicken spread	1 serving (2 oz)	88	2	10	23	9	13	11	30	15
Poultry salad spread	1 tbsp	26	1	2	7	3	4	3	9	4
Roast beef spread	.25 cup	127	2	9	33	14	18	15	43	22
Oscar Mayer Chicken, Beef, and Pork Sandwich Spread	1 oz	66	4	5	17	7	9	8	22	11
Bologna										
Beef bologna	1 slice (1 oz)	88	1	8	23	9	12	11	30	15
Beef and pork bologna	1 oz	87	2	7	23	9	12	11	30	15
Low-fat beef and pork bologna	1 slice (1 oz)	64	1	5	16	7	9	8	22	11
Pork bologna	1 slice (1 oz)	70	0	6	18	7	10	9	24	12
Pork, turkey, and beef bologna	1 oz	94	2	8	24	10	13	11	32	16
Light turkey and pork bologna	1 oz	59	1	5	15	6	8	7	20	10
Lebanon beef bologna	1 oz	52	0	3	13	6	7	6	18	9
Louis Rich turkey bologna	1 oz	52	1	4	13	5	7	6	18	9
Oscar Mayer Beef, Pork, and Chicken Bologna	1 oz	89	1	8	23	9	13	11	30	15
Oscar Mayer Beef Bologna	1 slice (1 oz)	88	1	8	23	9	13	11	30	15
Oscar Mayer Light Beef Bologna	1 slice (1 oz)	56	2	4	14	6	8	7	19	10
Oscar Mayer Fat Free Beef Bologna	1 oz	22	2	0	6	2	3	3	8	4
Oscar Mayer Light Beef, Pork, and Chicken Bologna	1 slice (1 oz)	57	2	4	15	6	8	7	19	10
Oscar Mayer Wisconsin Made Ring Bologna	1 oz	88	1	8	23	9	12	11	30	15
Oscar Mayer Smokies Link Sausage	1 link (43 g)	130	1	12	33	14	18	16	44	22
Oscar Mayer Beef Smokies	1 link (43 g)	127	1	11	33	14	18	15	43	22
Oscar Mayer Cheese Smokies	1 link (43 g)	130	1	12	34	14	18	16	44	22
Oscar Mayer Little Pork Smokies	1 link (9 g)	27	0	2	7	3	4	3	9	5

FOOD	AMOUNT	CAL	CARBS	FAT	WALK	RUN	BIKE	SWIM	YOGA	DANCE
Oscar Mayer Little Cheese Pork/Turkey Smokies	1 link (9 g)	28	0	3	7	3	4	3	10	5
Chicken/Pork/Beef Bologna	1 oz	76	2	6	20	8	11	9	26	13
Chicken/Pork Bologna	1 oz	94	1	9	24	10	13	11	32	16
Chicken										
Oven-roasted chicken breast roll	1 serving (2 oz)	75	1	4	19	8	11	9	26	13
Fat-free mesquite-flavored chicken breast	1 oz	22	1	0	6	2	3	3	7	4
Louis Rich Classic Carving Board Chicken Breast	1 oz	27	1	0	7	3	4	3	9	5
Louis Rich Oven Roasted Deluxe Chicken Breast	1 oz	28	1	1	7	3	4	3	10	5
Louis Rich Whjte Oven Roasted Chicken Breast	1 oz	36	1	2	9	4	5	4	12	6
Oscar Mayer Honey Glazed Chicken Breast	1 oz	28	1	0	7	3	4	3	10	5
Oscar Mayer Oven Roasted Fat Free Chicken Breast	1 oz	24	0	0	6	3	3	3	8	4
Perdue Short Cuts Honey Roasted Grilled Chicken Breast Filets	1 filet	80	5	1	21	9	11	10	27	14
Corned Beef										
Jellied corned beef	1 slice (1 oz)	43	0	2	11	5	6	5	15	7
Corned beef brisket	3 oz	213	0	16	55	23	30	26	72	36
Chef-Mate Canned Corned Beef Hash	1 cup	486	29	30	125	52	69	59	165	83
Hormel Canned Corned Beef Hash	1 cup	387	22	24	100	41	55	47	132	66
Ham										
Chopped ham	1 slice	50	0	4	13	5	7	6	17	9
Extra-lean sliced ham	3 slices (63 g)	69	2	2	18	7	10	8	24	12
Sliced ham (11% fat)	1 slice (1 oz)	91	2	5	24	10	13	11	31	16
Minced ham	2 oz	149	1	12	38	16	21	18	51	25
Ham salad spread	1 tbsp	32	2	2	8	3	5	4	11	5
Ham and cheese loaf or roll	1 slice (1 oz)	67	1	5	17	7	10	8	23	11

FOOD	AMOUNT	CAL	CARBS	FAT	WALK	RUN	BIKE	SWIM	YOGA	DANCE
Ham and cheese spread	1 tbsp	37	0	3	9	4	5	4	13	6
Smoked honey ham	1 oz	34	2	1	9	4	5	4	12	6
Prosciutto	2 slices (30 g)	70	0	5	18	7	10	9	24	12
Oscar Mayer Ham and Cheese Loaf	1 oz	66	1	5	17	7	9	8	22	11
Oscar Mayer Chopped Ham	1 slice (1 oz)	50	1	3	13	5	7	6	17	9
Oscar Mayer 96% Fat Free Ham	1 oz	29	1	1	7	3	4	4	10	5
Oscar Mayer Ham	1 oz	29	0	1	7	3	4	4	10	5
Oscar Mayer Ham with Honey	1 oz	31	1	1	8	3	4	4	11	5
Oscar Mayer Smoked Ham	1 oz	28	0	1	7	3	4	3	10	5
Oscar Mayer Fat Free Smoked Ham	1 oz	20	1	0	5	2	3	2	7	3
Pork										
Pork olive loaf	2 slices (2 oz)	134	5	9	35	14	19	16	46	23
Pork and beef peppered loaf	2 slices (2 oz)	84	3	4	22	9	12	10	29	14
Pork and beef pepperoni	15 slices (1 oz)	135	1	12	35	14	19	16	46	23
Pork pickle and pimento loaf	1 slice (38 g)	86	3	6	22	9	12	10	29	15
Pork picnic loaf	2 slices (2 oz)	132	3	9	34	14	19	16	45	22
Pork/beef sandwich spread	1 tbsp	35	2	3	9	4	5	4	12	6
Scrapple	2 oz	119	8	8	31	13	17	15	41	20
Oscar Mayer Pork/Beef/ Chicken Sandwich Spread	1 oz	66	4	5	17	7	9	8	22	11
Oscar Mayer Olive Loaf	1 oz	74	2	6	19	8	10	9	25	13
Spam										
Hormel Spam	1 oz	87	1	8	22	9	12	11	30	15
Hormel Lite Spam	1 oz	53	0	4	14	6	8	6	18	9
Pastrami										
Turkey pastrami	2 slices (2 oz)	70	2	2	18	7	10	9	24	12
Cured beef pastrami	2 slices (2 oz)	82	0	3	21	9	12	10	28	14

FOOD	AMOUNT	CAL	CARBS	FAT	WALK	RUN	BIKE	SWIM	YOGA	DANCE
98% fat-free beef pastrami	6 slices (2 oz)	54	1	1	14	6	8	7	18	9
Pâté										
Chicken liver pâté	1 tbsp	26	1	2	7	3	4	3	9	4
Pâté de foie gras	1 tbsp	60	1	6	15	6	9	7	20	10
Salami										
Beef salami	1 oz	73	1	6	19	8	10	9	25	12
Cooked beef and pork salami	1 oz	71	1	6	18	8	10	9	24	12
Turkey salami	1 oz	43	0	3	11	5	6	5	15	7
Dry or hard pork salami	1 oz	114	0	9	29	12	16	14	39	19
Dry or hard beef/pork salami	3 slices (1 oz)	104	1	8	27	11	15	13	35	18
Italian pork salami	1 oz	119	0	10	31	13	17	14	40	20
Louis Rich Turkey Salami	1 serving	41	0	3	11	4	6	5	14	7
Louis Rich Turkey Salami Cotto	1 oz	42	0	3	11	4	6	5	14	7
Oscar Mayer Beef Salami Cotto	2 slices (46 g)	95	1	7	24	10	13	12	32	16
Oscar Mayer Beef, Pork, and Chicken Salami Cotto	2 slices (46 g)	113	1	9	29	12	16	14	38	19
Oscar Mayer Genoa Salami	3 slices (1 oz)	105	0	9	27	11	15	13	36	18
Oscar Mayer Hard Salami	3 slices (1 oz)	99	0	8	26	11	14	12	34	17
Turkey										
Turkey breast	1 oz	29	1	0	7	3	4	4	10	5
Smoked 97% fat-free lemon-pepper turkey breast	1 slice (1 oz)	27	0	0	7	3	4	3	9	5
Turkey ham	1 oz	35	1	1	9	4	5	4	12	6
Extra-lean turkey ham	1 oz	33	0	1	9	4	5	4	11	6
Louis Rich Turkey Ham	1 oz	32	0	1	8	3	4	4	11	5
Louis Rich Turkey Bacon	1 oz	70	0	6	18	7	10	9	24	12
Light meat turkey roll	1 oz	42	0	2	11	4	6	5	14	7
Light and dark meat turkey roll	1 oz	42	1	2	11	4	6	5	14	7
Hormel Turkey Pepperoni	1 oz	68	1	3	18	7	10	8	23	12
Louis Rich Oven Roasted White Turkey Breast	1 oz	28	1	1	7	3	4	3	9	5
Louis Rich Smoked Sliced White Turkey Breast	1 oz	28	1	1	7	3	4	3	10	5

FOOD	AMOUNT	CAL	CARBS	FAT	WALK	RUN	BIKE	SWIM	YOGA	DANCE
Louis Rich Honey Roasted Fat Free Turkey	1 oz	29	1	0	7	3	4	4	10	5
Louis Rich Oven Roasted Fat Free Turkey Breast	1 oz	24	1	0	6	3	3	3	8	4
Louis Rich Smoked Turkey Sausage	1 oz	45	1	3	12	5	6	5	15	8
Louis Rich Smoked Carving Board Turkey Breast	1 slice	21	0	0	5	2	3	3	7	4
Louis Rich Smoked Fat Free Turkey Breast	1 serving (2 oz)	52	1	0	13	6	7	6	18	9
Oscar Mayer Fat Free Smoked Turkey Breast	1 oz	22	1	0	6	2	3	3	7	4
White rotisserie turkey	1 oz	31	2	1	8	3	4	4	11	5
Soy Deli										
Lightlife Smart Deli Bologna	4 slices (57 g)	60	0	0	15	6	9	7	20	10
Lightlife Smart Deli Turkey	4 slices (57 g)	80	4	0	21	9	11	10	27	14
Lightlife Original Smart Ground	.33 cup	80	7	1	21	9	11	10	27	14
Lightlife Taco Smart Ground	.33 cup	70	5	0	18	7	10	9	24	12
Lightlife Smart Ham	4 slices (57 g)	90	5	0	23	10	13	11	31	15
Yves Veggie Bologna	4 slices (62 g)	80	4	1	21	9	11	10	27	14
Yves Veggie Salami	4 slices (62 g)	90	5	0	23	10	13	11	31	15
Yves Veggie Ground Round	.33 cup	60	5	1	15	6	9	7	20	10
Yves Veggie Turkey	4 slices (62 g)	90	4	2	23	10	13	11	31	15
Hot Dogs (57g unless noted)										
■ Beef										
Beef frank	1 frank	188	2	17	48	20	27	23	64	32
Low-fat beef frank	1 frank	133	1	11	34	14	19	16	45	23
Beef/pork frank	1 frank	174	1	16	45	19	25	21	59	30
Low-fat beef/pork frank	1 frank	88	3	6	23	9	12	11	30	15
Fat-free beef/pork/turkey frank	1 frank	62	6	1	16	7	9	8	21	11
Ball Park Beef Frank	1 frank	180	3	16	46	19	26	22	61	31
Ball Park Nonfat Frank	1 frank (50 g)	40	4	0	10	4	6	5	14	7

FOOD	AMOUNT	CAL	CARBS	FAT	WALK	RUN	BIKE	SWIM	YOGA	DANCE
Boar's Head Beef Frank	1 frank	160	1	14	41	17	23	19	54	27
Boar's Head Lite Beef Frank	1 frank (45 g)	90	0	6	23	10	13	11	31	15
Boar's Head Skinless Beef Frank	1 frank (45 g)	120	0	11	31	13	17	15	41	20
Healthy Choice Beef Frank	1 frank (50 g)	70	7	3	18	7	10	9	24	12
Hebrew National Beef Frank	1 frank (49 g)	150	1	14	39	16	21	18	51	26
Hebrew National 97% Fat Free Beef Frank	1 frank (49 g)	45	3	2	12	5	6	5	15	8
Hebrew National Cocktail Beef Frank	5 links (57 g)	180	1	16	46	19	26	22	61	31
Hebrew National 1/4 lb Beef Dinner Frank	1 frank (113 g)	350	1	32	90	37	50	43	119	60
Hebrew National Beef Franks in a Blanket	5 franks (81 g)	290	8	24	75	31	41	35	99	49
Hebrew National Reduced Fat Beef Frank	1 frank (49 g)	120	0	10	31	13	17	15	41	20
Oscar Mayer Beef Frank	1 frank (45 g)	147	1	14	38	16	21	18	50	25
Oscar Mayer Bun-Length Wiener	1 frank	185	2	17	48	20	26	22	63	31
Oscar Mayer Fat-Free Wiener	1 frank (50 g)	39	3	0	10	4	6	5	13	7
Oscar Mayer Light Wiener	1 frank	110	2	8	28	12	16	13	37	19
Hormel Wrangles Beef Frank	1 frank	162	1	14	42	17	23	20	55	28
Oscar Mayer XXL Beef Frank	1 frank (76 g)	240	1	23	62	26	34	29	82	41

■ Chicken

FOOD	AMOUNT	CAL	CARBS	FAT	WALK	RUN	BIKE	SWIM	YOGA	DANCE
Chicken frank	1 frank	146	4	11	38	16	21	18	50	25

■ Turkey

FOOD	AMOUNT	CAL	CARBS	FAT	WALK	RUN	BIKE	SWIM	YOGA	DANCE
Turkey frank	1 frank	129	1	10	33	14	18	16	44	22
Butcher Boy Turkey Frank	1 serving	134	3	10	34	14	19	16	46	23
Louis Rich Turkey Frank	1 frank (45 g)	101	1	8	26	11	14	12	34	17
Louis Rich Turkey Cheese Frank	1 frank (45 g)	109	1	9	28	12	15	13	37	19
Oscar Mayer Turkey Cheese Hot Dog	1 frank (45 g)	143	1	13	37	15	20	17	49	24

FOOD	AMOUNT	CAL	CARBS	FAT	WALK	RUN	BIKE	SWIM	YOGA	DANCE
■ Pork										
Pork frank	1 link (76 g)	204	0	18	53	22	29	25	70	35
■ Mixed meat										
Baked beans with franks	1 cup	368	40	17	95	39	52	45	125	63
Ball Park Light Frank	1 frank (50 g)	100	3	7	26	11	14	12	34	17
Boar's Head Natural Casing Pork and Beef Frank	1 frank	150	0	14	39	16	21	18	51	26
Boar's Head Skinless Pork and Beef Frank	1 frank	150	0	14	39	16	21	18	51	26
Louis Rich Turkey and Chicken Frank	1 frank (45 g)	85	2	6	22	9	12	10	29	14
Louis Rich Turkey and Chicken Cheese Frank	1 frank (45 g)	90	2	7	23	10	13	11	31	15
Oscar Mayer Pork/Turkey Wiener	1 frank (45 g)	147	1	13	38	16	21	18	50	25
Oscar Mayer Light Pork, Turkey, Beef Wiener	1 frank	111	2	8	29	12	16	13	38	19
■ Meatless										
Meatless frank	1 frank (70 g)	163	5	10	42	17	23	20	55	28
Meatless sausage	1 link	64	2	5	16	7	9	8	22	11
Meatless breaded and fried chicken	1 cup, pieces	393	14	21	101	42	56	48	134	67
Meatless fish sticks	3 sticks	244	8	15	63	26	35	30	83	42
Meatless luncheon slices	3 thin slices	79	2	5	20	8	11	10	27	13
Meatless meatballs	1 cup	284	12	13	73	30	40	35	97	48
Soy burger	1 patty	125	9	4	32	13	18	15	43	21
Vegetarian fillets	1 fillet (3 oz)	246	8	15	63	26	35	30	84	42
Meatless sandwich spread	1 tbsp	22	1	1	6	2	3	3	7	4
Vegetarian meatloaf	1 slice (2 oz)	110	4	5	28	12	16	13	37	19
Meatless bacon	3 strips	46	1	4	12	5	7	6	16	8
Meatless bacon bits	1 tbsp	33	2	2	9	4	5	4	11	6
■ Salads										
Homemade coleslaw	.5 cup	41	7	2	11	4	6	5	14	7
Homemade potato salad	1 cup	358	28	21	92	38	51	43	122	61

FOOD	AMOUNT	CAL	CARBS	FAT	WALK	RUN	BIKE	SWIM	YOGA	DANCE
Canned sauerkraut	1 cup	27	6	0	7	3	4	3	9	5
Tuna salad	1 cup	383	19	19	99	41	54	47	130	65
Coleslaw	.5 cup	41	7	2	11	4	6	5	14	7
Chicken salad	.5 cup	200	0	11	52	21	28	24	68	34
Low-fat tuna salad	1 cup	240	6	5	62	26	34	29	82	41
Black bean salad	4 oz	130	19	4	34	14	18	16	44	22
Four-bean salad	4 oz	120	26	1	31	13	17	15	41	20
■ **Pickles**										
Vlasic Kosher Dill Spears	1 oz	5	1	0	1	1	1	1	2	1

Poultry

Chicken

■ Chicken Breast with Skin

FOOD	AMOUNT	CAL	CARBS	FAT	WALK	RUN	BIKE	SWIM	YOGA	DANCE
Roasted chicken breast with skin	.5 breast, bone removed	193	0	8	50	21	27	23	66	33
Fried, batter-dipped chicken breast with skin	.5 breast, bone removed	364	13	18	94	39	52	44	124	62
Fried, floured chicken breast with skin	.5 breast, bone removed	218	2	9	56	23	31	27	74	37
Stewed chicken breast with skin	.5 breast, bone removed	202	0	8	52	22	29	25	69	34
■ **Skinless Chicken Breast**										
Fried chicken breast, no skin	.5 breast, bone removed	161	0	4	41	17	23	20	55	27
Roasted chicken breast, no skin	.5 breast, bone removed	142	0	3	37	15	20	17	48	24
Stewed chicken breast, no skin	.5 breast, bone removed	143	0	3	37	15	20	17	49	24
Fat-free mesquite-flavored chicken breast	2 slices (95 g)	34	1	0	9	4	5	4	12	6
Louis Rich Oven Roasted Deluxe Chicken Breast	1 oz	28	1	1	7	3	4	3	10	5

FOOD	AMOUNT	CAL	CARBS	FAT	WALK	RUN	BIKE	SWIM	YOGA	DANCE
Oscar Mayer Honey Glazed Chicken Breast	1 oz	28	1	0	7	3	4	3	10	5
Perdue Short Cuts Honey Roasted Grilled Chicken Breast Filets	1 filet	80	5	1	21	9	11	10	27	14
■ **Chicken Drumstick with Skin**										
Fried, batter-dipped drumstick with skin	1 drumstick, bone removed	193	6	11	50	21	27	23	66	33
Fried, floured drumstick with skin	1 drumstick, bone removed	120	1	7	31	13	17	15	41	20
Roasted drumstick with skin	1 drumstick, bone removed	112	0	6	29	12	16	14	38	19
Stewed drumstick with skin	1 drumstick, bone removed	116	0	6	30	12	16	14	39	20
■ **Chicken Drumstick, No Skin**										
Fried drumstick, no skin	1 drumstick, bone removed	82	0	3	21	9	12	10	28	14
Roasted drumstick, no skin	1 drumstick, bone removed	76	0	2	20	8	11	9	26	13
Stewed drumstick, no skin	1 drumstick, bone removed	78	0	3	20	8	11	9	27	13
■ **Chicken Thigh with Skin**										
Fried, batter-dipped chicken thigh with skin	1 thigh, bone removed	238	8	14	61	25	34	29	81	41
Fried, floured chicken thigh with skin	1 thigh, bone removed	162	2	9	42	17	23	20	55	28
Roasted chicken thigh with skin	1 thigh, bone removed	153	0	10	39	16	22	19	52	26

FOOD	AMOUNT	CAL	CARBS	FAT	WALK	RUN	BIKE	SWIM	YOGA	DANCE
Stewed chicken thigh with skin	1 thigh, bone removed	158	0	10	41	17	22	19	54	27
■ Chicken Thigh, No Skin										
Fried chicken thigh, no skin	1 thigh, bone removed	113	1	5	29	12	16	14	38	19
Roasted chicken thigh, no skin	1 thigh, bone removed	109	0	6	28	12	15	13	37	19
Stewed chicken thigh, no skin	1 thigh, bone removed	107	0	5	28	11	15	13	36	18
■ Chicken Wing with Skin										
Fried, batter-dipped chicken wing with skin	1 wing, no bone	159	5	11	41	17	23	19	54	27
Fried, floured chicken wing with skin	1 wing, no bone	104	1	7	27	11	15	13	35	18
Roasted chicken wing with skin	1 wing, no bone	99	0	7	26	11	14	12	34	17
Stewed chicken wing with skin	1 wing, no bone	100	0	7	26	11	14	12	34	17
■ Chicken Wing, No Skin										
Fried chicken wing, no skin	1 wing, no bone	42	0	2	11	4	6	5	14	7
Roasted chicken wing, no skin	1 wing, no bone	43	0	2	11	5	6	5	15	7
Stewed chicken wing, no skin	1 wing, no bone	43	0	2	11	5	6	5	15	7
■ Other Chicken										
Canned chicken liver pâté	1 oz	57	2	4	15	6	8	7	19	10
Pan-fried chicken liver	1 oz	48	0	2	12	5	7	6	16	8
Chicken liver, simmered	1 oz	47	0	2	12	5	7	6	16	8
Chicken hearts, simmered	1 oz	52	0	2	13	6	7	6	18	9
Roasted chicken capon with skin	4 oz (includes bone)	256	0	13	66	27	36	31	87	44
Stewed dark meat chicken, no skin	4 oz (includes bone)	289	0	17	74	31	41	35	98	49

FOOD	AMOUNT	CAL	CARBS	FAT	WALK	RUN	BIKE	SWIM	YOGA	DANCE
Stewed light meat chicken, no skin	4 oz (includes bone)	239	0	9	62	25	34	29	81	41
Stewed chicken with skin	4 oz (includes bone)	319	0	21	82	34	45	39	109	54
Roasted dark meat chicken, no skin	4 oz (includes bone)	199	0	10	51	21	28	24	68	34
Roasted light meat chicken, no skin	4 oz (includes bone)	171	0	5	44	18	24	21	58	29
Roasted chicken with skin	4 oz (includes bone)	250	0	15	64	27	35	30	85	43
Canned chicken with broth	1 cup	377	2	17	97	40	54	46	128	64
Breaded and fried meatless chicken	1 cup pieces	393	14	21	101	42	56	48	134	67
Arby's Chicken Tenders	3 pieces	434	32	21	112	46	62	53	148	74
Burger King Chicken Tenders	4 pieces	170	10	9	44	18	24	21	58	29
Health Is Wealth Chicken Nuggets	4 nuggets	150	9	6	39	16	21	18	51	26
Health Is Wealth Chicken Tenders	3 tenders	130	11	3	34	14	18	16	44	22
McDonald's Chicken McNuggets	4 pieces	170	10	10	44	18	24	21	58	29
Perdue Rotisserie Chicken, White Meat	3 oz (bone removed)	140	0	7	36	15	20	17	48	24
Perdue Rotisserie Chicken, Dark Meat	3 oz (bone removed)	180	0	13	46	19	26	22	61	31
Wendy's Chicken Nuggets	4 nuggets	180	10	11	46	19	26	22	61	31
Turkey										
■ **Fryer-Roasters**										
Roasted back with skin	4 oz (includes bone)	228	0	11	59	24	32	28	78	39
Roasted back, no skin	4 oz (includes bone)	190	0	6	49	20	27	23	65	32
Roasted breast with skin	4 oz (includes bone)	171	0	4	44	18	24	21	58	29

FOOD	AMOUNT	CAL	CARBS	FAT	WALK	RUN	BIKE	SWIM	YOGA	DANCE
Roasted breast, no skin	4 oz (includes bone)	151	0	1	39	16	21	18	51	26
Roasted dark meat with skin	4 oz (includes bone)	204	0	8	53	22	29	25	69	35
Roasted dark meat, no skin	4 oz (includes bone)	181	0	5	47	19	26	22	62	31
Roasted light meat with skin	4 oz (includes bone)	184	0	5	47	20	26	22	63	31
Roasted light meat, no skin	4 oz (includes bone)	157	0	1	40	17	22	19	53	27
Roasted leg with skin	1 leg (bone removed)	416	0	13	107	44	59	51	141	71
Roasted leg, no skin	1 leg (bone removed)	356	0	8	92	38	50	43	121	61
Roasted wing with skin	1 wing (bone removed)	186	0	9	48	20	26	23	63	32
Roasted wing, no skin	1 wing (bone removed)	98	0	2	25	10	14	12	33	17
■ **Fast Food Turkey**										
Boston Market Roasted Turkey	5 oz	180	0	3	46	19	26	22	61	31
Cousins Subs Turkey Breast Sub	1 7½" sub	537	50	28	138	57	76	65	183	91
Denny's Roast Turkey and Stuffing	14 oz	388	38	3	100	41	55	47	132	66
Subway 6" Turkey Breast Sub	1 sub	280	46	5	72	30	40	34	95	48
Schlotzky's Deli Original Turkey Breast Sandwich	1 small sandwich	574	54	24	148	61	81	70	195	98
Schlotzky's Deli Original Turkey Breast Sandwich	1 medium sandwich	799	79	31	206	85	113	97	272	136
■ **Turkey Products**										
Battered, fried turkey patties	1 patty (3.33 oz)	266	15	17	69	28	38	32	90	45
Battered, fried turkey stick	1 stick (2.25 oz)	179	11	11	46	19	25	22	61	30

FOOD	AMOUNT	CAL	CARBS	FAT	WALK	RUN	BIKE	SWIM	YOGA	DANCE
Cooked ground turkey	4 oz	263	0	15	68	28	37	32	89	45
Cooked turkey bacon	1 oz	61	1	4	16	6	9	7	21	10
Turkey frank	1 frank	102	1	8	26	11	14	12	35	17
Canned turkey with broth	1 cup	220	0	9	57	23	31	27	75	37
Louis Rich Smoked Turkey Sausage	1 oz	45	1	3	12	5	6	5	15	8
Louis Rich Turkey Bologna	1 serving	52	1	4	13	5	7	6	18	9
Louis Rich Turkey Salami	1 serving	41	0	3	11	4	6	5	14	7
Louis Rich Oven Roasted White Turkey Breast	1 oz	28	1	1	7	3	4	3	9	5
Louis Rich Smoked Sliced White Turkey Breast	1 oz	28	1	1	7	3	4	3	10	5
Louis Rich Honey Roasted Fat Free Turkey	1 oz	29	1	0	7	3	4	4	10	5
Louis Rich Oven Roasted Fat Free Turkey Breast	1 oz	24	1	0	6	3	3	3	8	4
Oscar Mayer Oven Roasted White Turkey Breast	1 slice	30	1	1	8	3	4	4	10	5
Frozen Entrées										
Birds Eye Voila Garlic Chicken	1 cup, cooked	240	21	8	62	26	34	29	82	41
Birds Eye Voila Chicken Fajita	1 cup, cooked	150	13	6	39	16	21	18	51	26
Birds Eye Voila Three Cheese Chicken	1 cup, cooked	210	21	8	54	22	30	26	71	36
Birds Eye Voila Chicken Stir-Fry	1 cup, cooked	160	22	3	41	17	23	19	54	27
Birds Eye Voila Garden Herb Chicken	1 cup, cooked	280	30	11	72	30	40	34	95	48
Birds Eye Voila Pesto Chicken Primavera	1 cup, cooked	210	24	7	54	22	30	26	71	36
Birds Eye Voila Teriyaki Chicken	1 cup, cooked	250	44	3	64	27	35	30	85	43
Birds Eye Voila Reduced Carb Chicken and Sausage Tuscano	1 cup, cooked	170	10	8	44	18	24	21	58	29
Birds Eye Voila Reduced Carb Roasted Garlic Chicken and Vegetables	1 cup, cooked	120	13	3	31	13	17	15	41	20
Birds Eye Voila Reduced Carb Chicken Teriyaki and Vegetables	1 cup, cooked	150	15	3	39	16	21	18	51	26

FOOD	AMOUNT	CAL	CARBS	FAT	WALK	RUN	BIKE	SWIM	YOGA	DANCE
Birds Eye Voila Reduced Carb Down Home Chicken and Vegetables	1 cup, cooked	180	17	5	46	19	26	22	61	31
Healthy Choice Asiago Chicken Portobello	1 meal (12.5 oz)	330	47	6	85	35	47	40	112	56
Healthy Choice Blackened Chicken	1 meal (11 oz)	300	36	6	77	32	43	36	102	51
Healthy Choice Chicken Enchilada Dinner	1 meal (9 oz)	310	46	7	80	33	44	38	105	53
Healthy Choice Chicken Teriyaki	1 meal (11 oz)	270	37	6	70	29	38	33	92	46
Healthy Choice Country Herb Chicken	1 meal (11.35 oz)	280	37	6	72	30	40	34	95	48
Healthy Choice Grilled Chicken with Smokehouse BBQ Sauce	1 meal (12 oz)	370	59	6	95	39	52	45	126	63
Healthy Choice Mesquite Chicken BBQ	1 meal (10.5 oz)	300	44	5	77	32	43	36	102	51
Healthy Choice Sesame Chicken Dinner	1 meal (10.8 oz)	330	38	8	85	35	47	40	112	56
Healthy Choice Sweet and Sour Chicken	1 meal (11 oz)	340	54	7	88	36	48	41	116	58
Healthy Choice Chicken Broccoli Alfredo	1 meal (11.5 oz)	300	34	7	77	32	43	36	102	51
Healthy Choice Chicken Parmigiana	1 meal (11 oz)	320	40	9	82	34	45	39	109	55
Healthy Choice Country Breaded Chicken	1 meal (10.6 oz)	370	55	9	95	39	52	45	126	63
Healthy Choice Honey Glazed Chicken	1 meal (11 oz)	320	46	6	82	34	45	39	109	55
Healthy Choice Chicken Tuscany	1 meal (10.6 oz)	330	42	9	85	35	47	40	112	56
Healthy Choice Grilled Basil Chicken	1 meal (10.6 oz)	290	33	7	75	31	41	35	99	49
Healthy Choice Roasted Chicken Breast	1 meal (11 oz)	280	32	8	72	30	40	34	95	48
Healthy Choice Grilled Chicken Caesar	1 meal (10 oz)	290	42	7	75	31	41	35	99	49
Healthy Choice Cajun Style Chicken and Shrimp	1 meal (10.4 oz)	240	32	4	62	26	34	29	82	41
Healthy Choice Roasted Chicken Chardonnay	1 meal (10.6 oz)	280	32	7	72	30	40	34	95	48

FOOD	AMOUNT	CAL	CARBS	FAT	WALK	RUN	BIKE	SWIM	YOGA	DANCE
Healthy Choice Chicken Margherita	1 meal (10 oz)	340	25	8	88	36	48	41	116	58
Healthy Choice Creamy Herb Roasted Chicken	1 meal (10 oz)	220	35	5	57	23	31	27	75	37
Healthy Choice Grilled Chicken Baja	1 meal (10 oz)	270	33	5	70	29	38	33	92	46
Healthy Choice Grilled Chicken Marinara	1 meal (10 oz)	280	37	5	72	30	40	34	95	48
Healthy Choice Princess Chicken	1 meal (10.75 oz)	310	41	7	80	33	44	38	105	53
Healthy Choice Roasted Chicken Marsala	1 meal (10.4 oz)	240	23	6	62	26	34	29	82	41
Healthy Choice Oriental Style Chicken	1 meal (8.5 oz)	240	28	5	62	26	34	29	82	41
Healthy Choice Cheesy Rice and Chicken	1 meal (9 oz)	230	33	4	59	24	33	28	78	39
Healthy Choice Chicken Carbonara	1 meal (9 oz)	310	39	7	80	33	44	38	105	53
Healthy Choice Chicken Fettuccini Alfredo	1 meal (8.5 oz)	280	28	7	72	30	40	34	95	48
Healthy Choice Country Glazed Chicken	1 meal (8.5 oz)	230	29	5	59	24	33	28	78	39
Healthy Choice Grilled Chicken and Mashed Potatoes	1 meal (8.5 oz)	230	22	7	59	24	33	28	78	39
Healthy Choice Homestyle Chicken and Pasta	1 meal (9 oz)	270	32	6	70	29	38	33	92	46
Healthy Choice Breaded Chicken Breast Strips and Macaroni and Cheese	1 meal (8 oz)	290	35	5	75	31	41	35	99	49
Healthy Choice Chicken Breast and Vegetables	1 meal (10.5 oz)	230	29	5	59	24	33	28	78	39
Healthy Choice Familiar Favorites Chicken Enchiladas	1 meal (11.3 oz)	360	59	7	93	38	51	44	122	61
Healthy Choice Chicken Piccata	1 meal (9 oz)	270	40	5	70	29	38	33	92	46
Healthy Choice Grilled Chicken Breast and Pasta	1 meal (9 oz)	240	25	6	62	26	34	29	82	41
Healthy Choice Mandarin Chicken	1 meal (10 oz)	280	43	4	72	30	40	34	95	48
Healthy Choice Familiar Favorites Sesame Chicken	1 meal (9 oz)	260	34	6	67	28	37	32	88	44
Healthy Choice Traditional Turkey Breasts	1 meal (10.5 oz)	330	50	5	85	35	47	40	112	56

FOOD	AMOUNT	CAL	CARBS	FAT	WALK	RUN	BIKE	SWIM	YOGA	DANCE
Healthy Choice Grilled Turkey Breast	1 meal (10 oz)	250	31	5	64	27	35	30	85	43
Healthy Choice Roast Turkey Breast	1 meal (8.5 oz)	230	25	6	59	24	33	28	78	39
Healthy Choice Slow-Roasted Turkey Breast and Mashed Potatoes	1 meal (8.5 oz)	200	19	5	52	21	28	24	68	34
Weight Watchers Smart Ones Teriyaki Chicken and Vegetable Bowl	1 package (297 g)	270	46	3	70	29	38	33	92	46
Weight Watchers Smart Ones Stuffed Turkey Breast	1 package (283 g)	290	42	6	75	31	41	35	99	49
Weight Watchers Smart Ones Lemon Herb Chicken Piccata	1 package (255 g)	250	36	5	64	27	35	30	85	43
Weight Watchers Smart Ones Honey Dijon Chicken	1 package (241 g)	220	38	4	57	23	31	27	75	37
Weight Watchers Smart Ones Fiesta Chicken	1 package (241 g)	250	45	2	64	27	35	30	85	43
Weight Watchers Smart Ones Chicken Oriental	1 package (255 g)	230	39	3	59	24	33	28	78	39
Other Poultry										
Roasted duck with skin	4 oz (includes bone)	377	0	32	97	40	53	46	128	64
Roasted duck, no skin	4 oz (includes bone)	225	0	13	58	24	32	27	77	38
Roasted goose with skin	4 oz (includes bone)	342	0	25	88	36	49	42	116	58
Roasted goose, no skin	4 oz (includes bone)	267	0	14	69	28	38	32	91	45
Pâté de foie gras (canned goose liver pâté)	1 oz	131	1	12	34	14	19	16	45	22
Cooked pheasant	4 oz (bone removed)	277	0	14	71	29	39	34	94	47
Cooked quail	4 oz (bone removed)	262	0	16	68	28	37	32	89	45
Cornish game hen with skin	1 bird, whole	668	0	47	172	71	95	81	227	114
Cornish game hen, no skin	1 bird, whole	295	0	9	76	31	42	36	100	50

FOOD	AMOUNT	CAL	CARBS	FAT	WALK	RUN	BIKE	SWIM	YOGA	DANCE

Beef

Braised Brisket

■ ¼″ Trim

FOOD	AMOUNT	CAL	CARBS	FAT	WALK	RUN	BIKE	SWIM	YOGA	DANCE
Whole brisket, any grade	5 oz	547	0	45	141	58	78	67	186	93
Whole brisket, lean only, any grade	5 oz	344	0	18	89	37	49	42	117	59
Point half, any grade	5 oz	574	0	49	148	61	81	70	195	98
Point half, lean only, any grade	5 oz	371	0	22	96	40	53	45	126	63

■ ⅛″ Trim

FOOD	AMOUNT	CAL	CARBS	FAT	WALK	RUN	BIKE	SWIM	YOGA	DANCE
Flat half, average all grades	5 oz	410	0	26	106	44	58	50	139	70
Flat half, average all grades, lean only	5 oz	278	0	9	72	30	39	34	95	47
Flat half, choice	5 oz	423	0	28	109	45	60	51	144	72
Flat half, choice, lean only	5 oz	288	0	10	74	31	41	35	98	49
Flat half, select	5 oz	398	0	25	103	42	56	48	135	68
Flat half, select, lean only	5 oz	268	0	7	69	29	38	33	91	46
Point half, average all grades	5 oz	496	0	39	128	53	70	60	169	84
Whole brisket, average all grades	5 oz	470	0	35	121	50	67	57	160	80

■ 0″ Trim

FOOD	AMOUNT	CAL	CARBS	FAT	WALK	RUN	BIKE	SWIM	YOGA	DANCE
Flat half, average all grades	5 oz	302	0	11	78	32	43	37	103	51
Flat half, average all grades, lean only	5 oz	291	0	10	75	31	41	35	99	50
Flat half, choice	5 oz	314	0	13	81	33	45	38	107	53
Flat half, choice, lean only	5 oz	301	0	11	78	32	43	37	102	51
Flat half, select	5 oz	291	0	10	75	31	41	35	99	50
Flat half, select, lean only	5 oz	281	0	8	72	30	40	34	96	48
Point half, average all grades	5 oz	508	0	40	131	54	72	62	173	87
Point half, average all grades, lean only	5 oz	346	0	20	89	37	49	42	118	59
Whole brisket, average all grades	5 oz	413	0	28	106	44	59	50	140	70
Whole brisket, average all grades, lean only	5 oz	310	0	14	80	33	44	38	105	53

FOOD	AMOUNT	CAL	CARBS	FAT	WALK	RUN	BIKE	SWIM	YOGA	DANCE
Braised Chuck Blade Roast										
■ **¼″ Trim**										
Average all grades	5 oz	356	0	19	92	38	50	43	121	61
Average all grades, lean only	5 oz	356	0	19	92	38	50	43	121	61
Choice	5 oz	515	0	40	133	55	73	63	175	88
Choice, lean only	5 oz	373	0	20	96	40	53	45	127	64
Select	5 oz	463	0	33	119	49	66	56	157	79
Select, lean only	5 oz	337	0	16	87	36	48	41	115	57
■ **0″ Trim**										
Average all grades, lean only	5 oz	359	0	19	93	38	51	44	122	61
Choice	5 oz	494	0	37	127	53	70	60	168	84
Choice, lean only	5 oz	376	0	21	97	40	53	46	128	64
Select	5 oz	444	0	31	114	47	63	54	151	76
Select, lean only	5 oz	338	0	17	87	36	48	41	115	58
■ **½″ Trim**										
Prime	5 oz	592	0	48	153	63	84	72	201	101
Prime, lean only	5 oz	452	0	29	116	48	64	55	154	77
■ **⅛″ Trim**										
Average all grades	5 oz	484	0	36	125	52	69	59	165	82
Choice	5 oz	510	0	39	131	54	72	62	173	87
Select	5 oz	452	0	32	116	48	64	55	154	77
Beef Flank										
■ **Braised—0″ Trim**										
Choice, lean only	5 oz	337	0	18	87	36	48	41	115	57
■ **Broiled—0″ Trim**										
Average all grades	5 oz	267	0	12	69	28	38	32	91	45
Average all grades, lean only	5 oz	264	0	11	68	28	37	32	90	45
Choice	5 oz	287	0	13	74	31	41	35	98	49
Choice lean only	5 oz	275	0	12	71	29	39	33	94	47
Select	5 oz	254	0	10	65	27	36	31	86	43
Select, lean only	5 oz	253	0	9	65	27	36	31	86	43
Beef Rib										
■ **Broiled Whole Ribs—½″ Trim**										
Prime	5 oz	579	0	50	149	62	82	70	197	99
Prime, lean only	5 oz	398	0	27	103	42	56	48	135	68

FOOD	AMOUNT	CAL	CARBS	FAT	WALK	RUN	BIKE	SWIM	YOGA	DANCE
■ **Broiled Whole Ribs—¼″ Trim**										
Average all grades	5 oz	486	0	39	125	52	69	59	165	83
Average all grades, lean only	5 oz	317	0	17	82	34	45	39	108	54
Choice	5 oz	511	0	42	132	54	72	62	174	87
Choice, lean only	5 oz	337	0	20	87	36	48	41	115	57
Select	5 oz	459	0	36	118	49	65	56	156	78
Select, lean only	5 oz	293	0	15	76	31	42	36	100	50
Prime	5 oz	557	0	47	144	59	79	68	189	95
Prime, lean only	5 oz	398	0	27	103	42	56	48	135	68
■ **Broiled Whole Ribs—⅛″ Trim**										
Average all grades	5 oz	470	0	38	121	50	67	57	160	80
Choice	5 oz	500	0	40	129	53	71	61	170	85
Prime	5 oz	548	0	46	141	58	78	67	186	93
Select	5 oz	447	0	34	115	48	63	54	152	76
■ **Roasted Whole Ribs—½″ Trim**										
Prime	5 oz	604	0	52	156	64	86	73	205	103
Prime, lean only	5 oz	415	0	28	107	44	59	50	141	71
■ **Roasted Whole Ribs—¼″ Trim**										
Average all grades	5 oz	508	0	41	131	54	72	62	173	87
Average all grades, lean only	5 oz	325	0	18	84	35	46	40	111	55
Choice	5 oz	534	0	44	138	57	76	65	182	91
Choice, lean only	5 oz	345	0	20	89	37	49	42	117	59
Select	5 oz	477	0	38	123	51	68	58	162	81
Select, lean only	5 oz	302	0	15	78	32	43	37	103	51
Prime	5 oz	581	0	49	150	62	82	71	198	99
Prime, lean only	5 oz	415	0	28	107	44	59	50	141	71
■ **Roasted Whole Ribs—⅛″ Trim**										
Average all grades	5 oz	498	0	40	128	53	71	61	169	85
Choice	5 oz	518	0	42	134	55	73	63	176	88
Prime	5 oz	568	0	48	146	60	81	69	193	97
Select	5 oz	469	0	36	121	50	67	57	160	80
■ **Broiled Rib Eye (Small End)—0″ Trim**										
Average all grades	5 oz	351	0	21	90	37	50	43	119	60
Choice	5 oz	376	0	24	97	40	53	46	128	64
Choice, lean only	5 oz	291	0	13	75	31	41	35	99	50

FOOD	AMOUNT	CAL	CARBS	FAT	WALK	RUN	BIKE	SWIM	YOGA	DANCE
Select	5 oz	327	0	18	84	35	46	40	111	56
Select, lean only	5 oz	258	0	9	66	27	37	31	88	44
■ **Broiled Rib (Small End)—½" Trim**										
Prime	5 oz	517	0	41	133	55	73	63	176	88
Prime, lean only	5 oz	369	0	22	95	39	52	45	126	63
■ **Broiled Rib (Small End)—¼" Trim**										
Prime	5 oz	513	0	41	132	55	73	62	174	87
Prime, lean only	5 oz	369	0	22	95	39	52	45	126	63
■ **Broiled Rib (Small End)—⅛" Trim**										
Average all grades	5 oz	413	0	28	106	44	59	50	140	70
Average all grades, lean only	5 oz	277	0	11	71	29	39	34	94	47
Choice	5 oz	432	0	31	111	46	61	53	147	74
Choice, lean only	5 oz	287	0	13	74	31	41	35	98	49
Prime	5 oz	503	0	40	130	54	71	61	171	86
Select	5 oz	395	0	26	102	42	56	48	134	67
Select, lean only	5 oz	267	0	9	69	28	38	32	91	45
■ **Broiled Rib (Small End)—0" Trim**										
Average all grades	5 oz	354	0	21	91	38	50	43	120	60
Average all grades, lean only	5 oz	274	0	11	71	29	39	33	93	47
Choice	5 oz	443	0	32	114	47	63	54	151	75
Choice, lean only	5 oz	320	0	17	82	34	45	39	109	55
Select	5 oz	405	0	28	104	43	57	49	138	69
Select, lean only	5 oz	281	0	12	72	30	40	34	96	48
■ **Roasted Rib (Small End)—½" Trim**										
Prime	5 oz	596	0	51	154	63	85	73	203	102
Prime, lean only	5 oz	432	0	30	111	46	61	53	147	74
■ **Roasted Rib (Small End)—¼" Trim**										
Average all grades	5 oz	493	0	40	127	53	70	60	168	84
Average all grades, lean only	5 oz	310	0	16	80	33	44	38	105	53
Choice	5 oz	521	0	43	134	55	74	63	177	89
Choice, lean only	5 oz	329	0	19	85	35	47	40	112	56
Prime	5 oz	592	0	51	153	63	84	72	201	101
Prime, lean only	5 oz	432	0	30	111	46	61	53	147	74
Select	5 oz	470	0	37	121	50	67	57	160	80
Select, lean only	5 oz	288	0	14	74	31	41	35	98	49

FOOD	AMOUNT	CAL	CARBS	FAT	WALK	RUN	BIKE	SWIM	YOGA	DANCE
■ Roasted Rib (Small End)—⅛″ Trim										
Average all grades	5 oz	484	0	39	125	52	69	59	165	82
Choice	5 oz	510	0	41	131	54	72	62	173	87
Prime	5 oz	584	0	50	151	62	83	71	199	99
Select	5 oz	459	0	36	118	49	65	56	156	78
■ Broiled Ribs (Large End)—½″ Trim										
Prime	5 oz	604	0	54	156	64	86	73	205	103
Prime, lean only	5 oz	417	0	30	107	44	59	51	142	71
■ Broiled Ribs (Large End)—¼″ Trim										
Average all grades	5 oz	493	0	40	127	53	70	60	168	84
Average all grades, lean only	5 oz	318	0	18	82	34	45	39	108	54
Choice	5 oz	521	0	44	134	55	74	63	177	89
Choice, lean only	5 oz	341	0	21	88	36	48	41	116	58
Prime	5 oz	586	0	51	151	62	83	71	199	100
Prime, lean only	5 oz	417	0	30	107	44	59	51	142	71
Select	5 oz	460	0	37	119	49	65	56	156	78
Select, lean only	5 oz	293	0	15	76	31	42	36	100	50
■ Broiled Ribs (Large End)—⅛″ Trim										
Average all grades	5 oz	480	0	39	124	51	68	58	163	82
Choice	5 oz	525	0	44	135	56	74	64	179	89
Prime	5 oz	574	0	50	148	61	81	70	195	98
Select	5 oz	460	0	37	119	49	65	56	156	78
■ Roasted Ribs (Large End)—½″ Trim										
Prime	5 oz	578	0	49	149	62	82	70	197	98
Prime, lean only	5 oz	402	0	26	104	43	57	49	137	68
■ Roasted Ribs (Large End)—¼″ Trim										
Average all grades, lean only	5 oz	337	0	19	87	36	48	41	115	57
Choice	5 oz	544	0	45	140	58	77	66	185	93
Choice, lean only	5 oz	355	0	21	91	38	50	43	121	60
Prime	5 oz	571	0	48	147	61	81	69	194	97
Prime, lean only	5 oz	402	0	26	104	43	57	49	137	68
Select	5 oz	483	0	38	124	51	69	59	164	82
Select, lean only	5 oz	312	0	16	80	33	44	38	106	53
■ Roasted Ribs (Large End)—⅛″ Trim										
Average all grades	5 oz	504	0	40	130	54	71	61	171	86
Choice	5 oz	537	0	44	138	57	76	65	183	91

FOOD	AMOUNT	CAL	CARBS	FAT	WALK	RUN	BIKE	SWIM	YOGA	DANCE
Prime	5 oz	558	0	46	144	59	79	68	190	95
Select	5 oz	473	0	37	122	50	67	58	161	81
■ **Roasted Ribs (Large End)—0″ Trim**										
Average all grades, lean only	5 oz	338	0	19	87	36	48	41	115	58
Choice	5 oz	528	0	43	136	56	75	64	180	90
Choice, lean only	5 oz	359	0	21	93	38	51	44	122	61
Select	5 oz	470	0	36	121	50	67	57	160	80
Select, lean only	5 oz	312	0	16	80	33	44	38	106	53
■ **Braised Short Ribs**										
Choice	5 oz	669	0	60	172	71	95	81	228	114
Choice, lean only	5 oz	419	0	26	108	45	59	51	143	71
Broiled Full Cut Round										
■ **¼″ Trim**										
Choice	5 oz	341	0	19	88	36	48	41	116	58
Choice, lean only	5 oz	271	0	10	70	29	38	33	92	46
Select	5 oz	317	0	17	82	34	45	39	108	54
Select, lean only	5 oz	244	0	7	63	26	35	30	83	42
■ **⅛″ Trim**										
Choice	5 oz	334	0	18	86	36	47	41	114	57
Select	5 oz	310	0	16	80	33	44	38	105	53
Round Tip Roast										
■ **½″ Trim**										
Prime	5 oz	403	0	27	104	43	57	49	137	69
Prime, lean only	5 oz	302	0	14	78	32	43	37	103	51
■ **¼″ Trim**										
Average all grades	5 oz	332	0	19	86	35	47	40	113	57
Average all grades, lean only	5 oz	263	0	10	68	28	37	32	89	45
Choice	5 oz	351	0	21	90	37	50	43	119	60
Choice, lean only	5 oz	267	0	10	69	28	38	32	91	45
Prime	5 oz	389	0	25	100	41	55	47	132	66
Prime, lean only	5 oz	302	0	14	78	32	43	37	103	51
Select	5 oz	320	0	17	82	34	45	39	109	55
Select, lean only	5 oz	256	0	9	66	27	36	31	87	44
■ **⅛″ Trim**										
Average all grades	5 oz	311	0	16	80	33	44	38	106	53
Choice	5 oz	324	0	18	84	35	46	39	110	55

FOOD	AMOUNT	CAL	CARBS	FAT	WALK	RUN	BIKE	SWIM	YOGA	DANCE
Select	5 oz	298	0	15	77	32	42	36	101	51
■ **0″ Trim**										
Average all grades	5 oz	267	0	12	69	28	38	32	91	45
Average all grades, lean only	5 oz	247	0	9	64	26	35	30	84	42
Choice	5 oz	278	0	13	72	30	39	34	95	47
Choice, lean only	5 oz	250	0	9	64	27	35	30	85	43
Select	5 oz	257	0	11	66	27	36	31	87	44
Select, lean only	5 oz	212	0	6	55	23	30	26	72	36
Pan-Fried Top Round										
■ **¼″ Trim**										
Choice	5 oz	393	0	22	101	42	56	48	134	67
Choice, lean only	5 oz	322	0	12	83	34	46	39	110	55
Broiled Top Round										
■ **½″ Trim**										
Prime	5 oz	337	0	17	87	36	48	41	115	57
Prime, lean only	5 oz	305	0	13	79	32	43	37	104	52
■ **¼″ Trim**										
Prime	5 oz	325	0	15	84	35	46	40	111	55
Prime, lean only	5 oz	305	0	13	79	32	43	37	104	52
■ **⅛″ Trim**										
Average all grades	5 oz	301	0	13	78	32	43	37	102	51
Average all grades, lean only	5 oz	263	0	8	68	28	37	32	89	45
Choice	5 oz	318	0	15	82	34	45	39	108	54
Choice, lean only	5 oz	274	0	9	71	29	39	33	93	47
Prime	5 oz	320	0	14	82	34	45	39	109	55
Select	5 oz	285	0	11	73	30	40	35	97	49
Select, lean only	5 oz	251	0	7	65	27	36	31	85	43
■ **0″ Trim**										
Average all grades	5 oz	264	0	8	68	28	37	32	90	45
Average all grades, lean only	5 oz	264	0	8	68	28	37	32	90	45
Choice	5 oz	284	0	10	73	30	40	35	97	48
Choice, lean only	5 oz	280	0	10	72	30	40	34	95	48
Select	5 oz	251	0	7	65	27	36	31	85	43
Select, lean only	5 oz	250	0	6	64	27	35	30	85	43

FOOD	AMOUNT	CAL	CARBS	FAT	WALK	RUN	BIKE	SWIM	YOGA	DANCE
Braised Top Round										
■ ¼" Trim										
Average all grades	5 oz	352	0	16	91	37	50	43	120	60
Average all grades, lean only	5 oz	291	0	8	75	31	41	35	99	50
Choice	5 oz	369	0	18	95	39	52	45	126	63
Choice, lean only	5 oz	302	0	9	78	32	43	37	103	51
Select	5 oz	332	0	14	86	35	47	40	113	57
Select, lean only	5 oz	278	0	7	72	30	39	34	95	47
■ ⅛" Trim										
Average all grades	5 oz	338	0	14	87	36	48	41	115	58
Choice	5 oz	355	0	16	91	38	50	43	121	60
Select	5 oz	320	0	12	82	34	45	39	109	55
■ 0" Trim										
Average all grades	5 oz	297	0	9	77	32	42	36	101	51
Average all grades, lean only	5 oz	283	0	7	73	30	40	34	96	48
Choice	5 oz	307	0	10	79	33	44	37	104	52
Choice, lean only	5 oz	294	0	8	76	31	42	36	100	50
Select	5 oz	284	0	8	73	30	40	35	97	48
Select, lean only	5 oz	270	0	6	70	29	38	33	92	46
Simmered Crosscut Shank										
■ ¼" Trim										
Choice	5 oz	373	0	21	96	40	53	45	127	64
Choice, lean only	5 oz	285	0	9	73	30	40	35	97	49
Broiled Porterhouse Steak										
■ ¼" Trim										
Average all grades	8 oz	747	0	59	193	80	106	91	254	127
Average all grades, lean only	8 oz	477	0	24	123	51	68	58	162	81
Choice	8 oz	776	0	63	200	83	110	94	264	132
Choice, lean only	8 oz	488	0	26	126	52	69	59	166	83
Select	8 oz	706	0	53	182	75	100	86	240	120
Select, lean only	8 oz	461	0	22	119	49	65	56	157	79
■ ⅛" Trim										
Choice	8 oz	679	0	50	175	72	96	83	231	116
Average all grades	8 oz	674	0	50	174	72	96	82	229	115
Select	8 oz	667	0	48	172	71	95	81	227	114

FOOD	AMOUNT	CAL	CARBS	FAT	WALK	RUN	BIKE	SWIM	YOGA	DANCE
■ **0″ Trim**										
Average all grades	8 oz	627	0	43.8	162	67	89	76	213	107
Average all grades, lean only	8 oz	481	0	25	124	51	68	59	164	82
Choice	8 oz	642	0	45.7	165	68	91	78	218	109
Choice, lean only	8 oz	508	0	29	131	54	72	62	173	87
Select	8 oz	606	0	41	156	65	86	74	206	103
Select, lean only	8 oz	440	0	20	113	47	62	54	150	75
Broiled T-Bone Steak										
■ **¼″ Trim**										
Average all grades	8 oz	695	0	52	179	74	99	85	236	118
Average all grades, lean only	8 oz	459	0	22	118	49	65	56	156	78
Choice	8 oz	731	0	57	188	78	104	89	249	125
Choice, lean only	8 oz	465	0	23	120	50	66	57	158	79
Select	8 oz	638	0	45	164	68	90	78	217	109
Select, lean only	8 oz	449	0	20	116	48	64	55	153	76
■ **⅛″ Trim**										
Choice	8 oz	649	0	46	167	69	92	79	221	111
Average all grades	8 oz	636	0	44	164	68	90	77	216	108
Select	8 oz	602	0	40	155	64	85	73	205	103
■ **0″ Trim**										
Average all grades	8 oz	561	0	36	145	60	80	68	191	96
Average all grades, lean only	8 oz	429	0	20	111	46	61	52	146	73
Choice	8 oz	586	0	39	151	62	83	71	199	100
Choice, lean only	8 oz	449	0	22	116	48	64	55	153	76
Select	8 oz	522	0	32	135	56	74	64	178	89
Select, lean only	8 oz	402	0	17	104	43	57	49	137	68
Roasted Tenderloin										
■ **¼″ Trim**										
Average all grades	5 oz	471	0	36	121	50	67	57	160	80
Average all grades; lean only	5 oz	315	0	16	81	34	45	38	107	54
Choice	5 oz	481	0	37	124	51	68	59	164	82
Choice, lean only	5 oz	328	0	18	85	35	47	40	112	56
Prime	5 oz	501	0	40	129	53	71	61	170	85
Prime, lean only	5 oz	362	0	22	93	39	51	44	123	62
Select	5 oz	460	0	35	119	49	65	56	156	78
Select, lean only	5 oz	300	0	15	77	32	43	36	102	51

FOOD	AMOUNT	CAL	CARBS	FAT	WALK	RUN	BIKE	SWIM	YOGA	DANCE
■ ⅛" Trim										
Average all grades	5 oz	460	0	35	119	49	65	56	156	78
Choice	5 oz	470	0	36	121	50	67	57	160	80
Prime	5 oz	487	0	38	126	52	69	59	166	83
Select	5 oz	449	0	34	116	48	64	55	153	76
Broiled Tenderloin										
■ ¼" Trim										
Prime	5 oz	450	0	33	116	48	64	55	153	77
Prime, lean only	5 oz	329	0	18	85	35	47	40	112	56
■ ⅛" Trim										
Average all grades	5 oz	379	0	24	98	40	54	46	129	65
Average all grades, lean only	5 oz	284	0	12	73	30	40	35	97	48
Choice	5 oz	388	0	25	100	41	55	47	132	66
Choice, lean only	5 oz	293	0	13	76	31	42	36	100	50
Prime	5 oz	437	0	32	113	47	62	53	149	74
Select	5 oz	372	0	23	96	40	53	45	127	63
Select, lean only	5 oz	275	0	11	71	29	39	33	94	47
■ 0" Trim										
Average all grades	5 oz	310	0	16	80	33	44	38	105	53
Average all grades, lean only	5 oz	274	0	11	71	29	39	33	93	47
Choice	5 oz	328	0	18	85	35	47	40	112	56
Choice, lean only	5 oz	293	0	13	76	31	42	36	100	50
Select	5 oz	291	0	14	75	31	41	35	99	50
Select, lean only	5 oz	254	0	9	65	27	36	31	86	43
Broiled Short Loin, Tenderloin										
■ ½" Trim										
Prime	5 oz	452	0	33	116	48	64	55	154	77
Prime, lean only	5 oz	329	0	18	85	35	47	40	112	56
Roasted Short Loin, Tenderloin										
■ ½" Trim										
Prime	5 oz	508	0	41	131	54	72	62	173	87
Prime, lean only	5 oz	362	0	22	93	39	51	44	123	62
Broiled Top Loin										
■ ½" Trim										
Prime	5 oz	481	0	37	124	51	68	59	164	82
Prime, lean only	5 oz	348	0	19	90	37	49	42	118	59

FOOD	AMOUNT	CAL	CARBS	FAT	WALK	RUN	BIKE	SWIM	YOGA	DANCE
■ ¼" Trim										
Prime	5 oz	459	0	34	118	49	65	56	156	78
Prime, lean only	5 oz	348	0	19	90	37	49	42	118	59
■ ⅛" Trim										
Average all grades	5 oz	375	0	24	97	40	53	46	128	64
Choice	5 oz	395	0	26	102	42	56	48	134	67
Prime	5 oz	440	0	31	113	47	62	54	150	75
Select	5 oz	355	0	21	91	38	50	43	121	60
Average all grades, lean only	5 oz	268	0	10	69	29	38	33	91	46
Choice, lean only	5 oz	285	0	12	73	30	40	35	97	49
Select, lean only	5 oz	251	0	8	65	27	36	31	85	43
■ 0" Trim										
Average all grades	5 oz	274	0	11	71	29	39	33	93	47
Average all grades, lean only	5 oz	258	0	9	66	27	37	31	88	44
Choice	5 oz	291	0	13	75	31	41	35	99	50
Choice, lean only	5 oz	273	0	11	70	29	39	33	93	47
Select	5 oz	256	0	9	66	27	36	31	87	44
Select, lean only	5 oz	244	0	7	63	26	35	30	83	42
Pan-Fried Top Sirloin										
■ ¼" Trim										
Choice	5 oz	463	0	32	119	49	66	56	157	79
Choice, lean only	5 oz	338	0	16	87	36	48	41	115	58
■ ⅛" Trim										
Choice	5 oz	444	0	30	114	47	63	54	151	76
Broiled Top Sirloin										
■ ⅛" Trim										
Average all grades	5 oz	345	0	20	89	37	49	42	117	59
Choice	5 oz	365	0	22	94	39	52	44	124	62
Select	5 oz	327	0	18	84	35	46	40	111	56
Average all grades, lean only	5 oz	253	0	8	65	27	36	31	86	43
Choice, lean only	5 oz	266	0	10	69	28	38	32	90	45
Select, lean only	5 oz	241	0	7	62	26	34	29	82	41
■ 0" Trim										
Average all grades	5 oz	301	0	14	78	32	43	37	102	51
Average all grades, lean only	5 oz	260	0	8	67	28	37	32	88	44
Choice	5 oz	311	0	15	80	33	44	38	106	53

FOOD	AMOUNT	CAL	CARBS	FAT	WALK	RUN	BIKE	SWIM	YOGA	DANCE
Choice, lean only	5 oz	267	0	9	69	28	38	32	91	45
Select	5 oz	293	0	13	76	31	42	36	100	50
Select, lean only	5 oz	251	0	7	65	27	36	31	85	43
Roasted Bottom Sirloin, Tri-Tip										
■ **0″ Trim**										
Average all grades	5 oz	295	0	16	76	31	42	36	100	50
Average all grades, lean only	5 oz	258	0	12	66	27	37	31	88	44
Choice	5 oz	310	0	18	80	33	44	38	105	53
Choice, lean only	5 oz	274	0	14	71	29	39	33	93	47
Select	5 oz	281	0	14	72	30	40	34	96	48
Select, lean only	5 oz	254	0	10	65	27	36	31	86	43
Ground Beef										
■ **Nonspecific Fat %**										
Frozen ground beef patties	3 oz patty	240	0	17	62	26	34	29	82	41
Fried hamburger patty	100 g	235	0	14	61	25	33	29	80	40
■ **70% Lean/30% Fat**										
Baked ground beef loaf	3 oz	205	0	13	53	22	29	25	70	35
Pan-broiled beef patty	3 oz patty	202	0	13	52	22	29	25	69	34
■ **85% Lean/15% Fat**										
Baked ground beef loaf	3 oz	204	0	12	53	22	29	25	69	35
Pan-broiled beef patty	3 oz patty	197	0	12	51	21	28	24	67	34
■ **95% Lean/5% Fat**										
Baked ground beef loaf	3 oz patty	148	0	5	38	16	21	18	50	25
Pan-broiled beef patty	3 oz patty	139	0	5	36	15	20	17	47	24
■ **Other Beef Products**										
Braised beef liver	3 oz	162	4	4	42	17	23	20	55	28
Pan-fried beef liver	3 oz	149	4	4	38	16	21	18	51	25
Simmered beef kidneys	3 oz	134	0	4	35	14	19	16	46	23
Simmered tongue	3 oz	241	0	19	62	26	34	29	82	41
Canned corned beef	3 oz	212	0	13	55	23	30	26	72	36
Cooked beef breakfast strips	3 slices (34 g)	153	0	12	39	16	22	19	52	26
Cooked corned beef	3 oz	213	0	16	55	23	30	26	72	36
Jellied corned beef	1 slice (1 oz)	43	0	2	11	5	6	5	15	7
Pastrami	2 slices (2 oz)	82	0	3	21	9	12	10	28	14

FOOD	AMOUNT	CAL	CARBS	FAT	WALK	RUN	BIKE	SWIM	YOGA	DANCE
Smoked cured beef sausage	1 sausage (43 g)	134	1	12	35	14	19	16	46	23
Beef salami	1 oz	73	1	6	19	8	10	9	25	12
Beef frank	1 frank	188	2	17	48	20	27	23	64	32
Light beef frank	1 frank (45 g)	90	0	6	23	10	13	11	31	15
Boar's Head Lean Corned Beef Round	2 oz	80	0	3	21	9	11	10	27	14
Boar's Head First Cut Lean Corned Beef Brisket	2 oz	80	0	4	21	9	11	10	27	14
Hillshire Farm Corned Beef	1 oz	31	1	0	8	3	4	4	11	5
Oscar Mayer Corned Beef	.6 oz	17	0	0	4	2	2	2	6	3
Dinty Moore Canned Corned Beef	2 oz	130	0	8	34	14	18	16	44	22
Braised Chuck Arm Pot Roast										
■ 0″ Trim										
Average all grades	5 oz	422	0	27	109	45	60	51	144	72
Choice, lean only	5 oz	301	0	11	78	32	43	37	102	51
Select	5 oz	402	0	25	104	43	57	49	137	68
Select, lean only	5 oz	277	0	8	71	29	39	34	94	47
■ ½″ Trim										
Prime	5 oz	555	0	44	143	59	79	68	189	95
Prime, lean only	5 oz	371	0	19	96	40	53	45	126	63
■ ⅛″ Trim										
Average all grades	5 oz	429	0	27	111	46	61	52	146	73
Average all grades, lean only	5 oz	304	0	10	78	32	43	37	103	52
Choice	5 oz	439	0	28	113	47	62	53	149	75
Choice, lean only	5 oz	318	0	12	82	34	45	39	108	54
Select	5 oz	419	0	26	108	45	59	51	143	71
Select, lean only	5 oz	291	0	9	75	31	41	35	99	50
Braised Bottom Round										
■ ½″ Trim										
Prime	5 oz	422	0	27	109	45	60	51	144	72
Prime, lean only	5 oz	354	0	18	91	38	50	43	120	60
■ ⅛″ Trim										
Average all grades	5 oz	351	0	17	90	37	50	43	119	60
Average all grades, lean only	5 oz	307	0	11	79	33	44	37	104	52

FOOD	AMOUNT	CAL	CARBS	FAT	WALK	RUN	BIKE	SWIM	YOGA	DANCE
Choice	5 oz	361	0	18	93	38	51	44	123	61
Choice, lean only	5 oz	324	0	13	84	35	46	39	110	55
Select	5 oz	341	0	16	88	36	48	41	116	58
Select, lean only	5 oz	291	0	9	75	31	41	35	99	50
■ 0″ Trim										
Average all grades	5 oz	317	0	13	82	34	45	39	108	54
Average all grades, lean only	5 oz	304	0	11	78	32	43	37	103	52
Choice	5 oz	327	0	14	84	35	46	40	111	56
Choice, lean only	5 oz	317	0	13	82	34	45	39	108	54
Select	5 oz	308	0	11	79	33	44	37	105	52
Select, lean only	5 oz	293	0	9	76	31	42	36	100	50
Roasted Bottom Round										
■ ⅛″ Trim										
Average all grades	5 oz	310	0	17	80	33	44	38	105	53
Choice	5 oz	317	0	18	82	34	45	39	108	54
Choice, lean only	5 oz	254	0	10	65	27	36	31	86	43
Select	5 oz	301	0	15	78	32	43	37	102	51
Select, lean only	5 oz	233	0	7	60	25	33	28	79	40
■ 0″ Trim										
Average all grades	5 oz	266	0	11	69	28	38	32	90	45
Average all grades, lean only	5 oz	251	0	9	65	27	36	31	85	43
Choice	5 oz	283	0	13	73	30	40	34	96	48
Choice, lean only	5 oz	263	0	11	68	28	37	32	89	45
Select	5 oz	248	0	9	64	26	35	30	84	42
Select, lean only	5 oz	240	0	8	62	26	34	29	82	41
Roasted Eye of Round										
■ ½″ Trim										
Prime	1 piece, cooked, excluding refuse	355	0	21	91	38	50	43	121	60
Prime, lean only	1 piece, cooked, excluding refuse	281	0	12	72	30	40	34	96	48
■ ⅛″ Trim										
Average all grades	5 oz	295	0	14	76	31	42	36	100	50
Average all grades, lean only	5 oz	240	0	7	62	26	34	29	82	41

FOOD	AMOUNT	CAL	CARBS	FAT	WALK	RUN	BIKE	SWIM	YOGA	DANCE
Choice	5 oz	301	0	14	78	32	43	37	102	51
Choice, lean only	5 oz	248	0	8	64	26	35	30	84	42
Select	5 oz	290	0	13	75	31	41	35	99	49
Select, lean only	5 oz	231	0	6	60	25	33	28	79	39
■ 0″ Trim										
Average all grades	5 oz	239	0	7	62	25	34	29	81	41
Average all grades, lean only	5 oz	230	0	6	59	24	33	28	78	39
Choice	5 oz	236	0	7	61	25	33	29	80	40
Choice, lean only	5 oz	230	0	6	59	24	33	28	78	39
Select	5 oz	240	0	7	62	26	34	29	82	41
Select, lean only	5 oz	231	0	6	60	25	33	28	79	39
Chuck Clod Roast										
■ ¼″ Trim										
Average all grades	5 oz	344	0	22	89	37	49	42	117	59
Average all grades, lean only	5 oz	246	0	10	63	26	35	30	84	42
Choice	5 oz	344	0	22	89	37	49	42	117	59
Choice, lean only	5 oz	253	0	11	65	27	36	31	86	43
Select	5 oz	345	0	22	89	37	49	42	117	59
Select, lean only	5 oz	236	0	8	61	25	33	29	80	40
■ 0″ Trim										
Average all grades	5 oz	294	0	15	76	31	42	36	100	50
Average all grades, lean only	5 oz	244	0	9	63	26	35	30	83	42
Choice	5 oz	307	0	17	79	33	44	37	104	52
Choice, lean only	5 oz	243	0	10	63	26	34	30	83	41
Select	5 oz	278	0	12	72	30	39	34	95	47
Select, lean only	5 oz	244	0	8	63	26	35	30	83	42
Braised Chuck Clod Steak										
■ ¼″ Trim										
Average all grades	5 oz	386	0	25	99	41	55	47	131	66
Average all grades, lean only	5 oz	268	0	10	69	29	38	33	91	46
Choice	5 oz	386	0	25	99	41	55	47	131	66
Choice, lean only	5 oz	274	0	11	71	29	39	33	93	47
Select	5 oz	385	0	25	99	41	55	47	131	66
Select, lean only	5 oz	260	0	9	67	28	37	32	88	44
■ 0″ Trim										
Average all grades	5 oz	312	0	15	80	33	44	38	106	53

FOOD	AMOUNT	CAL	CARBS	FAT	WALK	RUN	BIKE	SWIM	YOGA	DANCE
Average all grades, lean only	5 oz	273	0	10	70	29	39	33	93	47
Choice	5 oz	328	0	17	85	35	47	40	112	56
Choice, lean only	5 oz	274	0	11	71	29	39	33	93	47
Select	5 oz	291	0	12	75	31	41	35	99	50
Select, lean only	5 oz	271	0	10	70	29	38	33	92	46
Broiled Chuck Mock Tender Steak										
■ 0″ Trim										
Average all grades	5 oz	227	0	8	59	24	32	28	77	39
Average all grades, lean only	5 oz	227	0	8	59	24	32	28	77	39
Choice	5 oz	229	0	8	59	24	32	28	78	39
Choice, lean only	5 oz	229	0	8	59	24	32	28	78	39
Select	5 oz	226	0	7	58	24	32	27	77	39
Select, lean only	5 oz	223	0	7	57	24	32	27	76	38
Broiled Chuck Top Blade										
■ 0″ Trim										
Average all grades	5 oz	307	0	17	79	33	44	37	104	52
Average all grades, lean only	5 oz	288	0	14	74	31	41	35	98	49
Choice	5 oz	322	0	18	83	34	46	39	110	55
Choice, lean only	5 oz	308	0	17	79	33	44	37	105	52
Select	5 oz	284	0	14	73	30	40	35	97	48
Select, lean only	5 oz	261	0	11	67	28	37	32	89	44
Broiled Inside Skirt Steak										
■ 0″ Trim										
Average all grades	5 oz	312	0	17	80	33	44	38	106	53
Average all grades, lean only	5 oz	291	0	14	75	31	41	35	99	50
Broiled Outside Skirt Steak										
■ 0″ Trim										
Average all grades	5 oz	362	0	24	93	39	51	44	123	62
Average all grades, lean only	5 oz	331	0	20	85	35	47	40	113	56
Frozen entrees										
Birds Eye Voila Beef Steak and Garlic Potato	1 cup, cooked	190	22	7	49	20	27	23	65	32
Birds Eye Voila Reduced Carb Teriyaki Beef and Vegetables	1 cup, cooked	160	15	4	41	17	23	19	54	27
Healthy Choice Beef Stroganoff	1 meal (11 oz)	330	40	9	85	35	47	40	112	56

FOOD	AMOUNT	CAL	CARBS	FAT	WALK	RUN	BIKE	SWIM	YOGA	DANCE
Healthy Choice Char-Broiled Beef Patty	1 meal (11 oz)	310	37	9	80	33	44	38	105	53
Healthy Choice Oven-Roasted Beef	1 meal (10.15 oz)	280	33	7	72	30	40	34	95	48
Healthy Choice Salisbury Steak	1 meal (12.5 oz)	360	45	9	93	38	51	44	122	61
Healthy Choice Beef Pot Roast	1 meal (11 oz)	320	39	9	82	34	45	39	109	55
Healthy Choice Beef Tips Portabello	1 meal (11.25 oz)	280	28	8	72	30	40	34	95	48
Healthy Choice Boneless Beef Ribs with Classic BBQ Sauce	1 meal (11 oz)	360	47	9	93	38	51	44	122	61
Healthy Choice Meatloaf	1 meal (12 oz)	300	36	9	77	32	43	36	102	51
Healthy Choice Mushroom Roasted Beef	1 meal (11 oz)	280	28	8	72	30	40	34	95	48
Healthy Choice Salisbury Steak and Mashed Potatoes	1 meal (8 oz)	210	21	6	54	22	30	26	71	36
Healthy Choice Grilled Steak in Roasted Garlic Sauce	1 meal (10 oz)	240	46	7	62	26	34	29	82	41
Healthy Choice Oriental Style Beef	1 meal (10.6 oz)	300	27	9	77	32	43	36	102	51
Healthy Choice Beef Merlot	1 meal (10 oz)	240	26	8	62	26	34	29	82	41
Healthy Choice Grilled Whiskey Steak	1 meal (9.5)	300	46	5	77	32	43	36	102	51
Healthy Choice Beef Teriyaki	1 meal (9.5)	310	46	7	80	33	44	38	105	53
Healthy Choice Sirloin Beef Tips and Mushroom Sauce	1 meal (8 oz)	270	35	6	70	29	38	33	92	46
Weight Watchers Smart Ones Salisbury Steak, Macaroni and Cheese	1 package (269 g)	260	26	7	67	28	37	32	88	44
Weight Watchers Smart Ones Three Cheese and Italian Style Meatballs	1 package (127 g)	290	43	7	75	31	41	35	99	49
Beef Jerky										
Beef jerky	1 piece	82	2	5	21	9	12	10	28	14
Jack Link's Jumbo Kippered Beef Teriyaki Steak	2 oz	160	10	2	41	17	23	19	54	27
Slim Jim Twin Pack Spicy Smoked Snack	1 package (55 g)	290	4	26	75	31	41	35	99	49

FOOD	AMOUNT	CAL	CARBS	FAT	WALK	RUN	BIKE	SWIM	YOGA	DANCE
Slim Jim Beef Jerky	1 package (19 g)	80	2	5	21	9	11	10	27	14

Pork

Pork Leg

FOOD	AMOUNT	CAL	CARBS	FAT	WALK	RUN	BIKE	SWIM	YOGA	DANCE
Roasted pork leg	3 oz	232	0	15	60	25	33	28	79	40
Roasted pork leg (rump half)	3 oz	214	0	12	55	23	30	26	73	36
Roasted pork leg (rump half), fat removed	3 oz	175	0	7	45	19	25	21	60	30
Roasted pork leg (shank half)	3 oz	246	0	17	63	26	35	30	84	42
Roasted pork leg (shank half), fat removed	3 oz	183	0	9	47	19	26	22	62	31
Roasted pork leg, fat removed	3 oz	179	0	8	46	19	25	22	61	30

Pork Loin

■ Blade

FOOD	AMOUNT	CAL	CARBS	FAT	WALK	RUN	BIKE	SWIM	YOGA	DANCE
Broiled/braised pork loin blade (chop), bone in	3 oz	272	0	21	70	29	39	33	93	46
Broiled/braised pork loin blade (chop), bone in, fat removed	3 oz	199	0	12	51	21	28	24	68	34
Pan-fried pork loin blade (chop), bone in	3 oz	291	0	24	75	31	41	35	99	50
Pan-fried pork loin blade (chop), bone in, fat removed	3 oz	205	0	13	53	22	29	25	70	35
Roasted pork loin blade (roasts), bone in	3 oz	275	0	21	71	29	39	33	94	47
Roasted pork loin blade (roasts), bone in, fat removed	3 oz	210	0	13	54	22	30	26	71	36

■ Center Loin

FOOD	AMOUNT	CAL	CARBS	FAT	WALK	RUN	BIKE	SWIM	YOGA	DANCE
Broiled/braised pork center loin (chop), bone in	3 oz	204	0	11	53	22	29	25	69	35
Broiled/braised pork center loin (chop), bone in, fat removed	3 oz	172	0	7	44	18	24	21	58	29
Pan-fried pork, center loin (chop), bone in	3 oz	235	0	14	61	25	33	29	80	40
Pan-fried pork, center loin (chop), bone in, fat removed	3 oz	197	0	9	51	21	28	24	67	34
Roasted pork center loin (roasts), bone in	3 oz	199	0	11	51	21	28	24	68	34

FOOD	AMOUNT	CAL	CARBS	FAT	WALK	RUN	BIKE	SWIM	YOGA	DANCE
Roasted pork center loin (roasts), bone in, fat removed	3 oz	169	0	8	44	18	24	21	57	29
John Morrell Frozen Barbecued Center-Cut Pork Chop	4.5 oz	230	7	9	59	24	33	28	78	39
■ Center Rib										
Broiled pork loin, center rib (chops), boneless	3 oz	221	0	13	57	24	31	27	75	38
Broiled pork loin, center rib (chops), boneless, fat removed	3 oz	184	0	9	47	20	26	22	62	31
Broiled/braised pork loin center rib (chop), bone in	3 oz	224	0	13	58	24	32	27	76	38
Broiled/braised pork loin center rib (chop), bone in, fat removed	3 oz	186	0	8	48	20	26	23	63	32
Pan-fried pork loin, center rib (chop), bone in	3 oz	225	0	14	58	24	32	27	77	38
Pan-fried pork loin, center rib (chop), bone in, fat removed	3 oz	185	0	9	48	20	26	23	63	32
Pan-fried pork loin, center rib (chops), boneless	3 oz	232	0	15	60	25	33	28	79	40
Pan-fried pork loin, center rib (chops), boneless, fat removed	3 oz	190	0	10	49	20	27	23	65	32
Roasted pork loin center rib (roasts), bone in	3 oz	217	0	13	56	23	31	26	74	37
Roasted pork loin center rib (roasts), bone in, fat removed	3 oz	190	0	9	49	20	27	23	65	32
Roasted pork loin, center rib (roasts), boneless	3 oz	214	0	13	55	23	30	26	73	36
Roasted pork loin, center rib (roasts), boneless, fat removed	3 oz	182	0	9	47	19	26	22	62	31
■ Sirloin										
Broiled pork sirloin (chop), boneless	3 oz	177	0	7	46	19	25	22	60	30
Broiled pork sirloin (chop), boneless, fat removed	3 oz	164	0	6	42	17	23	20	56	28
Broiled/braised pork sirloin (chop), bone in	3 oz	220	0	14	57	23	31	27	75	38
Broiled/braised pork sirloin (chop), bone in, fat removed	3 oz	181	0	9	47	19	26	22	62	31
Roasted pork sirloin (roasts), bone in	3 oz	222	0	14	57	24	31	27	76	38
Roasted pork sirloin (roasts), bone in, fat removed	3 oz	184	0	9	47	20	26	22	63	31

FOOD	AMOUNT	CAL	CARBS	FAT	WALK	RUN	BIKE	SWIM	YOGA	DANCE
Roasted pork sirloin (roasts), boneless	3 oz	176	0	8	45	19	25	21	60	30
Roasted pork sirloin (roasts), boneless, fat removed	3 oz	168	0	7	43	18	24	20	57	29
■ **Top Loin**										
Broiled pork top loin (chop), boneless	3 oz	154	0	5	40	16	22	19	52	26
Broiled pork top loin (chop), boneless, fat removed	3 oz	141	0	4	36	15	20	17	48	24
Pan-fried pork top loin (chop), boneless	3 oz	218	0	13	56	23	31	27	74	37
Pan-fried pork, top loin (chop), boneless, fat removed	3 oz	191	0	9	49	20	27	23	65	33
Roasted pork top loin (roasts), boneless	3 oz	192	0	10	49	20	27	23	65	33
Roasted pork top loin (roasts), boneless, fat removed	3 oz	165	0	6	43	18	23	20	56	28
■ **Tenderloin**										
Broiled pork tenderloin	3 oz	171	0	7	44	18	24	21	58	29
Broiled pork tenderloin, fat removed	3 oz	159	0	5	41	17	23	19	54	27
Roasted pork tenderloin	3 oz	147	0	5	38	16	21	18	50	25
Roasted pork tenderloin, fat removed	3 oz	139	0	4	36	15	20	17	47	24
Hormel Teriyaki-Flavored Pork Tenderloin	4 oz	133	5	3	34	14	19	16	45	23
John Morrell Frozen Barbecued Pork Tenderloin	100 g	153	4	6	39	16	22	19	52	26
■ **Nonspecific Loin**										
Roasted/braised/broiled pork loin	3 oz	211	0	12	54	22	30	26	72	36
Roasted/braised/broiled pork loin, fat removed	3 oz	178	0	8	46	19	25	22	60	30
Hormel Always Tender Boneless Pork Loin	4 oz	162	1	8	42	17	23	20	55	28
Hormel Always Tender Center Cut Pork Chops	4 oz	187	1	11	48	20	27	23	64	32
John Morrell Frozen Barbecued Pork Loin	5 slices	150	5	6	39	16	21	18	51	26
Swanson Frozen Pork Loin	10.75 oz	280	27	12	72	30	40	34	95	48

FOOD	AMOUNT	CAL	CARBS	FAT	WALK	RUN	BIKE	SWIM	YOGA	DANCE
Shoulder										
Broiled pork, Boston shoulder (steaks)	3 oz	220	0	14	57	23	31	27	75	38
Broiled pork, Boston shoulder (steaks), fat removed	3 oz	193	0	11	50	21	27	23	66	33
Cured pork, shoulder blade roll	3 oz	229	0	19	59	24	32	28	78	39
Roasted cured pork shoulder, arm picnic	3 oz	238	0	18	61	25	34	29	81	41
Roasted cured pork, arm picnic, fat removed	3 oz	144	0	6	37	15	20	18	49	25
Roasted pork shoulder, arm picnic	3 oz	269	0	20	69	29	38	33	91	46
Roasted pork shoulder, arm picnic, fat removed	3 oz	194	0	11	50	21	28	24	66	33
Roasted pork, Boston shoulder (roasts)	3 oz	229	0	16	59	24	32	28	78	39
Roasted pork, Boston shoulder (roasts), fat removed	3 oz	197	0	12	51	21	28	24	67	34
Roasted whole pork shoulder	3 oz	248	0	18	64	26	35	30	84	42
Roasted whole pork shoulder, fat removed	3 oz	196	0	12	51	21	28	24	67	33
Cook's Smoked Super Trim Whole Picnic Shoulder	3 oz	160	1	13	41	17	23	19	54	27
Ribs										
Braised pork spareribs	3 oz	337	0	26	87	36	48	41	115	57
Roasted pork back ribs	3 oz	314	0	20	81	33	45	38	107	53
Roasted pork country-style ribs	3 oz	279	0	22	72	30	40	34	95	48
Roasted pork country-style ribs, fat removed	3 oz	210	0	13	54	22	30	26	71	36
John Morrell Frozen Barbecued Pork Ribs	4.75 oz	240	8	17	62	26	34	29	82	41
Lloyd's Babyback Ribs with Barbecue Sauce	3 ribs	350	17	23	90	37	50	43	119	60
Lloyd's Spareribs with Barbecue Sauce	3 ribs	380	13	27	98	40	54	46	129	65
Ham										
Boneless cured extra-lean ham (steak)	1 slice (2 oz)	70	0	2	18	7	10	9	24	12
Canned extra-lean ham	3 oz	102	0	4	26	11	14	12	35	17
Canned ham	1 cup	162	0	11	42	17	23	20	55	28

FOOD	AMOUNT	CAL	CARBS	FAT	WALK	RUN	BIKE	SWIM	YOGA	DANCE
Cured ham	3 oz	209	0	16	54	22	30	25	71	36
Cured ham patties	1 patty (65 g)	205	1	18	53	22	29	25	70	35
Cured ham, center slice	3 oz	173	0	11	45	18	25	21	59	29
Cured ham, fat removed	3 oz	125	0	5	32	13	18	15	43	21
Roasted boneless extra-lean ham	3 oz	123	1	5	32	13	17	15	42	21
Roasted boneless ham	3 oz	151	0	8	39	16	21	18	51	26
Serrano ham	4 oz	320	0	18	82	34	45	39	109	55
Bauemschinken	4 oz	240	0	16	62	26	34	29	82	41
Berkshire smoked ham	3 oz	120	4	5	31	13	17	15	41	20
Honey-glazed ham	3 oz	105	3	3	27	11	15	13	36	18
D&W Gourmet Lite Ham	3 oz	75	2	2	19	8	11	9	26	13
Healthy Choice Deli Thin Sliced Ham	6 slices	60	1	2	15	6	9	7	20	10
Healthy Choice Deli Thin Sliced Honey Ham	6 slices	60	2	2	15	6	9	7	20	10
Healthy Choice Deli Thin Sliced Honey Mustard Ham	6 slices	60	3	2	15	6	9	7	20	10
Healthy Choice Deli Thin Sliced Virginia Ham	5 slices	60	2	2	15	6	9	7	20	10
Healthy Choice Hearty Deli Thin Sliced Ham	1 slice	30	1	1	8	3	4	4	10	5
Healthy Choice Hearty Deli Thin Sliced Honey Ham	1 slice	30	1	1	8	3	4	4	10	5
Healthy Choice Hearty Deli Thin Sliced Virginia Ham	1 slice	30	1	1	8	3	4	4	10	5
Healthy Choice Honey-Cured Ham	1 slice	30	1	1	8	3	4	4	10	5
Healthy Choice Regular Sliced Ham	1 slice	30	1	1	8	3	4	4	10	5
Healthy Choice Regular Sliced Honey Ham	1 slice	30	1	1	8	3	4	4	10	5
Healthy Choice Regular Sliced Variety Ham Pack	1 slice	30	1	1	8	3	4	4	10	5
Healthy Choice Thin Sliced Honey Ham	5 slices	60	2	2	15	6	9	7	20	10
Healthy Choice Thin Sliced Honey Maple Ham	6 slices	60	3	2	15	6	9	7	20	10
Hormel Cure 81 Ham	3 oz	90	0	3	23	10	13	11	31	15

FOOD	AMOUNT	CAL	CARBS	FAT	WALK	RUN	BIKE	SWIM	YOGA	DANCE
Hormel Prosciutto	3 oz	266	0	21	69	28	38	32	90	45
Bacon										
Grilled Canadian bacon	2 slices	87	1	4	22	9	12	11	30	15
Microwaved cured bacon	3 slices	114	0	8	29	12	16	14	39	19
Pan-fried cured bacon	1 slice, cooked	126	0	10	32	13	18	15	43	21
Pan-fried/roasted bacon	3 slices	130	0	10	34	14	18	16	44	22
Boar's Head Extra Lean Canadian Bacon	2 oz	70	1	3	18	7	10	9	24	12
Hormel Canadian-Style Bacon	2 oz	68	1	3	18	7	10	8	23	12
Hormel 50% Less Fat Bacon Bits	1 tsp	30	0	2	8	3	4	4	10	5
Hormel Bacon Bits	1 tbsp	30	0	2	8	3	4	4	10	5
Hormel Bacon Pieces	1 oz	94	2	5	24	10	13	11	32	16
Oscar Mayer Bacon	1 slice	70	0	6	18	7	10	9	24	12
Sausage										
Italian pork sausage	1 link (91 g)	230	1	18	59	24	33	28	78	39
Pork and bacon sausage	2 links	100	1	9	26	11	14	12	34	17
Pork bratwurst	1 link (109 g)	270	1	22	70	29	38	33	92	46
Pork sausage	1 oz	109	2	32	28	12	15	13	37	19
Hickory Farms Safari Sausage	1 oz	98	1	9	25	10	14	12	33	17
Jimmy Dean Hot Sausage	1 oz	123	0	12	32	13	17	15	42	21
Jimmy Dean Light Pork Sausage	1.2 oz	80	1	7	21	9	11	10	27	14
Jimmy Dean Pork Sausage	1 oz	120	1	11	31	13	17	15	41	20
Oscar Mayer Pork Sausage links	1 oz	96	0	9	25	10	14	12	33	16
Owen's Country Style Pork Sausage	1 oz	143	0	13	37	15	20	17	49	24
Owen's Hot Country Style Pork Sausage	1 oz	143	0	13	37	15	20	17	49	24
Tyson Country Pork Sausage	1 oz	90	0	8	23	10	13	11	31	15
Other Pork										
Braised pork tongue	3 oz	230	0	16	59	24	33	28	78	39
Cooked breakfast strips	3 slices	156	0	12	40	17	22	19	53	27
Cured pork fat	3 oz	492	0	52	127	52	70	60	167	84
Cured salt pork	3 oz	636	0	68	164	68	90	77	216	108

FOOD	AMOUNT	CAL	CARBS	FAT	WALK	RUN	BIKE	SWIM	YOGA	DANCE
Ground pork	3 oz	252	0	18	65	27	36	31	86	43
Pickled pork's feet	3 oz	174	0	14	45	19	25	21	59	30
Pork stew meat	4 oz (raw)	160	0	6	41	17	23	19	54	27
Pork bologna	1 oz	69	0	6	18	7	10	8	23	12
Pork cutlets	3 oz	194	0	14	50	21	28	24	66	33
Baken-ets Fried Pork Skins	9 pieces	80	0	5	21	9	11	10	27	14
Baken-ets Hot 'n Spicy Fried Pork Skins	9 pieces	80	<1	5	21	9	11	10	27	14
Baken-ets Chili Limon Fried Pork Skins	9 pieces	70	0	5	18	7	10	9	24	12
Baken-ets Sweet 'n Tangy BBQ Fried Pork Skins	9 pieces	80	1	5	21	9	11	10	27	14
Baken-ets Pork Cracklins	8 pieces	90	<1	6	23	10	13	11	31	15
Baken-ets Hot 'n Spicy Pork Cracklins	8 pieces	80	<1	5	21	9	11	10	27	14
Banquet Pork Cutlet Entrée	1 entrée	420	38	25	108	45	60	51	143	72
Campbell's Pork and Beans in Tomato Sauce	.5 cup	130	24	2	34	14	18	16	44	22
Chun King Frozen Sweet and Sour Pork Entrée	13 oz	400	78	5	103	43	57	49	136	68
Cook's Hickory Smoked Pork Hocks	1 oz	89	2	7	23	9	13	11	30	15
Healthy Choice Duos Country Breaded Pork and Potatoes	1 meal	280	38	6	72	30	40	34	95	48
Healthy Choice Apple Glazed Pork Medallions	1 meal (10.8 oz)	310	46	6	80	33	44	38	105	53
Hormel Frozen Breaded Pork Steak	3 oz	218	11	15	56	23	31	27	74	37
LaChoy Canned Chow Mein Bi-Pack	.75 cup	80	7	3	21	9	11	10	27	14
LaChoy Canned Sweet and Sour Pork	.75 cup	250	48	4	64	27	35	30	85	43
La Choy Frozen Spicy Pork Egg Roll	1 roll	196	23	9	51	21	28	24	67	33
La Choy Sweet and Sour Pork Entrée	1 cup	241	43	6	62	26	34	29	82	41
Lean Cuisine Pork with Cherry Sauce	1 package (8.25 oz)	260	41	4	67	28	37	32	88	44
Marie Callendar Country Fried Pork Chop	15 oz	550	50	27	142	59	78	67	187	94

FOOD	AMOUNT	CAL	CARBS	FAT	WALK	RUN	BIKE	SWIM	YOGA	DANCE
South Beach Diet Savory Pork with Pecans and Green Beans	1 package	260	13	13	67	28	37	32	88	44
Spam Luncheon Meat	2 oz	180	1	16	46	19	26	22	61	31
Spam Light Luncheon Meat	3 oz	161	1	12	41	17	23	20	55	27
Tyson Deluxe Pork Pattie	6.5 oz	370	48	14	95	39	52	45	126	63

Lamb, Veal, and Game Meat

Lamb

■ Roasted Whole Leg—⅛″ Trim

FOOD	AMOUNT	CAL	CARBS	FAT	WALK	RUN	BIKE	SWIM	YOGA	DANCE
Australian	4 oz	276	0	17	71	29	39	34	94	47
Australian, lean only	4 oz	215	0	9	55	23	30	26	73	37
Domestic, choice	4 oz	273	0	16	70	29	39	33	93	47
New Zealand	4 oz	264	0	16	68	28	37	32	90	45

■ Roasted Whole Leg—¼″ Trim

FOOD	AMOUNT	CAL	CARBS	FAT	WALK	RUN	BIKE	SWIM	YOGA	DANCE
Domestic, choice	4 oz	292	0	19	75	31	41	36	99	50
Domestic, choice, lean only	4 oz	216	0	9	56	23	31	26	73	37

■ Broiled Leg, Bone In, Center Slice—⅛″ Trim

FOOD	AMOUNT	CAL	CARBS	FAT	WALK	RUN	BIKE	SWIM	YOGA	DANCE
Australian	4 oz	243	0	13	63	26	34	30	83	41
Australian, lean only	4 oz	207	0	9	53	22	29	25	70	35

■ Roasted Leg, Sirloin Half—⅛″ Trim

FOOD	AMOUNT	CAL	CARBS	FAT	WALK	RUN	BIKE	SWIM	YOGA	DANCE
Australian	4 oz	318	0	22	82	34	45	39	108	54
Australian, lean only	4 oz	243	0	12	63	26	34	30	83	41
Domestic, choice	4 oz	321	0	22	83	34	46	39	109	55

■ Roasted Leg, Sirloin Half—¼″ Trim

FOOD	AMOUNT	CAL	CARBS	FAT	WALK	RUN	BIKE	SWIM	YOGA	DANCE
Domestic, choice	4 oz	330	0	23	85	35	47	40	112	56
Domestic, choice, lean only	4 oz	231	0	10	60	25	33	28	79	39

■ Roasted Leg, Shank Half—⅛″ Trim

FOOD	AMOUNT	CAL	CARBS	FAT	WALK	RUN	BIKE	SWIM	YOGA	DANCE
Australian	4 oz	261	0	15	67	28	37	32	89	44
Australian, lean only	4 oz	206	0	8	53	22	29	25	70	35
Domestic, choice	4 oz	245	0	13	63	26	35	30	83	42

■ Roasted Leg, Shank Half—¼″ Trim

FOOD	AMOUNT	CAL	CARBS	FAT	WALK	RUN	BIKE	SWIM	YOGA	DANCE
Domestic, choice	4 oz	254	0	14	65	27	36	31	86	43
Domestic, choice, lean only	4 oz	203	0	8	52	22	29	25	69	35

■ Broiled Sirloin Chop—⅛″ Trim

FOOD	AMOUNT	CAL	CARBS	FAT	WALK	RUN	BIKE	SWIM	YOGA	DANCE
Australian	4 oz	266	0	16	69	28	38	32	90	45

FOOD	AMOUNT	CAL	CARBS	FAT	WALK	RUN	BIKE	SWIM	YOGA	DANCE
Australian, lean only	4 oz	212	0	9	55	23	30	26	72	36
■ **Broiled Loin Chop—⅛″ Trim**										
Australian	4 oz	247	0	14	64	26	35	30	84	42
Australian, lean only	4 oz	217	0	10	56	23	31	26	74	37
Domestic, choice	4 oz	336	0	23	87	36	48	41	114	57
New Zealand	4 oz	334	0	24	86	36	47	41	114	57
■ **Broiled Loin Chop—¼″ Trim**										
Domestic, choice	4 oz	357	0	26	92	38	51	43	121	61
Domestic, choice, lean only	4 oz	244	0	11	63	26	35	30	83	42
■ **Roasted Loin Chop—⅛″ Trim**										
Domestic, choice	4 oz	328	0	24	85	35	47	40	112	56
■ **Roasted Loin Chop—¼″ Trim**										
Domestic, choice	4 oz	349	0	27	90	37	50	42	119	59
Domestic, choice, lean only	4 oz	228	0	11	59	24	32	28	78	39
■ **Roasted Rib—⅛″ Trim**										
Australian	4 oz	313	0	23	81	33	44	38	106	53
Australian, lean only	4 oz	237	0	13	61	25	34	29	81	40
Domestic, choice	4 oz	385	0	31	99	41	55	47	131	66
New Zealand	4 oz	358	0	29	92	38	51	44	122	61
■ **Roasted Rib—¼″ Trim**										
Domestic, choice	4 oz	406	0	34	105	43	58	49	138	69
Domestic, choice, lean only	4 oz	262	0	15	68	28	37	32	89	45
■ **Broiled Rib—⅛″ Trim**										
Domestic, Choice	4 oz	384	0	30	99	41	54	47	131	65
■ **Broiled Rib—¼″ Trim**										
Domestic, choice	4 oz	408	0	33	105	43	58	50	139	70
Domestic, choice, lean only	4 oz	266	0	15	69	28	38	32	90	45
■ **Braised Whole Shoulder—⅛″ Trim**										
Domestic, choice	4 oz	382	0	27	98	41	54	46	130	65
New Zealand	4 oz	386	0	27	99	41	55	47	131	66
■ **Braised Whole Shoulder—¼″ Trim**										
Domestic, choice	4 oz	389	0	28	100	41	55	47	132	66
Domestic, choice, lean only	4 oz	320	0	18	82	34	45	39	109	55
■ **Broiled Whole Shoulder—⅛″ Trim**										
Domestic, choice	4 oz	303	0	21	78	32	43	37	103	52

FOOD	AMOUNT	CAL	CARBS	FAT	WALK	RUN	BIKE	SWIM	YOGA	DANCE
■ Broiled Whole Shoulder—¼″ Trim										
Domestic, choice	4 oz	314	0	22	81	33	45	38	107	53
Domestic, choice, lean only	4 oz	237	0	12	61	25	34	29	81	40
■ Roasted Whole Shoulder—⅛″ Trim										
Domestic, choice	4 oz	304	0	22	78	32	43	37	103	52
■ Roasted Whole Shoulder—¼″ Trim										
Domestic, choice	4 oz	312	0	23	80	33	44	38	106	53
Domestic, choice, lean only	4 oz	231	0	12	60	25	33	28	79	39
■ Braised Arm—⅛″ Trim										
Australian	4 oz	351	0	23	90	37	50	43	119	60
Australian, lean only	4 oz	269	0	12	69	29	38	33	91	46
Domestic, choice	4 oz	381	0	26	98	41	54	46	130	65
■ Braised Arm—¼″ Trim										
Domestic, choice	4 oz	391	0	27	101	42	55	48	133	67
Domestic, choice, lean only	4 oz	315	0	16	81	34	45	38	107	54
■ Broiled Arm—⅛″ Trim										
Domestic, choice	4 oz	304	0	20	78	32	43	37	103	52
■ Broiled Arm—¼″ Trim										
Domestic, choice	4 oz	318	0	22	82	34	45	39	108	54
Domestic, choice, lean only	4 oz	226	0	10	58	24	32	27	77	39
■ Roasted Arm—⅛″ Trim										
Domestic, choice	4 oz	302	0	21	78	32	43	37	103	51
■ Roasted Arm—¼″ Trim										
Domestic, choice	4 oz	315	0	23	81	34	45	38	107	54
Domestic, choice, lean only	4 oz	217	0	10	56	23	31	26	74	37
■ Braised Shoulder Blade—⅛″ Trim										
Domestic, choice	4 oz	383	0	27	99	41	54	47	130	65
■ Braised Shoulder Blade—¼″ Trim										
Domestic, choice	4 oz	390	0	28	101	42	55	47	133	66
Domestic, choice, lean only	4 oz	325	0	19	84	35	46	40	111	55
■ Broiled Shoulder Blade—⅛″ Trim										
Australian	4 oz	329	0	25	85	35	47	40	112	56
Domestic, choice	4 oz	302	0	21	78	32	43	37	103	51
■ Broiled Shoulder Blade—¼″ Trim										
Domestic, choice	4 oz	314	0	23	81	33	45	38	107	53
Domestic, choice, lean only	4 oz	238	0	13	61	25	34	29	81	41

FOOD	AMOUNT	CAL	CARBS	FAT	WALK	RUN	BIKE	SWIM	YOGA	DANCE
■ Roasted Shoulder Blade—⅛″ Trim										
Domestic, choice	4 oz	305	0	22	79	32	43	37	104	52
■ Roasted Shoulder Blade—¼″ Trim										
Domestic, choice	4 oz	318	0	23	82	34	45	39	108	54
Domestic, choice, lean only	4 oz	236	0	13	61	25	33	29	80	40
■ Braised Lamb Cubes (for Stews and Kabobs)										
Domestic, choice, 1/4″ Trim	4 oz	252	0	10	65	27	36	31	86	43
Domestic, choice, 1/4″ Trim, lean only	4 oz	210	0	8	54	22	30	26	71	36
■ Braised Foreshank—⅛″ Trim										
Australian	4 oz	267	0	16	69	28	38	32	91	45
Australian, lean only	4 oz	186	0	6	48	20	26	23	63	32
New Zealand	4 oz	292	0	18	75	31	41	36	99	50
■ Braised Foreshank—¼″ Trim										
Domestic, choice	4 oz	275	0	15	71	29	39	33	94	47
Domestic, choice, lean only	4 oz	211	0	7	54	22	30	26	72	36
■ Other Lamb										
Broiled ground lamb	3 oz	241	0	17	62	26	34	29	82	41
Braised lamb tongue	3 oz	234	0	17	60	25	33	28	80	40
Veal										
■ Leg (Top Round)										
Braised	4 oz	238	0	7	61	25	34	29	81	41
Braised, lean only	4 oz	229	0	6	59	24	32	28	78	39
Pan-fried and breaded	4 oz	258	11	10	66	27	37	31	88	44
Pan-fried and breaded, lean only	4 oz	233	11	7	60	25	33	28	79	40
Pan-fried (not breaded)	4 oz	238	0	9	61	25	34	29	81	41
Pan-fried (not breaded), lean only	4 oz	207	0	5	53	22	29	25	70	35
Roasted	4 oz	181	0	5	47	19	26	22	62	31
Roasted, lean only	4 oz	169	0	4	44	18	24	21	57	29
■ Loin										
Braised	4 oz	321	0	19	83	34	46	39	109	55
Braised, lean only	4 oz	255	0	10	66	27	36	31	87	43
Roasted	4 oz	245	0	14	63	26	35	30	83	42
Roasted, lean only	4 oz	198	0	8	51	21	28	24	67	34

FOOD	AMOUNT	CAL	CARBS	FAT	WALK	RUN	BIKE	SWIM	YOGA	DANCE
■ **Rib**										
Braised	4 oz	284	0	14	73	30	40	35	97	48
Braised, lean only	4 oz	246	0	9	63	26	35	30	84	42
Roasted	4 oz	258	0	16	66	27	37	31	88	44
Roasted, lean only	4 oz	200	0	8	52	21	28	24	68	34
■ **Whole Shoulder**										
Braised	4 oz	258	0	11	66	27	37	31	88	44
Braised, lean only	4 oz	225	0	7	58	24	32	27	77	38
Roasted	4 oz	208	0	10	54	22	30	25	71	35
Roasted, lean only	4 oz	192	0	7	49	20	27	23	65	33
■ **Arm**										
Braised	4 oz	267	0	12	69	28	38	32	91	45
Braised, lean only	4 oz	227	0	6	59	24	32	28	77	39
Roasted	4 oz	207	0	9	53	22	29	25	70	35
Roasted, lean only	4 oz	185	0	7	48	20	26	23	63	32
■ **Blade**										
Braised	4 oz	254	0	11	65	27	36	31	86	43
Braised, lean only	4 oz	224	0	7	58	24	32	27	76	38
Roasted	4 oz	210	0	10	54	22	30	26	71	36
Roasted, lean only	4 oz	193	0	8	50	21	27	23	66	33
■ **Sirloin**										
Braised	4 oz	285	0	15	73	30	40	35	97	49
Braised, lean only	4 oz	231	0	7	60	25	33	28	79	39
Roasted	4 oz	228	0	12	59	24	32	28	78	39
Roasted, lean only	4 oz	190	0	7	49	20	27	23	65	32
■ **Braised, Boneless Breast**										
Whole breast	4 oz	301	0	19	78	32	43	37	102	51
Whole breast, lean only	4 oz	246	0	11	63	26	35	30	84	42
Plate half	4 oz	319	0	21	82	34	45	39	109	54
Plate half, lean only	4 oz	280	0	16	72	30	40	34	95	48
■ **Veal Shank**										
Braised	4 oz	216	0	7	56	23	31	26	73	37
Braised, lean only	4 oz	200	0	5	52	21	28	24	68	34
■ **Braised Veal Cubes (for Stew)**										
Leg and shoulder meat, lean only	4 oz	212	0	5	55	23	30	26	72	36

FOOD	AMOUNT	CAL	CARBS	FAT	WALK	RUN	BIKE	SWIM	YOGA	DANCE
■ **Other Veal**										
Cooked ground veal	4 oz	194	0	9	50	21	28	24	66	33
Braised veal tongue	3 oz	172	0	9	44	18	24	21	59	29
Game Meat										
■ **Bison**										
Roasted, lean only	4 oz	162	0	3	42	17	23	20	55	28
Ribeye, lean only, roasted	4 oz	200	0	6	52	21	28	24	68	34
Top round, lean only, broiled	4 oz	197	0	6	51	21	28	24	67	34
Braised chuck, shoulder clod, lean only	4 oz	218	0	6	56	23	31	27	74	37
Sirloin, lean only, broiled	4 oz	193	0	6	50	21	27	23	66	33
Pan-broiled ground bison	4 oz	269	0	17	69	29	38	33	91	46
■ **Deer**										
Roasted	4 oz	179	0	4	46	19	25	22	61	30
Broiled loin, lean only	4 oz	169	0	3	44	18	24	21	57	29
Braised shoulder clod, lean only	4 oz	216	0	4	56	23	31	26	73	37
Broiled tenderloin, lean only	4 oz	168	0	3	43	18	24	20	57	29
Broiled top round, lean only	4 oz	172	0	2	44	18	24	21	59	29
Pan-broiled ground deer	4 oz	211	0	9	54	22	30	26	72	36
■ **Elk**										
Roasted	4 oz	165	0	2	43	18	23	20	56	28
Broiled loin, lean only	4 oz	189	0	4	49	20	27	23	64	32
Broiled tenderloin, lean only	4 oz	183	0	4	47	19	26	22	62	31
Broiled round, lean only	4 oz	176	0	3	45	19	25	21	60	30
Pan-broiled ground elk	4 oz	218	0	10	56	23	31	27	74	37
■ **Other Game Meat**										
Antelope, cooked	4 oz	169	0	3	44	18	24	21	57	29
Bear, simmered	4 oz	293	0	15	76	31	42	36	100	50
Beaver, cooked	4 oz	240	0	8	62	26	34	29	82	41
Beefalo, roasted	4 oz	212	0	7	55	23	30	26	72	36
Wild boar, roasted	4 oz	181	0	5	47	19	26	22	62	31
Water buffalo, roasted	4 oz	148	0	2	38	16	21	18	50	25
Caribou, roasted	4 oz	189	0	5	49	20	27	23	64	32
Goat, roasted	4 oz	162	0	3	42	17	23	20	55	28
Moose, roasted	4 oz	151	0	1	39	16	21	18	51	26

FOOD	AMOUNT	CAL	CARBS	FAT	WALK	RUN	BIKE	SWIM	YOGA	DANCE
Wild rabbit, stewed	4 oz	195	0	4	50	21	28	24	66	33
Domesticated rabbit, stewed	4 oz	233	0	10	60	25	33	28	79	40
Domesticated rabbit, roasted	4 oz	223	0	9	57	24	32	27	76	38

Sauce and Gravy

Asian Sauces										
Hoisin sauce	2 oz	123	24	2	32	13	17	15	42	21
Plum sauce	1 oz	52	12	0	13	6	7	6	18	9
A Taste of Thai Coconut Milk	.33 cup	140	3	15	36	15	20	17	48	24
A Taste of Thai Light Coconut Milk	.33 cup	45	3	4	12	5	6	5	15	8
A Taste of Thai Pad Thai Sauce	2 tbsp	90	20	1	23	10	13	11	31	15
A Taste of Thai Peanut Satay Sauce	2 tbsp	80	9	5	21	9	11	10	27	14
Boyajian Toasted Sesame Oil	2 tbsp	120	0	4	31	13	17	15	41	20
Gold's Wasabi Sauce	1 tsp	15	1	2	4	2	2	2	5	3
Kikkoman Tempura Dipping Sauce	1 tsp	5	1	0	1	1	1	1	2	1
La Choy Plum Sauce	1 tbsp	25	6	0	6	3	4	3	8	4
La Choy Spicy Szechwan Stir-Fry Sauce	.25 cup	42	9	0	11	4	6	5	14	7
Lum Kum Kee Black Bean and Garlic Sauce	1 tbsp	30	3	1	8	3	4	4	10	5
Lum Kum Kee Hoisin Sauce	2 tbsp	100	22	1	26	11	14	12	34	17
BBQ Sauce										
Barbecue sauce	1 cup	188	32	5	48	20	27	23	64	32
Bull's Eye Original Barbecue Sauce	2 tbsp	60	13	0	15	6	9	7	20	10
Hunt's Chicken Sensations Barbecue Sauce	1 tbsp	35	3	3	9	4	5	4	12	6
Hunt's Original Barbecue Sauce	2 tbsp	50	13	0	13	5	7	6	17	9
KC Masterpiece Original Barbecue Sauce	2 tbsp	60	15	0	15	6	9	7	20	10
Kraft Barbecue Sauce	2 tbsp	40	11	0	10	4	6	5	14	7
Open Pit Original Barbecue Sauce	2 tbsp	50	11	1	13	5	7	6	17	9

FOOD	AMOUNT	CAL	CARBS	FAT	WALK	RUN	BIKE	SWIM	YOGA	DANCE
Cheese Sauce										
Cheese fondue	1 cup	492	8	29	127	52	70	60	167	84
Homemade cheese sauce	1 cup	479	13	36	123	51	68	58	163	82
Chef-Mate Sharp Cheddar Sauce	1 cup	532	7	46	137	57	75	65	181	91
Chef-Mate Golden Cheese Sauce	1 cup	554	9	46	143	59	79	67	189	94
Chef-Mate Basic Cheddar Sauce	1 cup	327	32	19	84	35	46	40	111	56
Cheez Whiz Original Cheese Dip	2 tbsp	90	4	7	23	10	13	11	31	15
Cheez Whiz Light	2 tbsp	80	6	4	21	9	11	10	27	14
Cheez Whiz Cheezin 'n Squeezin	2 tbsp	100	4	8	26	11	14	12	34	17
Digiorno 4 Cheese Sauce	.25 cup	160	3	15	41	17	23	19	54	27
La Victoria Cheddar Cheese Sauce	.25 cup	105	6	8	27	11	15	13	36	18
La Victoria Medium Nacho Cheese Sauce with Jalapeño Pepper	.25 cup	122	7	10	31	13	17	15	41	21
Nestlé Que Bueno Jalapeño Cheese Sauce	1 cup	325	31	19	84	35	46	40	111	55
Ortega Mild Nacho Cheese Sauce	1 cup	476	10	41	123	51	68	58	162	81
Ortega Nacho Cheese Sauce	1 cup	512	16	40	132	54	73	62	174	87
Velveeta Spread	1 oz	85	3	6	22	9	12	10	29	14
Velveeta Reduced Fat	1 oz	62	3	3	16	7	9	8	21	11
Fruit Salsa										
Newman's Own Pineapple Salsa	2 tbsp	15	3	0	4	2	2	2	5	3
Santa Barbara Peach and Chipotle Salsa	2 tbsp	10	2	0	3	1	1	1	3	2
Santa Barbara Mango and Peach Salsa	2 tbsp	15	4	0	4	2	2	2	5	3
Gravy										
■ **Beef Gravy**										
Canned beef gravy	1 cup	123	11	6	32	13	17	15	42	21
Instant beef gravy	1 serving (6.7 g)	25	4	1	6	3	4	3	8	4
Franco-American Beef Gravy	1 cup	100	12	4	26	11	14	12	34	17
Heinz Beef Gravy	1 cup	120	16	1	31	13	17	15	41	20

FOOD	AMOUNT	CAL	CARBS	FAT	WALK	RUN	BIKE	SWIM	YOGA	DANCE
McCormick Schilling Beef and Herb Gravy Mix	2 tsp	30	3	1	8	3	4	4	10	5
Pepperidge Farm Hearty Beef Gravy	1 package	146	21	2	38	16	21	18	50	25
■ **Chicken Gravy**										
Canned chicken gravy	1 cup	188	13	14	48	20	27	23	64	32
Heinz Chicken Gravy	1 cup	200	12	4	52	21	28	24	68	34
Pillsbury Chicken-Style Gravy Mix	2 tsp	10	3	0	3	1	1	1	3	2
Pillsbury Chicken-Style Gravy	.25 cup	20	4	0	5	2	3	2	7	3
■ **Turkey Gravy**										
Homemade turkey gravy	1 cup	100	12	4	26	11	14	12	34	17
Instant turkey gravy	1 serving (6.7 g)	27	4	1	7	3	4	3	9	5
Canned turkey gravy	1 cup	121	12	5	31	13	17	15	41	21
Trio turkey gravy mix	1 serving	29	6	0	7	3	4	4	10	5
■ **Fast Food and Restaurant Gravy**										
El Pollo Loco Gravy	1 oz	14	2	0	4	1	2	2	5	2
Hardee's Gravy	1 serving	20	3	0	5	2	3	2	7	3
Whataburger Peppered Gravy	3 oz	75	8	5	19	8	11	9	26	13
Shoney's Country Gravy	3 oz	114	6	10	29	12	16	14	39	19
Denny's Brown Gravy	1 oz	13	2	0	3	1	2	2	4	2
Denny's Chicken Gravy	1 oz	15	2	1	4	2	2	2	5	3
Boston Market Poultry Gravy	2 oz	25	4	1	6	3	4	3	9	4
Denny's Country Gravy	1 oz	17	2	1	4	2	2	2	6	3
Denny's Sausage Gravy	4 oz	126	6	10	32	13	18	15	43	21
■ **Other Gravies**										
Canned au jus gravy	1 cup	38	6	0	10	4	5	5	13	6
Canned mushroom gravy	1 cup	119	13	6	31	13	17	14	40	20
Onion gravy	1 cup	77	16	1	20	8	11	9	26	13
Pork gravy mix	1 tbsp	25	4	1	6	3	4	3	9	4
McCormick Schilling Onion Gravy Mix	2 tsp	20	3	1	5	2	3	2	7	3
Nestlé Chef-Mate Country Sausage Gravy	1 cup	384	16	31	99	41	54	47	131	65
Pillsbury Brown Gravy	.25 cup	10	3	0	3	1	1	1	3	2
Pillsbury Homestyle Gravy	.25 cup	10	3	0	3	1	1	1	3	2
Pillsbury Homestyle Gravy Mix	2 tsp	10	3	0	3	1	1	1	3	2

FOOD	AMOUNT	CAL	CARBS	FAT	WALK	RUN	BIKE	SWIM	YOGA	DANCE
Trio Southern Gravy Mix	1 tbsp	48	6	3	12	5	7	6	16	8
Trio Country Gravy Mix	1 tbsp	35	5	1	9	4	5	4	12	6
Mole Poblano										
Homemade mole poblano	2 oz	92	7	6	24	10	13	11	31	16
Mole poblano mix	1 oz	160	12	12	41	17	23	19	54	27
La Victoria Mole Poblano	2 oz	240	28	10	62	26	34	29	82	41
Pasta Sauce										
■ Traditional										
Spaghetti sauce	1 cup	185	28	6	48	20	26	23	63	32
Homemade tomato sauce	.5 cup	60	9	1	15	6	9	7	20	10
Meatless spaghetti sauce	4 oz	54	10	1	14	6	8	7	18	9
Tomato sauce	1 cup	78	18	1	20	8	11	10	27	13
Tomato mushroom sauce	1 cup	86	21	0	22	9	12	10	29	15
Tomato sauce with onions	1 cup	103	24	0	27	11	15	13	35	18
Tomato sauce with cheese	.5 cup	144	25	5	37	15	20	18	49	25
Prego traditional spaghetti sauce	1 cup	240	38	7	62	26	34	29	82	41
Healthy Choice Traditional Pasta Sauce	.5 cup	50	11	0	13	5	7	6	17	9
Del Monte Traditional Spaghetti Sauce	.5 cup	60	15	1	15	6	9	7	20	10
Ragu Smooth Pasta Sauce	1 cup	160	24	5	41	17	23	19	54	27
■ Meat										
Contadina Spicy Italian Sausage and Bell Pepper Sauce	.5 cup	100	9	5	26	11	14	12	34	17
Del Monte Spaghetti Meat Sauce	.5 cup	60	14	1	15	6	9	7	20	10
Prego Meatball Parmesan Hearty Meat Sauce	1 cup	320	30	14	82	34	45	39	109	55
Prego 3 Meat Supreme Hearty Meat Sauce	1 cup	340	26	20	88	36	48	41	116	58
Ragu Hearty Beef Flavored Pasta Sauce	.5 cup	130	19	5	34	14	18	16	44	22
■ Vegetable										
Tomato-vodka pasta sauce	.5 cup	180	8	14	46	19	26	22	61	31
Del Monte Green Peppers and Mushroom Spaghetti Sauce	.5 cup	80	16	1	21	9	11	10	27	14
Del Monte Mushroom Spaghetti Sauce	.5 cup	60	14	1	15	6	9	7	20	10

FOOD	AMOUNT	CAL	CARBS	FAT	WALK	RUN	BIKE	SWIM	YOGA	DANCE
Del Monte Tomato Basil Sauce	.5 cup	70	16	1	18	7	10	9	24	12
Healthy Choice Super Chunky Vegetable Primavera Sauce	.5 cup	45	9	0	12	5	6	5	15	8
Healthy Choice Sun Dried Tomato and Herb Sauce	.5 cup	60	12	1	15	6	9	7	20	10
Ragu Light Chunky Mushroom Pasta Sauce	.5 cup	50	11	0	13	5	7	6	17	9
Ragu Gardenstyle Chunky Pasta Sauce	.5 cup	120	18	4	31	13	17	15	41	20
Ragu Tomato and Herb Pasta Sauce	.5 cup	50	11	0	13	5	7	6	17	9
■ **Alfredo Sauce**										
Alfredo sauce	.5 cup	280	6	26	72	30	40	34	95	48
Contadina Alfredo Sauce	.5 cup	400	8	38	103	43	57	49	136	68
Contadina Light Alfredo Sauce	.5 cup	190	10	13	49	20	27	23	65	32
Digiorno Light Alfredo Sauce	.25 cup	140	9	9	36	15	20	17	48	24
Healthy Choice Creamy Alfredo 4 Cheese Sauce	.25 cup	45	3	3	12	5	6	5	15	8
Progresso Alfredo Sauce	.5 cup	340	6	30	88	36	48	41	116	58
■ **Bolognese**										
Homemade bolognese sauce	.5 cup	120	8	6	31	13	17	15	41	20
Contadina Bolognese Sauce	5 oz	130	0	7	34	14	18	16	44	22
■ **Marinara**										
Marinara sauce	1 cup	185	28	6	48	20	26	23	63	32
Contadina Marinara Sauce	.5 cup	80	8	4	21	9	11	10	27	14
Healthy Choice Marinara Wine Sauce	.5 cup	50	11	1	13	5	7	6	17	9
Prego Marinara Sauce	.5 cup	110	12	6	28	12	16	13	37	19
■ **Garlic**										
Del Monte Chunky Garlic and Herb Spaghetti Sauce	.5 cup	60	11	2	15	6	9	7	20	10
Del Monte Garlic and Onion Spaghetti Sauce	.5 cup	80	16	1	21	9	11	10	27	14
Healthy Choice Garlic and Herb Sauce	.5 cup	50	10	0	13	5	7	6	17	9
Healthy Choice Garlic and Onion Pasta Sauce	.5 cup	40	9	0	10	4	6	5	14	7
Healthy Choice Original Garlic and Herb Pasta Sauce	.5 cup	50	10	0	13	5	7	6	17	9

FOOD	AMOUNT	CAL	CARBS	FAT	WALK	RUN	BIKE	SWIM	YOGA	DANCE
■ Cheese										
Del Monte 4 Cheese Spaghetti Sauce	.5 cup	70	15	2	18	7	10	9	24	12
Ragu Hearty Parmesan Pasta Sauce	.5 cup	120	18	4	31	13	17	15	41	20
■ Light										
Ragu Light Pasta Sauce	.5 cup	50	11	0	13	5	7	6	17	9
Ragu Light, No Added Sugar Pasta Sauce	.5 cup	60	9	2	15	6	9	7	20	10
■ Pesto Sauce										
Contadina Pesto Sauce with Sun-Dried Tomatoes	.25 cup	250	6	24	64	27	35	30	85	43
Contadina Pesto Sauce with Basil	.25 cup	310	5	30	80	33	44	38	105	53
Digiorno Pesto Sauce	.25 cup	320	3	31	82	34	45	39	109	55
Bel Aria Alla Genovese Pesto	.25 cup	380	3	36	98	40	54	46	129	65
Pizza Sauce										
Contadina Pizza Sauce	.25 cup	30	6	0	8	3	4	4	10	5
Progresso Pizza Sauce	.25 cup	20	4	0	5	2	3	2	7	3
Salsa and Other Mexican Sauces										
Salsa	2 tbsp	9	2	0	2	1	1	1	3	2
Adobo fresco	1 cup	651	54	60	168	69	92	79	221	111
Homemade sofrito sauce	2 tbsp	71	2	5	18	8	10	9	24	12
Breakstone's Nonfat Creamy Salsa	2 tbsp	20	3	0	5	2	3	2	7	3
Guiltless Gourmet Picante Sauce	1 oz	8	1	0	2	1	1	1	3	1
Guiltless Gourmet Roasted Red Pepper Salsa	2 tbsp	10	2	0	3	1	1	1	3	2
Guiltless Gourmet Tomatillo Salsa	2 tbsp	10	2	0	3	1	1	1	3	2
Kraft Nonfat Salsa Dip	2 tbsp	20	3	0	5	2	3	2	7	3
La Victoria Hot Salsa Brava	2 tbsp	4	1	0	1	0	1	0	1	1
La Victoria Hot Salsa Victoria	2 tbsp	7	1	0	2	1	1	1	2	1
La Victoria Hot Salsa Ranchera	2 tbsp	9	2	0	2	1	1	1	3	2
La Victoria Mild or Medium Salsa Picante	2 tbsp	8	0	0	2	1	1	1	3	1
La Victoria Mild Salsa Suprema	2 tbsp	8	2	0	2	1	1	1	3	1

FOOD	AMOUNT	CAL	CARBS	FAT	WALK	RUN	BIKE	SWIM	YOGA	DANCE
La Victoria Medium Salsa Suprema	2 tbsp	8	1	0	2	1	1	1	3	1
La Victoria Mild Green Chile Salsa	2 tbsp	8	1	0	2	1	1	1	3	1
La Victoria Mild, Medium or Hot Thick 'n Chunky Salsa	2 tbsp	8	1	0	2	1	1	1	3	1
La Victoria Green Salsa Jalapeña	2 tbsp	10	1	0	2	1	1	1	3	2
La Victoria Red Salsa Jalapeña	2 tbsp	12	2	0	3	1	2	1	4	2
La Victoria Chunky Chili Dip	2 tbsp	9	2	0	2	1	1	1	3	2
La Victoria Enchilada Sauce	.25 cup	20	3	1	5	2	3	2	7	3
Old El Paso Cheese and Salsa Dip	2 tbsp	40	3	3	10	4	6	5	14	7
Old El Paso Hot Taco Salsa, Hot, Medium, Mild	2 tbsp	10	2	0	3	1	1	1	3	2
Old El Paso Green Chili Salsa	2 tbsp	10	2	0	3	1	1	1	3	2
Old El Paso Mild Enchilada Sauce	.25 cup	25	4	1	6	3	4	3	9	4
Old El Paso Picante Salsa	2 tbsp	10	2	0	3	1	1	1	3	2
Old El Paso Thick 'n Chunky Picante Sauce	2 tbsp	6	1	0	2	1	1	1	2	1
Ortega Thick and Chunky Salsa	2 tbsp	8	2	0	2	1	1	1	3	1
Pace Medium Chunky Salsa	2 tbsp	4	1	1	1	0	1	0	1	1
Pace Mild Chunky Salsa	2 tbsp	4	1	1	1	0	1	0	1	1
Pace Extra Thick 'n Chunky Picante Sauce	2 tsp	3	1	0	1	0	0	0	1	1
Santa Barbara Black Bean and Corn Salsa	2 tbsp	20	4	0	5	2	3	2	7	3
Santa Barbara Artichoke Salsa	2 tbsp	15	2	1	4	2	2	2	5	3
Santa Barbara Fire-Roasted Chili Salsa	2 tbsp	10	2	0	3	1	1	1	3	2
Tostitos Salsa Con Queso	2 tbsp	80	10	5	21	9	11	10	27	14
Tostitos Fire Roasted Tomato Salsa	2 tbsp	30	4	0	8	3	4	4	10	5
Tostitos Restaurant Style or Mild, Medium, or Hot Salsa	4 tbsp	30	6	0	8	3	4	4	10	5
Tostitos Monterey Jack Queso Party Bowl	2 tbsp	40	4	3	10	4	6	5	14	7

FOOD	AMOUNT	CAL	CARBS	FAT	WALK	RUN	BIKE	SWIM	YOGA	DANCE
Seafood Sauce										
Oyster sauce	1 oz	14	3	0	4	1	2	2	5	2
Del Monte Cocktail Sauce	.25 cup	100	24	0	26	11	14	12	34	17
Heinz Cocktail Sauce	.25 cup	60	14	0	15	6	9	7	20	10
Progresso Creamy Clam Sauce	.5 cup	110	8	6	28	12	16	13	37	19
Progresso Lobster Sauce	.5 cup	100	6	7	26	11	14	12	34	17
Progresso Red Clam Sauce	.5 cup	60	8	1	15	6	9	7	20	10
Progresso White Clam Sauce	.5 cup	140	5	10	36	15	20	17	48	24
Soy and Teriyaki Sauces										
Teriyaki sauce	1 oz	24	4	0	6	3	3	3	8	4
Chef-Mate Teriyaki	2 oz	73	13	2	19	8	10	9	25	12
Kikkoman Soy Sauce	1 tbsp	10	0	0	3	1	1	1	3	2
La Choy Hot Teriyaki Chun King Sauce	1 tbsp	17	3	0	4	2	2	2	6	3
La Choy Light Soy Sauce	1 tbsp	15	2	0	4	2	2	2	5	3
La Choy Light Teriyaki Sauce	1 tbsp	18	4	0	5	2	3	2	6	3
La Choy Mandarin Soy Sauce	.25 cup	35	8	0	9	4	5	4	12	6
La Choy Soy Sauce	1 tbsp	11	1	0	3	1	1	1	4	2
La Choy Teriyaki Sauce	.5 tsp	2	1	1	1	0	0	0	1	0
La Choy Teriyaki Sauce	.25 cup	47	11	0	12	5	7	6	16	8
Lum Kum Kee Soy Sauce	1 tbsp	10	1	0	3	1	1	1	3	2
Steak Sauce										
A-1 Bold Steak Sauce	1 tbsp	18	4	0	5	2	3	2	6	3
A-1 Steak Sauce	1 tbsp	18	4	0	5	2	3	2	6	3
Heinz 57 Steak Sauce	1 tbsp	15	4	0	4	2	2	2	5	3
Hunt's Steak Sauce	1 tbsp	10	2	0	3	1	1	1	4	2
Kikkoman Steak Sauce	1 tbsp	20	5	0	5	2	3	2	7	3
Peter Luger Steak Sauce	1 tbsp	30	7	0	8	3	4	4	10	5
Sweet and Sour Sauce										
Contadina Sweet and Sour Sauce	2 tbsp	40	8	1	10	4	6	5	14	7
Kikkoman Sweet and Sour Sauce	2 tbsp	35	9	0	9	4	5	4	12	6
La Choy Sweet and Sour Duck Sauce	1 tbsp	31	7	0	8	3	4	4	10	5
La Choy Sweet and Sour Sauce	.25 cup	69	18	0	18	7	10	8	23	12

FOOD	AMOUNT	CAL	CARBS	FAT	WALK	RUN	BIKE	SWIM	YOGA	DANCE
Taco Sauce										
Heinz Taco Sauce	1 tbsp	6	1	0	2	1	1	1	2	1
La Victoria Mild or Medium Red Taco Sauce	1 tbsp	7	1	0	2	1	1	1	2	1
La Victoria Mild or Medium Green Taco Sauce	1 tbsp	4	1	0	1	0	1	0	1	1
Old El Paso Extra Chunky Taco Sauce	1 tbsp	5	1	0	1	1	1	1	2	1
Tartar Sauce										
Hellman's Low Fat Tartar Sauce	2 tbsp	40	7	2	10	4	6	5	14	7
Hellman's Tartar Sauce	1 tbsp	70	0	8	18	7	10	9	24	12
Hellman's Tartar Sauce	2 tbsp	140	1	16	36	15	20	17	48	24
Worcestershire Sauce										
Worcestershire sauce	1 cup	184	54	0	47	20	26	22	63	31
Lea & Perrins Worcestershire Sauce	1 tsp	5	1	1	1	1	1	1	2	1
Other Sauces										
Homemade medium white sauce	.5 cup	184	11	13	47	20	26	22	63	31
Brown sauce	4 oz	57	7	3	15	6	8	7	19	10
Thick brown sauce	4 oz	100	6	8	26	11	14	12	34	17
Mushroom cream sauce	4 oz	265	4	27	68	28	38	32	90	45
Hot pepper sauce	1 oz	3	1	0	1	0	0	0	1	1
Chili tomato sauce	1 cup	284	54	1	73	30	40	35	97	48
Tabasco sauce	1 oz	3	0	0	1	0	0	0	1	1
Casbah Tahini Sauce Mix (prepared)	.25 cup	160	10	13	41	17	23	19	54	27
Chef-Mate Stir-Fry Sauce	4 oz	121	18	4	31	13	17	15	41	21
Chef-Mate Coney Island Hot Dog Sauce	4 oz	137	10	9	35	15	19	17	47	23
Green Giant Sloppy Joe Sauce	.25 cup	50	11	0	13	5	7	6	17	9
Gold's Horseradish Sauce	1 tsp	0	0	0	0	0	0	0	0	0
Gold's Horseradish Sauce with Beets	1 tsp	0	0	0	0	0	0	0	0	0
Hunt's Chicken Sensations Italian Garlic Sauce	1 tbsp	30	1	3	8	3	4	4	10	5
Hunt's Chicken Sensations Lemon Herb Sauce	1 tbsp	31	2	3	8	3	4	4	11	5

FOOD	AMOUNT	CAL	CARBS	FAT	WALK	RUN	BIKE	SWIM	YOGA	DANCE
Hunt's Chicken Sensations Southwestern Sauce	1 tbsp	27	1	3	7	3	4	3	9	5
Nestlé LJ Minor Creole Sauce	1 cup	99	15	3	26	11	14	12	34	17
Nestlé LJ Minor Lemon Sauce	2 tbsp	43	10	0	11	5	6	5	15	7
Schaller & Weber Creamy Horseradish Sauce	1 tsp	20	1	2	5	2	3	2	7	3
Tabasco Hot Pepper Sauce	.25 tsp	1	1	0	0	0	0	0	0	0
Tabasco Jalapeño Sauce	1 tsp	0	0	0	0	0	0	0	0	0
Sauce Mixes										
Bearnaise sauce mix	1 oz	101	17	3	26	11	14	12	34	17
Curry sauce mix	1 oz	120	14	6	31	13	17	15	41	20
Mushroom sauce mix	1 oz	98	15	3	25	10	14	12	33	17
Spaghetti sauce mix	1 oz	79	18	0	20	8	11	10	27	13
Spaghetti sauce mix with mushrooms	1 oz	85	14	3	22	9	12	10	29	14
Stroganoff sauce mix	1 oz	197	16	3	51	21	28	24	67	34
Sweet and sour sauce mix	1 oz	109	27	0	28	12	15	13	37	19
White sauce mix	1 oz	130	14	8	34	14	18	16	44	22
Sour cream sauce mix	1 oz	143	13	9	37	15	20	17	49	24
Kikkoman Sweet and Sour Sauce Mix	1.5 tbsp	60	14	0	15	6	9	7	20	10
Knorr Alfredo Sauce Mix	1 oz	115	13	5	30	12	16	14	39	20
McCormick Schilling Primavera Sauce Blend	1 tbsp	30	4	1	8	3	4	4	10	5
McCormick Schilling Spaghetti Sauce Mix	1 tbsp	25	5	0	6	3	4	3	9	4
McCormick Schilling Herb and Garlic Pasta Sauce Blend	1 tbsp	20	2	0	5	2	3	2	7	3
Trio Nacho Cheese Sauce Mix	1 oz	120	18	4	31	13	17	15	41	20
Condiments										
Hummus	1 tbsp	27	3	1	7	3	4	3	9	5
Tahini (sesame butter)	1 tbsp	89	3	8	23	10	13	11	30	15
French's Yellow Mustard	1 tsp	0	0	0	0	0	0	0	0	0
French's Honey Mustard	1 tsp	10	1	0	3	1	1	1	3	2
Grey Poupon Dijon Mustard	1 tsp	5	<1	0	1	1	1	1	2	1
Gulden's Spicy Brown Mustard	1 tsp	5	0	0	1	1	1	1	2	1
Heinz Ketchup	1 tbsp	15	4	0	4	2	2	2	5	3

FOOD	AMOUNT	CAL	CARBS	FAT	WALK	RUN	BIKE	SWIM	YOGA	DANCE
Hellman's Dijonnaise	1 tsp	5	1	0	1	1	1	1	2	1
Mayonnaise										
Hellman's Real Mayonnaise	1 tbsp	90	0	10	23	10	13	11	31	15
Hellman's Reduced Fat Mayonnaise	1 tbsp	20	2	2	5	2	3	2	7	3
Hellman's Light Mayonnaise	1 tbsp	45	<1	5	12	5	6	5	15	8

Fish and Shellfish

FOOD	AMOUNT	CAL	CARBS	FAT	WALK	RUN	BIKE	SWIM	YOGA	DANCE
Caviar										
Caviar, black and red	1 tbsp	40	1	3	10	4	6	5	14	7
Salmon roe	1 tbsp	40	0	2	10	4	6	5	14	7
Osetra caviar	1 tbsp	72	1	5	19	8	10	9	24	12
Roe (mixed species), raw	1 tbsp	20	0	1	5	2	3	2	7	3
Canned or Jarred Fish										
Anchovies canned in oil	1 oz, boneless	60	0	3	15	6	8	7	20	10
Season fillets of anchovies	6 pieces	25	0	1	6	3	4	3	9	4
Roland fillets of anchovies in olive oil	6 pieces	25	0	1	6	3	4	3	9	4
Atlantic cod, canned	3 oz	89	0	73	23	9	13	11	30	15
Jack mackerel, canned	3 oz	133	0	5	34	14	19	16	45	23
Gefilte fish	1 piece (65 g)	55	5	1	14	6	8	7	19	9
Pickled herring	1 oz, boneless	74	3	5	19	8	10	9	25	13
Kippered herring	1 oz, boneless	62	0	4	16	7	9	7	21	10
Salted mackerel	3 oz	259	0	21	67	28	37	32	88	44
Canned chum salmon	3 oz	120	0	5	31	13	17	15	41	20
Pink salmon, canned	3 oz	118	0	5	30	13	17	14	40	20
Sockeye salmon, canned	3 oz	130	0	6	34	14	18	16	44	22
Sardines, canned in oil	1 can (3.75 oz)	191	0	11	49	20	27	23	65	33
Season skinless boneless sardines canned in water	1 can (4.25 oz)	130	0	5	34	14	18	16	44	22
Season sardines in tomato sauce	1 can (4.375 oz)	180	2	10	46	19	26	22	61	31

FOOD	AMOUNT	CAL	CARBS	FAT	WALK	RUN	BIKE	SWIM	YOGA	DANCE
Light tuna, canned in oil	3 oz	168	0	7	43	18	24	20	57	29
Light tuna, canned in water	3 oz	99	0	1	26	11	14	12	34	17
White tuna, canned in oil	3 oz	158	0	7	41	17	22	19	54	27
White tuna, canned in water	3 oz	109	0	3	28	12	15	13	37	19
Bumblebee Chunk Light Tuna in Oil	2 oz	110	0	6	28	12	16	13	37	19
Bumblebee Chunk Light Tuna in Water	2 oz	60	0	5	15	6	9	7	20	10
Bumblebee Diet Chunk White Tuna in Water	2 oz	70	0	1	18	7	10	9	24	12
Chicken of the Sea Pink Salmon (in a pouch)	1 pouch (3 oz)	90	0	3	23	10	13	11	31	15
Ortiz Albacore Tuna Bonito in Olive Oil	.25 cup	160	0	11	41	17	23	19	54	27
Starkist Premium Chunk White Albacore Tuna in Water (in a pouch)	2 oz	80	0	1	21	9	11	10	27	14
Starkist Solid White Albacore Tuna in Spring Water	2 oz	70	0	1	18	7	10	9	24	12
Smoked Fish										
Haddock, smoked	3 oz, boneless	99	0	1	26	11	14	12	34	17
Sablefish, smoked	4 oz	73	0	6	19	8	10	9	25	12
Chinook salmon, smoked (lox)	3 oz	99	0	4	26	11	14	12	34	17
Smoked sturgeon	3 oz	147	0	4	38	16	21	18	50	25
Smoked whitefish	3 oz	92	0	1	24	10	13	11	31	16
Fish Salad										
Tuna salad	1 cup	383	19	19	99	41	54	47	130	65
Low-fat tuna salad	1 cup	240	6	5	62	26	34	29	82	41
Frozen Fish										
Sweet gefilte fish, from frozen loaf	1 slice (55 g)	80	7	4	21	9	11	10	27	14
Frozen Fish Entrees										
Frozen salmon nuggets	3 oz	240	16	13	62	26	34	29	82	41
Birds Eye Voila Garlic Shrimp	1 cup, cooked	220	27	8	57	23	31	27	75	37
Healthy Choice Herb Baked Fish	1 meal (10.9 oz)	360	55	8	93	38	51	44	122	61
Healthy Choice Lemon Pepper Fish	1 meal (10.7 oz)	280	49	5	72	30	40	34	95	48

FOOD	AMOUNT	CAL	CARBS	FAT	WALK	RUN	BIKE	SWIM	YOGA	DANCE
Healthy Choice Creamy Garlic Shrimp	1 meal (11.5 oz)	270	35	6	70	29	38	33	92	46
Healthy Choice Cajun Style Chicken and Shrimp	1 meal (10.4 oz)	240	32	4	62	26	34	29	82	41
Healthy Choice Tuna Casserole	1 meal (9 oz)	250	30	7	64	27	35	30	85	43
Weight Watchers Smart Ones Tuna Noodle Gratin	1 package (269 g)	270	38	7	70	29	38	33	92	46
Weight Watchers Smart Ones Shrimp Marinara	1 package (255 g)	180	28	2	46	19	26	22	61	31
Cooked Fish										
Freshwater bass, cooked	4 oz	165	0	5	43	18	23	20	56	28
Striped bass, cooked	4 oz	140	0	3	36	15	20	17	48	24
Sea bass, cooked	4 oz	140	0	3	36	15	20	17	48	24
Bluefish, cooked	4 oz	180	0	6	46	19	26	22	61	31
Butterfish, cooked	4 oz	211	0	12	54	22	30	26	72	36
Carp, cooked	4 oz	184	0	8	47	20	26	22	63	31
Farmed catfish, cooked	4 oz	172	0	9	44	18	24	21	59	29
Wild catfish, cooked	4 oz	119	0	3	31	13	17	14	40	20
Catfish, breaded and fried	4 oz	259	9	15	67	28	37	32	88	44
Cod (Pacific or Atlantic), cooked	4 oz	119	0	1	31	13	17	14	40	20
Atlantic croaker, breaded and fried	4 oz	250	9	14	64	27	35	30	85	43
Cusk, cooked	4 oz	127	0	99	33	14	18	15	43	22
Dolphinfish, cooked	1 fillet	123	0	1	32	13	17	15	42	21
Flatfish (flounder or sole), cooked	4 oz	132	0	2	34	14	19	16	45	22
Grouper, cooked	4 oz	133	0	1	34	14	19	16	45	23
Haddock, cooked	4 oz	127	0	1	33	14	18	15	43	22
Halibut (Atlantic or Pacific), cooked	4 oz	158	0	3	41	17	22	19	54	27
Greenland halibut	4 oz	270	0	20	70	29	38	33	92	46
Atlantic herring, cooked	4 oz	229	0	13	59	24	32	28	78	39
Pacific herring, cooked	4 oz	282	0	20	73	30	40	34	96	48
Ling, cooked	4 oz	125	0	1	32	13	18	15	43	21
Lingcod, cooked	4 oz	123	0	2	32	13	17	15	42	21
Atlantic mackerel, cooked	4 oz	296	0	20	76	32	42	36	101	50
Pacific or jack mackerel, cooked	4 oz	228	0	11	59	24	32	28	78	39

FOOD	AMOUNT	CAL	CARBS	FAT	WALK	RUN	BIKE	SWIM	YOGA	DANCE
King mackerel, cooked	4 oz	151	0	3	39	16	21	18	51	26
Spanish mackerel, cooked	4 oz	179	0	7	46	19	25	22	61	30
Milkfish, cooked	4 oz	215	0	10	55	23	30	26	73	37
Monkfish, cooked	4 oz	110	0	2	28	12	16	13	37	19
Striped mullet, cooked	4 oz	169	0	5	44	18	24	21	57	29
Atlantic ocean perch, cooked	4 oz	137	0	2	35	15	19	17	47	23
Perch (mixed species), cooked	4 oz	132	0	1	34	14	19	16	45	22
Ocean pout, cooked	4 oz	115	0	1	30	12	16	14	39	20
Northern pike, cooked	4 oz	128	0	1	33	14	18	16	44	22
Walleye pike, cooked	4 oz	134	0	2	35	14	19	16	46	23
Atlantic pollock, cooked	4 oz	133	0	1	34	14	19	16	45	23
Walleye pollock, cooked	4 oz	128	0	1	33	14	18	16	44	22
Florida pompano, cooked	4 oz	238	0	14	61	25	34	29	81	41
Pacific rockfish, cooked	4 oz	137	0	2	35	15	19	17	47	23
Orange roughy, cooked	4 oz	119	0	1	31	13	17	14	40	20
Sablefish, cooked	4 oz	282	0	22	73	30	40	34	96	48
Atlantic salmon (farmed), cooked	4 oz	233	0	14	60	25	33	28	79	40
Atlantic salmon (wild), cooked	4 oz	206	0	9	53	22	29	25	70	35
Chinook salmon, cooked	4 oz	261	0	15	67	28	37	32	89	44
Chum salmon, cooked	4 oz	174	0	5	45	19	25	21	59	30
Coho salmon (farmed), cooked	4 oz	201	0	9	52	21	29	24	68	34
Coho salmon (wild), cooked	4 oz	157	0	5	40	17	22	19	53	27
Pink salmon, cooked	4 oz	168	0	5	43	18	24	20	57	29
Sockeye salmon, cooked	4 oz	244	0	12	63	26	35	30	83	42
Scup, cooked	4 oz	153	0	4	39	16	22	19	52	26
Seatrout, cooked	4 oz	150	0	5	39	16	21	18	51	26
American shad, cooked	4 oz	285	0	20	73	30	40	35	97	49
Shark, batter-dipped and fried	4 oz	258	7	16	66	27	37	31	88	44
Sheepshead fish, cooked	4 oz	142	0	2	37	15	20	17	48	24
Rainbow smelt, cooked	4 oz	140	0	4	36	15	20	17	48	24
Snapper, cooked	4 oz	145	0	2	37	15	21	18	49	25
Spot, cooked	4 oz	179	0	7	46	19	25	22	61	30
Sturgeon, cooked	4 oz	153	0	6	39	16	22	19	52	26
White sucker, cooked	4 oz	134	0	3	35	14	19	16	46	23
Swordfish, cooked	4 oz	175	0	6	45	19	25	21	60	30
Tilefish, cooked	4 oz	166	0	5	43	18	24	20	56	28

FOOD	AMOUNT	CAL	CARBS	FAT	WALK	RUN	BIKE	SWIM	YOGA	DANCE
Rainbow trout (farmed), cooked	4 oz	191	0	8	49	20	27	23	65	33
Rainbow trout (wild), cooked	4 oz	169	0	7	44	18	24	21	57	29
Trout (mixed species), cooked	4 oz	215	0	10	55	23	30	26	73	37
Bluefin tuna, cooked	4 oz	208	0	7	54	22	30	25	71	35
Skipjack tuna, cooked	4 oz	149	0	1	38	16	21	18	51	25
Yellowfin tuna, cooked	4 oz	157	0	1	40	17	22	19	53	27
Yellowfin tuna, sesame crusted	6 oz	280	6	13	72	30	40	34	95	48
Turbot, cooked	4 oz	138	0	4	36	15	20	17	47	24
Whitefish (mixed species), cooked	4 oz	194	0	8	50	21	28	24	66	33
Whiting	4 oz	131	0	2	34	14	19	16	45	22
Wolffish	4 oz	139	0	3	36	15	20	17	47	24
Yellowtail	4 oz	211	0	8	54	22	30	26	72	36
Tilapia, cooked	4 oz	145	0	3	37	15	21	18	49	25
Shellfish										
Alaska king crab, cooked	1 leg	82	0	1	21	9	12	10	28	14
Blue crab, cooked	3 oz	87	0	2	22	9	12	11	30	15
Crab cake	1 cake (60 g)	93	0	5	24	10	13	11	32	16
Dungeness crab, cooked	3 oz	94	1	1	24	10	13	11	32	16
Queen crab	3 oz	98	0	1	25	10	14	12	33	17
Crayfish, cooked	3 oz	74	0	1	19	8	10	9	25	13
Northern lobster	3 oz	83	1	1	21	9	12	10	28	14
Spiny lobster	3 oz	122	3	2	31	13	17	15	41	21
Canned shrimp	10 shrimp	32	0	0	8	3	5	4	11	5
Breaded and fried shrimp	4 large shrimp	73	3	4	19	8	10	9	25	12
Cooked shrimp	4 large shrimp	22	0	0	6	2	3	3	7	4
Fried abalone	3 oz	161	9	6	41	17	23	20	55	27
Canned clams	1 cup	237	8	3	61	25	34	29	81	40
Breaded and fried clams	20 small clams	380	19	21	98	40	54	46	129	65
Cooked clams	20 small clams	281	10	4	72	30	40	34	96	48
Roland canned baby clams	0.5 cup	50	2	0	13	5	7	6	17	9

FOOD	AMOUNT	CAL	CARBS	FAT	WALK	RUN	BIKE	SWIM	YOGA	DANCE
Roland canned chopped clams	0.33 cup	45	0	0	12	5	6	5	15	8
Stuffed clams	1 clam (71 g)	120	14	5	31	13	17	15	41	20
Cooked mollusks	3 oz	134	1	1	35	14	19	16	46	23
Cooked mussels	3 oz	146	6	4	38	16	21	18	50	25
Cooked octopus	3 oz	139	4	2	36	15	20	17	47	24
Pacific oyster, raw	1 medium	40	2	1	10	4	6	5	14	7
Pacific oyster, cooked	1 medium	41	2	1	11	4	6	5	14	7
Eastern oyster (wild), raw	6 medium	57	3	2	15	6	8	7	19	10
Eastern oyster (wild), cooked (moist heat)	6 medium	58	3	2	15	6	8	7	20	10
Eastern oyster (wild), cooked (dry heat)	6 medium	42	3	1	11	4	6	5	14	7
Eastern oyster (farmed), raw	6 medium	50	5	1	13	5	7	6	17	9
Eastern oystern (farmed), cooked	6 medium	47	4	1	12	5	7	6	16	8
Breaded and fried eastern oysters	6 medium	173	10	11	45	18	25	21	59	29
Breaded and fried scallops	2 large	67	3	3	17	7	10	8	23	11
Steamed scallops	3 oz	95	0	1	24	10	13	12	32	16
Fried squid	3 oz	149	7	6	38	16	21	18	51	25
Baked/broiled conch	3 oz	66	1	1	17	7	9	8	22	11
Long John Silver's Battered Shrimp	1 piece	45	3	3	12	5	6	5	15	8
Buttered Lobster Bites (snack box)	4 oz	250	27	9	64	27	35	30	85	43
Red Lobster Grilled Jumbo Shrimp Dinner	1 serving	142	1	3	37	15	20	17	48	24
Red Lobster Jumbo Shrimp Cocktail Dinner	1 serving	228	2	4	59	24	32	28	78	39
Red Lobster Snow Crabs Legs	1 serving	262	0	5	68	28	37	32	89	45
Red Lobster Live Maine Lobster	1 serving	145	2	1	37	15	21	18	49	25
Red Lobster Rock Lobster Tail	1 serving	258	0	3	66	27	37	31	88	44
Red Lobster Lobster Chops	1 serving	321	0	9	83	34	46	39	109	55
Red Lobster King Crab Legs	1 serving	490	0	9	126	52	70	60	167	83
Fish Soups										
Homemade fish stock	100 g	17	0	1	4	2	2	2	6	3
Bouillabaisse	1 cup	90	10	4	23	10	13	11	31	15

FOOD	AMOUNT	CAL	CARBS	FAT	WALK	RUN	BIKE	SWIM	YOGA	DANCE
Shark-fin soup	1 cup	99	8	4	26	11	14	12	34	17
Condensed Manhattan Clam Chowder, prepared w/water	100 g	32	5	1	8	3	5	4	11	5
Condensed New England Clam Chowder, prepared w/water	100 g	39	5	1	10	4	6	5	13	7
Condensed New England Clam Chowder, prepared w/milk	100 g	66	7	3	17	7	9	8	22	11
Condensed Tomato Bisque, prepared w/milk	100 g	79	12	3	20	8	11	10	27	13
Au Bon Pain Clam Chowder	1 cup	220	20	13	57	23	31	27	75	37
Au Bon Pain Mediterranean Seafood Stew	1 cup	140	12	4	36	15	20	17	48	24
Boston Chowda Charleston Crab Soup	1 cup	320	16	23	82	34	45	39	109	55
Boston Chowda Lobster Bisque	1 cup	260	12	19	67	28	37	32	88	44
Boston Chowda New England Clam Chowder	1 cup	280	20	17	72	30	40	34	95	48
Boston Chowda Shrimp and Sausage Gumbo	1 cup	420	38	23	108	45	60	51	143	72
Cousins Subs New England Clam Chowder	large	234	39	4	60	25	33	28	80	40
Campbell's Condensed Manhattan Clam Chowder	4 oz	70	12	1	18	7	10	9	24	12
Denny's Clam Chowder	1 serving	624	55	42	161	66	89	76	212	106
Stouffer's Cajun Seasoned Stew	1 tsp	24	2	1	6	3	3	3	8	4
Progresso Healthy Classics New England Clam Chowder	100 g	48	8	1	12	5	7	6	16	8
Progresso Manhattan Clam Chowder	8 oz	110	17	2	28	12	16	13	37	19
Schlotzky's Boston Clam Chowder	1 cup	233	24	15	60	25	33	28	79	40
Schlotzky's Corn Chowder	1 cup	284	38	17	73	30	40	35	97	48
Other Seafood										
Eel, cooked	4 oz (boneless)	268	0	17	69	29	38	33	91	46
Surimi	3 oz	84	6	1	22	9	12	10	29	14
Fake crab (from surimi)	3 oz	87	0	1	22	9	12	11	30	15
Fake shrimp (from surimi)	3 oz	86	8	1	22	9	12	10	29	15
Fake scallops (from surimi)	3 oz	84	9	0	22	9	12	10	29	14
Meatless fish sticks	3 sticks	244	8	15	63	26	35	30	83	42

FOOD	AMOUNT	CAL	CARBS	FAT	WALK	RUN	BIKE	SWIM	YOGA	DANCE

Frozen and Canned Meals

Pasta Dinners

FOOD	AMOUNT	CAL	CARBS	FAT	WALK	RUN	BIKE	SWIM	YOGA	DANCE
Betty Crocker Bowl Appetit Herb Chicken Flavored Vegetable Rice	1 bowl	260	49	5	67	28	37	32	88	44
Hodgson Mill Whole Wheat Macaroni and Cheese Dinner	1 serving	263	48	3	68	28	37	32	89	45
Hamburger Helper Cheese-burger Macaroni	1 cup	320	30	4	82	34	45	39	109	55
Kraft Easy Mac Extreme Cheese	1 pouch	240	40	6	62	26	34	29	82	41
Kraft Deluxe Macaroni and Cheese Dinner with Original Cheddar Cheese Sauce	1 cup	320	46	9	82	34	45	39	109	55
Kraft Mac and Cheese, the Cheesiest	1 cup prepared	380	48	16	98	40	54	46	129	65
Kraft Macaroni and Cheese Dinner, Original	1 cup	259	48	3	67	28	37	32	88	44
Lipton Alfredo Egg Noodles in Creamy Sauce	1 cup	389	58	11	100	41	55	47	132	66
Wacky Mac	2 oz (⅙ package)	200	41	1	52	21	28	24	68	34

Frozen Soy and Veggie Burgers

■ Morningstar Farms

FOOD	AMOUNT	CAL	CARBS	FAT	WALK	RUN	BIKE	SWIM	YOGA	DANCE
Morningstar Farms Garden Vegetable Patties	1 patty	100	9	3	26	11	14	12	34	17
Morningstar Farms Deli Franks	1 frank	112	4	6	29	12	16	14	38	19
Morningstar Farms Burger Crumbles	.66 cup	80	4	3	21	9	11	10	27	14
Morningstar Farms Better'n Burgers	1 patty	100	6	2	26	11	14	12	34	17
Morningstar Farms Breakfast Links	2 links	80	3	3	21	9	11	10	27	14
Morningstar Farms Spicy Black Bean Burger	1 patty	140	15	4	36	15	20	17	48	24
Morningstar Farms Chik Patties	1 patty	150	16	6	39	16	21	18	51	26

■ Other Soy and Veggie Burgers

FOOD	AMOUNT	CAL	CARBS	FAT	WALK	RUN	BIKE	SWIM	YOGA	DANCE
Green Giant Harvest Burger	1 patty	138	7	4	36	15	20	17	47	24

FOOD	AMOUNT	CAL	CARBS	FAT	WALK	RUN	BIKE	SWIM	YOGA	DANCE
Loma Linda Meatless Big Franks	1 link	118	2	7	30	13	17	14	40	20
Natural Touch Garden Vegetable Burger	1 patty	119	10	4	31	13	17	14	40	20
Natural Touch Vegan Burger	1 patty	91	8	1	23	10	13	11	31	16
Canned Meals										
Armour Canned Beef Hash	1 serving	498	12	39	128	53	71	61	169	85
Canned beef stew	1 serving	220	16	12	57	23	31	27	75	37
Canned chili con carne with beans	1 cup	298	28	13	77	32	42	36	101	51
Canned macaroni and cheese	1 serving	200	28	6	52	21	28	24	68	34
Canned pasta with sliced franks in tomato aauce	1 serving	262	30	12	68	28	37	32	89	45
Chef Boyardee Canned Beef Ravioli in Tomato and Meat Sauce	1 serving	229	37	5	59	24	32	28	78	39
Chef Boyardee Canned Beefaroni	1 serving	184	31	3	48	20	26	22	63	31
Chef Boyardee Canned Mini Beef Ravioli in Tomato and Meat Sauce	1 serving	239	41	5	62	25	34	29	81	41
Chef Boyardee Canned Spaghetti and Meatballs in Tomato Sauce	1 serving	250	34	9	64	27	35	30	85	43
Chef Boyardee Canned Teenage Mutant Ninja Turtles Pasta and Mini Meatballs in Tomato Sauce	1 serving	227	34	7	58	24	32	28	77	39
Chef Mate Canned Corned Beef Hash	1 cup	486	29	30	125	52	69	59	165	83
Chef Mate Chili with Beans	1 cup	412	29	25	106	44	58	50	140	70
Chef Mate Chili without Beans	1 cup	430	18	32	111	46	61	52	146	73
Chun King Canned Sweet and Sour Vegetables, Fruit, and Sauce with Chicken	1 serving	165	32	2	43	18	23	20	56	28
Dinty Moore Canned Beef Stew	1 cup	222	16	13	57	24	31	27	75	38
El Rio Canned Chili Con Carne	1 serving	305	16	20	79	32	43	37	104	52
Hormel Canned Chili with Beans	1 cup	240	34	4	62	26	34	29	81	41
Hormel Canned Chili without Beans	1 cup	194	18	7	50	21	27	24	66	33

FOOD	AMOUNT	CAL	CARBS	FAT	WALK	RUN	BIKE	SWIM	YOGA	DANCE
Hormel Canned Roast Beef Hash	1 cup	385	23	24	99	41	55	47	131	66
Hormel Canned Turkey Chili with Beans	1 cup	203	26	3	52	22	29	25	69	35
Hormel Canned Vegetarian Chili with Beans	1 cup	205	38	1	53	22	29	25	70	35
Hormel Corn Beef Hash	1 cup	387	22	24	100	41	55	47	132	66
Nalley Canned Chili Con Carne	1 serving	281	12	8	72	30	40	34	96	48
Stagg Canned Classic Chili with Beans	1 cup	324	29	16	83	34	46	39	110	55
Stagg Canned Country Chili with Beans	1 cup	319	29	16	82	34	45	39	108	54
Stagg Canned Dynamite Chili with Beans	1 cup	333	31	15	86	36	47	41	113	57
Stagg Canned Ranchhouse Chili with Beans	1 cup	284	32	9	73	30	40	35	97	48
Stagg Canned Silverado Chili with Beans	1 cup	227	33	3	59	24	32	28	77	39
Sweet Sue Canned Chicken and Dumplings	1 serving	218	23	7	56	23	31	27	74	37
Frozen Breakfast Meals										
Frozen cinnamon swirl French toast with sausage	1 package	415	38	23	107	44	59	50	141	71
Frozen ham and cheese breakfast burrito	1 burrito	212	28	7	55	23	30	26	72	36
Frozen scrambled eggs and sausage with hash browns	1 package	361	17	27	93	38	51	44	123	62
Jimmy Dean Frozen Sausage Biscuit Breakfast Sandwich	1 sandwich	192	12	14	49	20	27	23	65	33
Sunny Fresh Frozen Egg and Cheese Biscuit Sandwich	1 serving	224	25	9	58	24	32	27	76	38
Sunny Fresh Frozen Egg, Ham and Cheese Biscuit Sandwich	1 serving	242	25	10	62	26	34	29	82	41
Sunny Fresh Frozen Bagel French Toast with Maple Syrup	1 serving	190	21	5	49	20	27	23	65	32
Sunny Fresh Frozen Stuff-Its Egg and Cheese Pockets	1 serving	147	15	8	38	16	21	18	50	25
Frozen Entrees										
Frozen spaghetti and meat sauce entrée	1 serving	255	43	3	66	27	36	31	87	43
Frozen beef pot pie	1 package	449	44	24	116	48	64	55	153	77

FOOD	AMOUNT	CAL	CARBS	FAT	WALK	RUN	BIKE	SWIM	YOGA	DANCE
Frozen chicken pot pie	1 serving	484	43	29	125	52	69	59	165	82
Frozen turkey pot pie	1 package	699	70	35	180	74	99	85	238	119
■ **Banquet—Beef and Veal**										
Banquet Extra Helping Meatloaf Dinner	1 package	612	34	40	158	65	87	74	208	104
Banquet Extra Helping Salisbury Steak Dinner	1 package	782	47	54	201	83	111	95	266	133
Banquet Salisbury Steak Meal	1 package	398	28	25	103	42	56	48	135	68
Banquet Sliced Beef Meal with Gravy, Mashed Potatoes and Peas	1 package	270	19	10	70	29	38	33	92	46
Banquet Veal Parmigiana, Mashed Potatoes, Peas and Sauce	1 package	362	35	19	93	39	51	44	123	62
■ **Banquet—Poultry**										
Banquet Chicken Pot Pie	1 serving	382	36	22	98	41	54	46	130	65
Banquet Original Fried Chicken Meal	1 package	470	35	27	121	50	67	57	160	80
Banquet Turkey and Gravy with Dressing, Mashed Potatoes and Corn	1 package	280	34	10	72	30	40	34	95	48
■ **Budget Gourmet**										
Budget Gourmet Italian Sausage Lasagna	1 package	456	40	24	118	49	65	55	155	78
Budget Gourmet Light and Healthy Salisbury Steak, Red Potato and Vegetables	1 package	261	34	6	67	28	37	32	89	45
Budget Gourmet Light and Healthy Teriyaki Chicken and Oriental Style Vegetable	1 package	317	52	4	82	34	45	39	108	54
Budget Gourmet Light French Recipe Chicken	1 package	178	9	6	46	19	25	22	61	30
Budget Gourmet Spinach au Gratin	1 package	222	11	17	57	24	31	27	75	38
■ **Hot Pockets**										
Hot Pockets Beef 'n Cheddar	1 piece	300	28	16	77	32	43	36	102	51
Hot Pockets Chicken, Broccoli and Cheddar Croissant	1 serving	301	39	11	78	32	43	37	102	51
Hot Pockets Ham 'n Cheese	1 piece	310	36	13	80	33	44	38	105	53
Hot Pockets Meatballs and Mozzarella	1 piece	330	42	14	85	35	47	40	112	56

FOOD	AMOUNT	CAL	CARBS	FAT	WALK	RUN	BIKE	SWIM	YOGA	DANCE
Hot Pockets Pepperoni Pizza	1 piece	360	44	17	93	38	51	44	122	61
Lean Pockets Glazed Chicken Supreme	1 package	464	68	12	120	49	66	56	158	79
■ **Lean Cuisine**										
Lean Cuisine Chicken a l'Orange with Sauce, Broccoli and Rice	1 package	268	39	2	69	29	38	33	91	46
Lean Cuisine Chicken and Vegetables with Vermicelli	1 package	252	32	6	65	27	36	31	86	43
Lean Cuisine Chicken Enchilada Suiza, Sour Cream Sauce and Mexican Style Rice	1 package	298	52	5	77	32	42	36	101	51
Lean Cuisine Glazed Chicken	1 package	210	25	4	54	22	30	26	71	36
Lean Cuisine Homestyle Beef Pot Roast	1 package	207	22	5	53	22	29	25	70	35
Lean Cuisine Homestyle Stuffed Cabbage, Meat, Tomato Sauce	1 package	199	26	6	51	21	28	24	68	34
Lean Cuisine Lunch Express Rice and Chicken Stir-Fry	1 package	270	40	7	70	29	38	33	92	46
Lean Cuisine Macaroni and Beef in Tomato Sauce	1 package	249	37	5	64	27	35	30	85	42
Lean Cuisine Oriental Beef with Vegetables and Rice	1 package	242	36	5	62	26	34	29	82	41
Lean Cuisine Roasted Turkey Breast	1 package	260	46	3	67	28	37	32	88	44
Lean Cuisine Spaghetti with Meat Sauce	1 package	280	48	4	72	30	40	34	95	48
Lean Cuisine Spaghetti with Meatballs and Sauce	1 package	299	40	8	77	32	42	36	102	51
Lean Cuisine Swedish Meatballs	1 package	280	32	7	72	30	40	34	95	48
■ **Marie Callender**										
Marie Callender's Beef Stroganoff and Noodles	1 package	600	59	27	155	64	85	73	204	102
Marie Callender's Chicken Pot Pie	1 cup	501	44	31	129	53	71	61	170	85
Marie Callender's Escalloped Noodles and Chicken	1 cup	397	38	21	102	42	56	48	135	68
Marie Callender's Turkey with Gravy and Dressing with Broccoli	1 package	504	52	19	130	54	72	61	171	86
■ **Patio**										
Patio Beef and Bean Burrito with Green Chili	1 burrito	325	44	12	84	35	46	40	110	55

FOOD	AMOUNT	CAL	CARBS	FAT	WALK	RUN	BIKE	SWIM	YOGA	DANCE
Patio Mexican Style Dinner—Tamale, Beef Enchilada, Chili Sauce, Beans and Rice	1 package	508	68	20	131	54	72	62	173	86
■ Stouffer's										
Stouffer's Baked Chicken Breast	1 package	250	20	10	64	27	35	30	85	43
Stouffer's Chicken Enchilada and Mexican Rice, Monterey Jack Cheese Sauce	1 package	376	48	15	97	40	53	46	128	64
Stouffer's Chicken Pie	1 package	572	37	37	147	61	81	70	194	97
Stouffer's Creamed Chipped Beef	1 package	435	18	30	112	46	62	53	148	74
Stouffer's Escalloped Chicken and Noodles	1 package	419	31	25	108	45	59	51	142	71
Stouffer's Frozen Creamed Spinach	1 cup	338	18	26	87	36	48	41	115	57
Stouffer's Large Stuffed Peppers	1 pepper with Sauce	180	21	7	46	19	26	22	61	31
Stouffer's Lasagna with Meat and Sauce	1 serving	277	26	11	71	29	39	34	94	47
Stouffer's Lunch Express Chicken Alfredo with Fettucini and Vegetables	1 package	373	33	19	96	40	53	45	127	63
Stouffer's Meatloaf	1 package	340	17	20	88	36	48	41	116	58
Stouffer's Salisbury Steak	1 package	370	27	18	95	39	52	45	126	63
Stouffer's White Meat Chicken Pot Pie	1 package	730	64	44	188	78	104	89	248	124
■ Tyson										
Tyson Beef Stir-Fry Kit	1 serving	433	71	5	112	46	61	53	147	74
Tyson Breaded Chicken Breast Patties	1 piece	180	12	11	46	19	26	22	61	31
Tyson Chicken Fajita Kit	1 serving	129	17	3	33	14	18	16	44	22
Tyson Chicken Mesquite with Barbecue Sauce, Corn, and Potatoes au Gratin	1 serving	321	45	8	83	34	46	39	109	55
Tyson Hot 'n Spicy Chicken Wings	3 pieces	220	1	15	57	23	31	27	75	37
Tyson Roasted Chicken with Garlic Sauce, Pasta and Vegetable Medley	1 package	214	22	7	55	23	30	26	73	36
■ Weight Watchers Smart Ones										
Weight Watchers Chicken Enchilada Suiza	1 package	283	33	10	73	30	40	34	96	48

FOOD	AMOUNT	CAL	CARBS	FAT	WALK	RUN	BIKE	SWIM	YOGA	DANCE
Weight Watchers Macaroni and Beef in Tomato Sauce	1 package	282	45	5	73	30	40	34	96	48
Weight Watchers On the Go Chicken, Broccoli and Cheddar Pocket	1 serving	266	40	6	69	28	38	32	91	45
Weight Watchers Smart Ones Broccoli and Cheddar Roasted Potatoes	1 package (283 g)	220	34	6	57	23	31	27	75	37
Weight Watchers Smart Ones Chicken Oriental	1 package (255 g)	230	39	3	59	24	33	28	78	39
Weight Watchers Smart Ones Fettuccini Alfredo	1 package (262 g)	290	45	6	75	31	41	35	99	49
Weight Watchers Smart Ones Fiesta Chicken	1 package (241 g)	250	45	2	64	27	35	30	85	43
Weight Watchers Smart Ones Honey Dijon Chicken	1 package (241 g)	210	38	4	54	22	30	26	71	36
Weight Watchers Smart Ones Lemon Herb Chicken Piccata	1 package (255 g)	250	36	5	64	27	35	30	85	43
Weight Watchers Smart Ones Penne Pollo	1 package (283 g)	280	39	6	72	30	40	34	95	48
Weight Watchers Smart Ones Radiatore Romano	1 package (294 g)	280	40	8	72	30	40	34	95	48
Weight Watchers Smart Ones Ravioli Florentine	1 package (241 g)	250	40	5	64	27	35	30	85	43
Weight Watchers Smart Ones Salisbury Steak, Macaroni and Cheese	1 package (269 g)	260	26	7	67	28	37	32	88	44
Weight Watchers Smart Ones Santa Fe Style Rice and Beans	1 package (283 g)	310	51	7	80	33	44	38	105	53
Weight Watchers Smart Ones Shrimp Marinara	1 package (255 g)	180	31	2	46	19	26	22	61	31
Weight Watchers Smart Ones Stuffed Turkey Breast	1 package (283 g)	290	42	6	75	31	41	35	99	49
Weight Watchers Smart Ones Swedish Meatballs	1 package (258 g)	270	35	5	70	29	38	33	92	46
Weight Watchers Smart Ones Teriyaki Chicken and Vegetable Bowl	1 package (297 g)	270	46	3	70	29	38	33	92	46
Weight Watchers Smart Ones Three Cheese and Italian Style Meatballs	1 package (127 g)	290	43	7	75	31	41	35	99	49
Weight Watchers Smart Ones Three Cheese Macaroni	1 package (255 g)	300	48	6	77	32	43	36	102	51

FOOD	AMOUNT	CAL	CARBS	FAT	WALK	RUN	BIKE	SWIM	YOGA	DANCE
Weight Watchers Smart Ones Traditional Lasagna with Meat Sauce	1 package (297 g)	300	43	6	77	32	43	36	102	51
Weight Watchers Smart Ones Tuna Noodle Gratin	1 package (269 g)	250	37	5	64	27	35	30	85	43
Weight Watchers Ultimate 200 Barbecue Glazed Chicken and Sauce with Mixed Vegetables	1 package	217	26	4	56	23	31	26	74	37
■ Amy's Organic										
Amy's Organic Asian Noodle Stir-Fry	1 meal (284 g)	290	50	7	75	31	41	35	99	49
Amy's Organic Beans, Rice and Cheddar Cheese Burrito	1 burrito (170 g)	280	43	8	72	30	40	34	95	48
Amy's Organic Black Bean and Vegetable Enchilada	1 enchilada (135 g)	170	26	5	44	18	24	21	58	29
Amy's Organic Black Bean Burrito	1 burrito (170 g)	280	54	8	72	30	40	34	95	48
Amy's Organic Black Bean Enchilada Dinner	1 meal (284 g)	320	55	8	82	34	45	39	109	55
Amy's Organic Black Bean Ranchero Breakfast Burrito	1 burrito (170 g)	230	38	6	59	24	33	28	78	39
Amy's Organic Broccoli Pot Pie with Cheddar Cheese Sauce	1 pot pie (213 g)	430	46	22	111	46	61	52	146	73
Amy's Organic Brown Rice and Black Peas Bowl	1 bowl (255 g)	290	38	11	75	31	41	35	99	49
Amy's Organic Brown Rice and Vegetable Bowl	1 bowl (283 g)	250	36	8	64	27	35	30	85	43
Amy's Organic Cheese Enchilada	1 enchilada (135 g)	210	18	12	54	22	30	26	71	36
Amy's Organic Cheese Enchilada Dinner	1 meal (255 g)	330	38	14	85	35	47	40	112	56
Amy's Organic Cheese Lasagna	1 lasagna (291 g)	390	35	20	101	42	55	47	133	66
Amy's Organic Chili and Corn Bread Dinner	1 meal (298 g)	340	59	6	88	36	48	41	116	58
Amy's Organic Country Dinner	1 meal (312 g)	390	60	12	101	42	55	47	133	66
Amy's Organic Country Vegetable Pie	1 pot pie (213 g)	370	47	16	95	39	52	45	126	63

FOOD	AMOUNT	CAL	CARBS	FAT	WALK	RUN	BIKE	SWIM	YOGA	DANCE
Amy's Organic Indian Mattar Paneer	1 meal (284 g)	320	54	8	82	34	45	39	109	55
Amy's Organic Indian Palek Paneer Bowl	1 bowl (283 g)	240	38	6	62	26	34	29	82	41
Amy's Organic Macaroni and Cheese	1 meal (255 g)	410	47	16	106	44	58	50	139	70
Amy's Organic Macaroni and Soy Cheese	1 meal (255 g)	370	42	15	95	39	52	45	126	63
Amy's Organic Mexican Casserole Bowl	1 bowl (269 g)	480	70	18	124	51	68	58	163	82
Amy's Organic Non-Dairy Beans and Rice Burrito	1 burrito (170 g)	280	48	6	72	30	40	34	95	48
Amy's Organic Non-Dairy Vegetable Pie	1 pot pie (213 g)	360	50	13	93	38	51	44	122	61
Amy's Organic Pesto Tortellini Bowl	1 meal (269 g)	470	58	19	121	50	67	57	160	80
Amy's Organic Stuffed Shells Bowl	1 bowl (283 g)	300	30	12	77	32	43	36	102	51
Amy's Organic Tofu Vegetable Lasagna	1 lasagna (269 g)	300	41	10	77	32	43	36	102	51
Amy's Organic Vegetable Lasagna	1 lasagna (269 g)	300	35	12	77	32	43	36	102	51
Amy's Organic Vegetable Shepherd's Pie	1 pot pie (227 g)	160	27	4	41	17	23	19	54	27
Amy's Organic Veggie Loaf	1 meal (284 g)	280	47	7	72	30	40	34	95	48
■ **Birds Eye**										
Birds Eye Voila! Beef Steak and Garlic Potato	1 cup, cooked	190	22	7	49	20	27	23	65	32
Birds Eye Voila! Chicken Fajita	1 cup, cooked	150	13	6	39	16	21	18	51	26
Birds Eye Voila! Chicken Stir-Fry	1 cup, cooked	160	22	3	41	17	23	19	54	27
Birds Eye Voila! Garden Herb Chicken	1 cup, cooked	280	30	11	72	30	40	34	95	48
Birds Eye Voila! Garlic Chicken	1 cup, cooked	240	21	8	62	26	34	29	82	41
Birds Eye Voila! Garlic Shrimp	1 cup, cooked	220	27	8	57	23	31	27	75	37
Birds Eye Voila! Pesto Chicken Primavera	1 cup, cooked	210	24	7	54	22	30	26	71	36

FOOD	AMOUNT	CAL	CARBS	FAT	WALK	RUN	BIKE	SWIM	YOGA	DANCE
Birds Eye Voila! Reduced Carb Chicken and Sausage Tuscano	1 cup, cooked	170	10	8	44	18	24	21	58	29
Birds Eye Voila! Reduced Carb Chicken Teriyaki and Vegetables	1 cup, cooked	150	15	3	39	16	21	18	51	26
Birds Eye Voila! Reduced Carb Down Home Chicken and Vegetables	1 cup, cooked	180	17	5	46	19	26	22	61	31
Birds Eye Voila! Reduced Carb Roasted Garlic Chicken and Vegetables	1 cup, cooked	120	13	3	31	13	17	15	41	20
Birds Eye Voila! Reduced Carb Teriyaki Beef and Vegetables	1 cup, cooked	160	15	4	41	17	23	19	54	27
Birds Eye Voila! Teriyaki Chicken	1 cup, cooked	250	44	3	64	27	35	30	85	43
Birds Eye Voila! Three Cheese Chicken	1 cup, cooked	210	21	8	54	22	30	26	71	36
■ **Healthy Choice**										
Healthy Choice Apple Glazed Pork Medallions	1 meal (10.8 oz)	310	46	6	80	33	44	38	105	53
Healthy Choice Asiago Chicken Portobello	1 meal (12.5 oz)	330	47	6	85	35	47	40	112	56
Healthy Choice Beef Merlot	1 meal (10 oz)	240	26	8	62	26	34	29	82	41
Healthy Choice Beef Pot Roast	1 meal (11 oz)	320	39	9	82	34	45	39	109	55
Healthy Choice Beef Stroganoff	1 meal (11 oz)	330	40	9	85	35	47	40	112	56
Healthy Choice Beef Teriyaki	1 meal (9.5)	310	46	7	80	33	44	38	105	53
Healthy Choice Beef Tips Portabello	1 meal (11.25 oz)	280	28	8	72	30	40	34	95	48
Healthy Choice Blackened Chicken	1 meal (11 oz)	300	36	6	77	32	43	36	102	51
Healthy Choice Boneless Beef Ribs with Classic BBQ Sauce	1 meal (11 oz)	360	47	9	93	38	51	44	122	61
Healthy Choice Breaded Chicken Breast Strips and Macaroni and Cheese	1 meal (8 oz)	290	35	5	75	31	41	35	99	49
Healthy Choice Cajun Style Chicken and Shrimp	1 meal (10.4 oz)	240	32	4	62	26	34	29	82	41

FOOD	AMOUNT	CAL	CARBS	FAT	WALK	RUN	BIKE	SWIM	YOGA	DANCE
Healthy Choice Cajun Style Chicken and Shrimp	1 meal (10.4 oz)	240	32	4	62	26	34	29	82	41
Healthy Choice Charbroiled Beef Patty	1 meal (11 oz)	310	37	9	80	33	44	38	105	53
Healthy Choice Cheddar Broccoli Potatoes	1 meal (10.5 oz)	280	41	7	72	30	40	34	95	48
Healthy Choice Cheesy Rice and Chicken	1 meal (9 oz)	230	33	4	59	24	33	28	78	39
Healthy Choice Chicken Breast and Vegetables	1 meal (10.5 oz)	230	29	5	59	24	33	28	78	39
Healthy Choice Chicken Broccoli Alfredo	1 meal (11.5 oz)	300	34	7	77	32	43	36	102	51
Healthy Choice Chicken Carbonara	1 meal (9 oz)	310	39	7	80	33	44	38	105	53
Healthy Choice Chicken Enchilada	1 meal (9 oz)	310	46	7	80	33	44	38	105	53
Healthy Choice Chicken Fettuccini Alfredo	1 meal (8.5 oz)	280	28	7	72	30	40	34	95	48
Healthy Choice Chicken Margherita	1 meal (10 oz)	340	25	8	88	36	48	41	116	58
Healthy Choice Chicken Parmigiana	1 meal (11 oz)	320	40	9	82	34	45	39	109	55
Healthy Choice Chicken Piccata	1 meal (9 oz)	270	40	5	70	29	38	33	92	46
Healthy Choice Chicken Teriyaki Dinner	1 meal (11 oz)	270	37	6	70	29	38	33	92	46
Healthy Choice Chicken Tuscany	1 meal (10.6 oz)	330	42	9	85	35	47	40	112	56
Healthy Choice Country Breaded Chicken	1 meal (10.6 oz)	370	55	9	95	39	52	45	126	63
Healthy Choice Country Glazed Chicken	1 meal (8.5 oz)	230	29	5	59	24	33	28	78	39
Healthy Choice Country Herb Chicken	1 meal (11.35 oz)	280	37	6	72	30	40	34	95	48
Healthy Choice Creamy Garlic Shrimp	1 meal (11.5 oz)	270	35	6	70	29	38	33	92	46
Healthy Choice Creamy Herb Roasted Chicken	1 meal (10 oz)	220	35	5	57	23	31	27	75	37
Healthy Choice Familiar Favorites Chicken Enchiladas	1 meal (11.3 oz)	360	59	7	93	38	51	44	122	61
Healthy Choice Familiar Favorites Sesame Chicken	1 meal (9 oz)	260	34	6	67	28	37	32	88	44

FOOD	AMOUNT	CAL	CARBS	FAT	WALK	RUN	BIKE	SWIM	YOGA	DANCE
Healthy Choice Fettuccini Alfredo	1 meal (8 oz)	240	36	6	62	26	34	29	82	41
Healthy Choice Grilled Basil Chicken	1 meal (10.6 oz)	290	33	7	75	31	41	35	99	49
Healthy Choice Grilled Chicken and Mashed Potatoes	1 meal (8.5 oz)	230	22	7	59	24	33	28	78	39
Healthy Choice Grilled Chicken Baja	1 meal (10 oz)	270	33	5	70	29	38	33	92	46
Healthy Choice Grilled Chicken Breast and Pasta	1 meal (9 oz)	240	25	6	62	26	34	29	82	41
Healthy Choice Grilled Chicken Caesar	1 meal (10 oz)	290	42	7	75	31	41	35	99	49
Healthy Choice Grilled Chicken Marinara	1 meal (10 oz)	280	37	5	72	30	40	34	95	48
Healthy Choice Grilled Chicken with Smokehouse BBQ Sauce	1 meal (12 oz)	370	59	6	95	39	52	45	126	63
Healthy Choice Grilled Steak in Roasted Garlic Sauce	1 meal (10 oz)	240	46	7	62	26	34	29	82	41
Healthy Choice Grilled Turkey Breast	1 meal (10 oz)	250	31	5	64	27	35	30	85	43
Healthy Choice Grilled Whiskey Steak	1 meal (9.5)	300	46	5	77	32	43	36	102	51
Healthy Choice Herb Baked Fish	1 meal (10.9 oz)	360	55	8	93	38	51	44	122	61
Healthy Choice Homestyle Chicken and Pasta	1 meal (9 oz)	270	32	6	70	29	38	33	92	46
Healthy Choice Honey Glazed Chicken	1 meal (11 oz)	320	46	6	82	34	45	39	109	55
Healthy Choice Lasagna Bake	1 meal (9 oz)	270	36	7	70	29	38	33	92	46
Healthy Choice Lemon Pepper Fish	1 meal (10.7 oz)	280	49	5	72	30	40	34	95	48
Healthy Choice Macaroni and Cheese	1 meal (9 oz)	270	40	6	70	29	38	33	92	46
Healthy Choice Mandarin Chicken	1 meal (10 oz)	280	43	4	72	30	40	34	95	48
Healthy Choice Manicotti with 3 Cheeses	1 meal (11 oz)	290	46	5	75	31	41	35	99	49
Healthy Choice Meatloaf	1 meal (12 oz)	300	36	9	77	32	43	36	102	51
Healthy Choice Mesquite Chicken BBQ	1 meal (10.5 oz)	300	44	5	77	32	43	36	102	51

FOOD	AMOUNT	CAL	CARBS	FAT	WALK	RUN	BIKE	SWIM	YOGA	DANCE
Healthy Choice Mushroom Roasted Beef	1 meal (11 oz)	280	28	8	72	30	40	34	95	48
Healthy Choice Oriental Style Beef	1 meal (10.6 oz)	300	27	9	77	32	43	36	102	51
Healthy Choice Oriental Style Chicken	1 meal (8.5 oz)	240	28	5	62	26	34	29	82	41
Healthy Choice Oven-Roasted Beef	1 meal (10.15 oz)	280	33	7	72	30	40	34	95	48
Healthy Choice Princess Chicken	1 meal (10.75 oz)	310	41	7	80	33	44	38	105	53
Healthy Choice Rigatoni with Broccoli and Chicken	1 meal (9 oz)	280	34	7	72	30	40	34	95	48
Healthy Choice Roast Turkey Breast	1 meal (8.5 oz)	230	25	6	59	24	33	28	78	39
Healthy Choice Roasted Chicken Breast	1 meal (11 oz)	280	32	8	72	30	40	34	95	48
Healthy Choice Roasted Chicken Chardonnay	1 meal (10.6)	280	32	7	72	30	40	34	95	48
Healthy Choice Roasted Chicken Marsala	1 meal (10.4 oz)	240	23	6	62	26	34	29	82	41
Healthy Choice Salisbury Steak	1 meal (12.5 oz)	360	45	9	93	38	51	44	122	61
Healthy Choice Salisbury Steak and Mashed Potatoes	1 meal (8 oz)	210	21	6	54	22	30	26	71	36
Healthy Choice Sesame Chicken Dinner	1 meal (10.8 oz)	330	38	8	85	35	47	40	112	56
Healthy Choice Sirloin Beef Tips and Mushroom Sauce	1 meal (8 oz)	270	35	6	70	29	38	33	92	46
Healthy Choice Slow-Roasted Turkey Breast and Mashed Potatoes	1 meal (8.5 oz)	200	19	5	52	21	28	24	68	34
Healthy Choice Spaghetti with Meat Sauce	1 meal (10 oz)	280	36	8	72	30	40	34	95	48
Healthy Choice Stuffed Pasta Shells	1 meal (11.15 oz)	290	40	6	75	31	41	35	99	49
Healthy Choice Sweet and Sour Chicken	1 meal (11 oz)	340	54	7	88	36	48	41	116	58
Healthy Choice Traditional Turkey Breasts	1 meal (10.5 oz)	330	50	5	85	35	47	40	112	56
Healthy Choice Tuna Casserole	1 meal (9 oz)	250	30	7	64	27	35	30	85	43

FOOD	AMOUNT	CAL	CARBS	FAT	WALK	RUN	BIKE	SWIM	YOGA	DANCE
■ **Other Brand Names**										
Barber Foods Chicken Cordon Bleu	1 serving	344	15	21	89	37	49	42	117	59
Fiesta Café Beef and Bean Chimichanga	1 package	422	56	12	109	45	60	51	144	72
Freezer Queen Gravy and Sliced Beef Meal	1 package	207	26	5	53	22	29	25	70	35
Green Giant Broccoli in Cheese Flavored Sauce	1 cup	113	15	4	29	12	16	14	38	19
Hanover Stir-Fry 2 White Rice and Vegetables with Oriental Soy Sauce	1 cup	130	27	0	34	14	18	16	44	22
Kid Cuisine Cosmic Chicken Nuggets, Macaroni and Cheese, Corn and Chocolate Pudding	1 package	524	53	27	135	56	74	64	178	89
Las Campanas Beef and Bean Burrito	1 serving	296	38	12	76	32	42	36	101	50
Marquez Primera Shredded Beef, Green Chili and Monterey Jack Burrito	1 package	324	40	12	83	34	46	39	110	55
Michelina's Spaghetti, Meatballs and Pomodoro Sauce	1 package	312	49	7	81	33	44	38	106	53
Red Baron Ham and Cheese Pockets	1 serving	356	36	17	92	38	50	43	121	61

Soup

Canned Soup										
Canned beef broth	1 cup	59	4	0	15	6	8	7	20	10
Bouillon	1 cup	20	2	1	5	2	3	2	7	3
Condensed black bean (prepared with water)	1 cup	116	20	2	30	12	16	14	39	20
Condensed cream of asparagus (prepared with water)	1 cup	85	11	4	22	9	12	10	29	14
Condensed cream of asparagus (prepared with milk)	1 cup	161	16	8	41	17	23	20	55	27
Condensed cream of mushroom (prepared with water	1 cup	129	9	9	33	14	18	16	44	22
Condensed cream of mushroom (prepared with milk)	1 cup	203	15	14	52	22	29	25	69	35

FOOD	AMOUNT	CAL	CARBS	FAT	WALK	RUN	BIKE	SWIM	YOGA	DANCE
Condensed cream of onion (prepared with water)	1 cup	107	13	5	28	11	15	13	36	18
Condensed cream of onion (prepared with milk)	1 cup	186	18	9	48	20	26	23	63	32
Condensed cream of potato (prepared with water)	1 cup	73	11	2	19	8	10	9	25	12
Condensed cream of potato (prepared with milk)	1 cup	149	17	6	38	16	21	18	51	25
Condensed cream of shrimp (prepared with water)	1 cup	90	8	5	23	10	13	11	31	15
Condensed cream of shrimp (prepared with milk)	1 cup	164	14	9	42	17	23	20	56	28
Condensed minestrone (prepared with water)	1 cup	82	11	3	21	9	12	10	28	14
Condensed mushroom barley (prepared with water)	1 cup	73	12	2	19	8	10	9	25	12
Condensed mushroom (prepared with water)	1 cup	96	11	5	25	10	14	12	33	16
Condensed onion (prepared with water)	1 cup	27	5	1	7	3	4	3	9	5
Condensed oyster stew (prepared with water)	1 cup	58	4	4	15	6	8	7	20	10
Condensed oyster stew (prepared with milk)	1 cup	135	10	8	35	14	19	16	46	23
Condensed pea (prepared with water)	1 cup	165	27	2	43	18	23	20	56	28
Condensed pea (prepared with milk)	1 cup	239	32	7	62	25	34	29	81	41
Condensed pepperpot (prepared with water)	1 cup	104	9	5	27	11	15	13	35	18
Condensed split pea with ham (prepared with water)	1 cup	190	28	4	49	20	27	23	65	32
Condensed tomato beef with noodles (prepared with water)	1 cup	139	21	4	36	15	20	17	47	24
Condensed tomato rice (prepared with water)	1 cup	119	22	3	31	13	17	14	40	20
Condensed tomato (prepared with milk)	1 cup	85	17	2	22	9	12	10	29	14
Condensed tomato (prepared with water)	1 cup	161	22	6	41	17	23	20	55	27
Condensed turkey noodle (prepared with water)	1 cup	68	9	2	18	7	10	8	23	12

FOOD	AMOUNT	CAL	CARBS	FAT	WALK	RUN	BIKE	SWIM	YOGA	DANCE
Condensed turkey vegetable (prepared with water)	1 cup	72	9	3	19	8	10	9	24	12
Condensed vegetable beef (prepared with water)	1 cup	78	10	2	20	8	11	9	27	13
Campbell's Condensed French Onion	4 oz	45	6	2	12	5	6	5	15	8
Campbell's Condensed 98% Fat Free Cream of Broccoli	4 oz	70	10	2	18	7	10	9	24	12
Campbell's Condensed 98% Fat Free Broccoli Cheese	4 oz	70	12	2	18	7	10	9	24	12
Campbell's Condensed Beef Consommé	4 oz	20	1	0	5	2	3	2	7	3
Campbell's Condensed Chicken Noodle Soup	4 oz	60	8	2	15	6	9	7	20	10
Campbell's Condensed Cream of Mushroom	4 oz	100	9	6	26	11	14	12	34	17
Campbell's Condensed Vegetable	4 oz	100	20	1	26	11	14	12	34	17
Campbell's Select Minestrone	8 oz	100	0	1	26	11	14	12	34	17
Campbell's Select Vegetable Medley	8 oz	100	21	1	26	11	14	12	34	17
Campbell's Select Chicken Alfredo	8 oz	210	15	12	54	22	30	26	71	36
Campbell's Soup at Hand Classic Tomato	1 container	140	31	0	36	15	20	17	48	24
Campbell's Soup at Hand Creamy Mushroom	1 container	120	10	7	31	13	17	15	41	20
Campbell's Chunky Chicken and Dumplings	8 oz	170	16	8	44	18	24	21	58	29
Campbell's Chunky Turkey Pot Pie	8 oz	190	15	10	49	20	27	23	65	32
Campbell's Chunky Hearty Bean and Ham	8 oz	180	30	2	46	19	26	22	61	31
Campbell's Chunky Classic Chicken Noodle Soup	8 oz	120	15	3	31	13	17	15	41	20
Health Valley Low Fat Chicken Broth	8 oz	35	0	2	9	4	5	4	12	6
Health Valley Fat Free Vegetable Broth	8 oz	20	5	0	5	2	3	2	7	3
Health Valley Organic Vegetable Broth	8 oz	15	4	0	4	2	2	2	5	3

FOOD	AMOUNT	CAL	CARBS	FAT	WALK	RUN	BIKE	SWIM	YOGA	DANCE
Health Valley Organic Potato & Leek	8 oz	70	15	0	18	7	10	9	24	12
Health Valley Nonfat 5 Bean Vegetable	8 oz	140	32	0	36	15	20	17	48	24
Health Valley Lentil and Carrot	8 oz	90	25	0	23	10	13	11	31	15
Health Valley Nonfat Minestrone	8 oz	90	21	0	23	10	13	11	31	15
Health Valley Organic Black Bean	8 oz	130	25	1	34	14	18	16	44	22
Health Valley Nonfat Black Bean and Vegetable	8 oz	110	24	0	28	12	16	13	37	19
Health Valley Nonfat Broccoli Carotene	8 oz	70	16	0	18	7	10	9	24	12
Health Valley Nonfat Carrot Pea	8 oz	110	17	0	28	12	16	13	37	19
Health Valley Nonfat Beef Broth	8 oz	20	0	0	5	2	3	2	7	3
Health Valley Nonfat Chicken Broth	8 oz	30	0	0	8	3	4	4	10	5
Manischewitz Clear Chicken with Matzo Ball	8 oz	160	18	8	41	17	23	19	54	27
Progresso Chicken Noodle	8 oz	90	9	2	23	10	13	11	31	15
Progresso Chicken and Wild Rice	8 oz	100	15	2	26	11	14	12	34	17
Progresso Sirloin Steak and Vegetable	8 oz	120	19	1	31	13	17	15	41	20
Progresso 99% Fat Free Minestrone	8 oz	110	19	1	28	12	16	13	37	19
Progresso French Onion	8 oz	50	9	2	13	5	7	6	17	9
Progresso Lentil	8 oz	140	22	2	36	15	20	17	48	24
Progresso Healthy Classics Tomato Garden	1 cup	98	22	1	25	10	14	12	33	17
Progresso Healthy Classics Split Pea	1 cup	180	30	2	46	19	26	22	61	31
Progresso Healthy Classics Garlic and Pasta	1 cup	100	20	1	26	11	14	12	34	17
Progresso Healthy Classics Chicken Noodle	1 cup	76	9	2	20	8	11	9	26	13
Progresso Healthy Classics Chicken Rice	1 cup	88	13	1	23	9	12	11	30	15
Progresso Healthy Classics Cream of Broccoli	1 cup	88	13	3	23	9	12	11	30	15

FOOD	AMOUNT	CAL	CARBS	FAT	WALK	RUN	BIKE	SWIM	YOGA	DANCE
Progresso Healthy Classics Lentil	1 cup	126	20	2	32	13	18	15	43	21
Progresso Healthy Classics Minestrone	1 cup	123	20	3	32	13	17	15	42	21
Progresso Healthy Classics Vegetable	1 cup	81	13	1	21	9	11	10	28	14
Progresso Healthy Classics Cream of Broccoli	1 cup	88	13	3	23	9	12	11	30	15
Swanson Clear Beef Broth	8 oz	20	1	1	5	2	3	2	7	3
Swanson Clear Chicken Broth	8 oz	30	1	2	8	3	4	4	10	5
Swanson Vegetable Broth	8 oz	20	3	1	5	2	3	2	7	3
Chowders and Bisques										
Condensed Manhattan clam chowder (prepared with water)	1 cup	78	12	2	20	8	11	9	27	13
Condensed New England clam chowder (prepared with water)	1 cup	164	7	7	42	17	23	20	56	28
Condensed New England clam chowder (prepared with milk)	1 cup	95	12	3	24	10	13	12	32	16
Condensed tomato bisque (prepared with milk)	1 cup	198	29	7	51	21	28	24	67	34
Condensed tomato bisque (prepared with water)	1 cup	124	24	3	32	13	18	15	42	21
Progresso Healthy Classics New England Clam Chowder	1 cup	117	20	2	30	12	17	14	40	20
Progresso Manhattan Clam Chowder	8 oz	110	17	2	28	12	16	13	37	19
Campbell's Condensed Manhattan Clam Chowder	4 oz	70	12	1	18	7	10	9	24	12
Mixes, Cubes, Instant Soups, Soup Bases										
Dry beef broth mix	1 packet	14	1	1	4	1	2	2	5	2
Beef broth cubes	1 cube	9	1	0	2	1	1	1	3	2
Dry chicken broth	1 tsp	5	0	0	1	1	1	1	2	1
Chicken broth cubes	1 cube	10	1	0	3	1	1	1	3	2
Cup Noodles Beef Flavor Soup	1 container	300	38	13	77	32	43	36	102	51
Herb-Ox Beef Bouillon	1 cube	5	1	0	1	1	1	1	2	1
Herb-Ox Chicken Bouillon	1 cube	5	1	0	1	1	1	1	2	1
Herb-Ox Vegetable Bouillon	1 cube	5	1	0	1	1	1	1	2	1
Kikkoman Aka Miso Soup Mix	1 serving	35	4	1	9	4	5	4	12	6

FOOD	AMOUNT	CAL	CARBS	FAT	WALK	RUN	BIKE	SWIM	YOGA	DANCE
Kikkoman Memmi Noodle Soup Base	2 tbsp	40	7	0	10	4	6	5	14	7
Kikkoman Instant Osuimono Broth	1 tbsp	25	5	0	6	3	4	3	9	4
Kikkoman Scallop-Flavored Seafood Soup Mix	1 tbsp	35	7	0	9	4	5	4	12	6
Kikkoman Shrimp-Flavored Seafood Soup Mix	1 tbsp	30	5	1	8	3	4	4	10	5
Kikkoman Shiro Miso Soup Mix	1 serving	35	4	1	9	4	5	4	12	6
Kikkoman Tofu Miso Soup Mix	1 serving	35	4	1	9	4	5	4	12	6
Kikkoman Tofu Spinach Miso Soup Mix	1 serving	35	4	1	9	4	5	4	12	6
Lipton Homestyle Pasta and Bean Soup Mix	1 serving	125	23	1	32	13	18	15	43	21
Lipton Recipe Secrets Onion Soup Mix	1 serving	18	4	0	5	2	3	2	6	3
Lipton Soup Secrets Noodle Soup with Extra Noodles Mix	1 serving	86	15	2	22	9	12	10	29	15
Lipton Soup Secrets Noodle Soup with Real Chicken Broth Mix	1 serving	62	9	2	16	7	9	8	21	11
Lipton Cup-A-Soup Broccoli and Cheese Mix	1 serving	67	9	3	17	7	10	8	23	11
Lipton Cup-A-Soup Hearty Chicken Noodle Soup Mix	1 serving	61	10	1	16	6	9	7	21	10
Lipton Cup-A-Soup Vegetable Soup Mix	1 serving	47	8	1	12	5	7	6	16	8
Lipton Cup-A-Soup Tomato Soup Mix	1 serving	95	20	1	24	10	13	12	32	16
Lipton Cup-A-Soup Green Pea Soup Mix	1 serving	75	12	1	19	8	11	9	26	13
Lipton Cup-A-Soup Cream of Mushroom Soup Mix	1 serving	60	10	2	15	6	9	7	20	10
Lipton Cup-A-Soup Fat Free Chicken Broth Mix	1 serving	18	3	0	5	2	3	2	6	3
Lipton Kettle Creations Lentil Soup Mix	1 serving	127	23	1	33	14	18	15	43	22
Lipton Recipe Secretes Savory Herb Soup with Garlic	1 serving	31	6	0	8	3	4	4	11	5
Ramen Oriental Noodle Soup Mix	1 serving	190	28	7	49	20	27	23	65	32

FOOD	AMOUNT	CAL	CARBS	FAT	WALK	RUN	BIKE	SWIM	YOGA	DANCE
Ramen Chicken Noodle Soup Mix	1 serving	188	27	5	48	20	27	23	64	32
Ramen Vegetable Curry Noodle Soup	1.5 oz	140	28	1	36	15	20	17	48	24
Ramen Vegetable Miso Noodle Soup	1.3 oz	130	25	1	34	14	18	16	44	22
Ramen Tomato Vegetable Noodle Soup	1.5 oz	150	31	1	39	16	21	18	51	26
Soups That Come in Boxes										
Imagine Organic Beef Broth	8 oz	20	1	1	5	2	3	2	7	3
Imagine Organic Vegetable Broth	8 oz	20	2	0	5	2	3	2	7	3
Imagine Creamy Butternut Squash	8 oz	90	18	2	23	10	13	11	31	15
Imagine Creamy Broccoli	8 oz	60	10	2	15	6	9	7	20	10
Imagine Creamy Chicken	8 oz	70	12	2	18	7	10	9	24	12
Imagine Creamy Portobello Mushroom	8 oz	80	10	3	21	9	11	10	27	14
Imagine Crab Bisque	8 oz	130	16	5	34	14	18	16	44	22
Imagine Lobster Bisque	8 oz	130	15	5	34	14	18	16	44	22
Imagine California Miso Broth	8 oz	35	5	1	9	4	5	4	12	6
Imagine Organic Soy Ginger Noodle Broth	8 oz	40	10	0	10	4	6	5	14	7
Chili										
Canned Chili Con Carne with Beans	1 cup	298	28	13	77	32	42	36	101	51
Chef Mate Chili with Beans	1 cup	412	29	25	106	44	58	50	140	70
Chef Mate Chili without Beans	1 cup	430	18	32	111	46	61	52	146	73
El Rio Canned Chili Con Carne	1 serving	305	16	20	79	32	43	37	104	52
Hormel Canned Chili with Beans	1 cup	240	34	4	62	26	34	29	81	41
Hormel Canned Chili without Beans	1 cup	194	18	7	50	21	27	24	66	33
Hormel Canned Turkey Chili with Beans	1 cup	203	26	3	52	22	29	25	69	35
Hormel Canned Vegetarian Chili with Beans	1 cup	205	38	1	53	22	29	25	70	35
Stagg Canned Classic Chili with Beans	1 cup	324	29	16	83	34	46	39	110	55
Stagg Canned Country Chili with Beans	1 cup	319	29	16	82	34	45	39	108	54

FOOD	AMOUNT	CAL	CARBS	FAT	WALK	RUN	BIKE	SWIM	YOGA	DANCE
Stagg Canned Dynamite Chili with Beans	1 cup	333	31	15	86	36	47	41	113	57
Stagg Canned Ranchhouse Chili with Beans	1 cup	284	32	9	73	30	40	35	97	48
Stagg Canned Silverado Chili with Beans	1 cup	227	33	3	59	24	32	28	77	39
Yves Veggie Chili	1 bowl entrée	240	37	1	62	26	34	29	82	41
Homemade Soup										
Homemade fish stock	1 cup	40	0	2	10	4	6	5	14	7
Bouillabaisse	1 cup	90	10	4	23	10	13	11	31	15
New England clam chowder	1 cup	260	16	17	67	28	37	32	88	44
Cream of tomato	1 cup	310	18	26	80	33	44	38	105	53
Minestrone	1 cup	120	18	4	31	13	17	15	41	20
Vegetarian chili	1 cup	140	23	4	36	15	20	17	48	24
Split pea	1 cup	250	35	7	64	27	35	30	85	43
Chicken noodle soup	1 cup	150	14	4	39	16	21	18	51	26
Chicken rice soup	1 cup	110	7	4	28	12	16	13	37	19
Shark-fin soup	1 cup	99	8	4	26	11	14	12	34	17
Frozen Soup										
Boston Chowda Charleston Crab Soup	1 cup	320	16	23	82	34	45	39	109	55
Boston Chowda Lobster Bisque	1 cup	260	12	19	67	28	37	32	88	44
Boston Chowda New England Clam Chowder	1 cup	280	20	17	72	30	40	34	95	48
Boston Chowda Shrimp and Sausage Gumbo	1 cup	420	38	23	108	45	60	51	143	72
Lean Cuisine 3 Bean Chili	4 oz	80	12	2	21	9	11	10	27	14
Marie Callender's Chili Entrée with Cornbread	8 oz	350	45	13	90	37	50	43	119	60
Moosewood Moroccan Stew	1 container (10 oz)	170	32	3	44	18	24	21	58	29
Moosewood Creamy Potato and Corn Soup	1 cup	160	26	5	41	17	23	19	54	27
Moosewood 2 Bean Chili	1 cup	190	31	5	49	20	27	23	65	32
Stouffer's Cajun Seasoned Stew	1 tsp	24	2	1	6	3	3	3	8	4

FOOD	AMOUNT	CAL	CARBS	FAT	WALK	RUN	BIKE	SWIM	YOGA	DANCE
Restaurant/Fast Food Soups and Stews										
Applebee's Onion Soup au Gratin	1 serving	150	8	n/a	39	16	21	18	51	26
Au Bon Pain Chicken Chili with Beans	1 cup	180	26	4	46	19	26	22	61	31
Au Bon Pain Black Bean Soup	1 cup	100	29	1	26	11	14	12	34	17
Au Bon Pain Mediterranean Seafood Stew	1 cup	140	12	4	36	15	20	17	48	24
Au Bon Pain Low Fat Garden Vegetable Soup	1 cup	50	9	1	13	5	7	6	17	9
Au Bon Pain Low Fat French Onion Soup	1 cup	80	12	3	21	9	11	10	27	14
Au Bon Pain Italian Wedding Soup	1 cup	100	12	4	26	11	14	12	34	17
Au Bon Pain Low Fat Chicken Noodle Soup	1 cup	100	14	2	26	11	14	12	34	17
Au Bon Pain Clam Chowder	1 cup	220	20	13	57	23	31	27	75	37
Au Bon Pain Potato Leek Soup	1 cup	190	19	12	49	20	27	23	65	32
Au Bon Pain Potato Cheese Soup	1 cup	160	16	9	41	17	23	19	54	27
Boston Market Chicken Chili	1 cup	220	21	7	57	23	31	27	75	37
Boston Market Chicken Noodle Soup	1 cup	130	12	5	34	14	18	16	44	22
Boston Market Potato Soup	1 cup	270	24	16	70	29	38	33	92	46
Boston Market Tomato Bisque	1 cup	280	16	23	72	30	40	34	95	48
Chick-Fil-A Small Hearty Breast of Chicken Soup	8.5 oz	140	18	4	36	15	20	17	48	24
Chick-Fil-A Large Hearty Breast of Chicken Soup	15.5 oz	250	32	7	64	27	35	30	85	43
Cousins Subs New England Clam Chowder	large	234	39	4	60	25	33	28	80	40
Cousins Subs Tomato Basil with Raviolini	large	151	30	1	39	16	21	18	51	26
Cousins Subs Vegetable Beef	large	110	18	3	28	12	16	13	37	19
Denny's Chili with Cheese Topping	11 oz	401	21	19	103	43	57	49	136	68
Denny's Clam Chowder	1 serving	624	55	42	161	66	89	76	212	106
Denny's Vegetable Beef Soup	1 cup	79	11	1	20	8	11	10	27	13
Denny's Split Pea Soup	1 cup	146	18	6	38	16	21	18	50	25

FOOD	AMOUNT	CAL	CARBS	FAT	WALK	RUN	BIKE	SWIM	YOGA	DANCE
Denny's Cream of Potato Soup	1 cup	222	23	12	57	24	31	27	76	38
Panera Bread Boston Clam Chowder	1 cup	200	19	11	52	21	28	24	68	34
Panera Bread French Onion Soup (with no cheese/croutons)	1 cup	80	12	3	21	9	11	10	27	14
Panera Bread French Onion Soup (with cheese/croutons)	1 cup	200	21	10	52	21	28	24	68	34
Panera Bread Vegetarian Roasted Tomato and Pepper Bisque	1 cup	260	19	20	67	28	37	32	88	44
Panera Bread Low Fat Vegetarian Garden Vegetable Soup	1 cup	90	17	1	23	10	13	11	31	15
Panera Bread Low Fat Chicken Noodle Soup	1 cup	100	15	2	26	11	14	12	34	17
P.F.Chang's Hot and Sour Soup	1 cup	56	2	4	14	6	8	7	19	10
P.F.Chang's Pin Rice Noodle Soup	1 cup	270	55	2	70	29	38	33	92	46
P.F.Chang's Wonton Soup	1 cup	52	4	3	13	6	7	6	18	9
Schlotzky's Boston Clam Chowder	1 cup	233	24	15	60	25	33	28	79	40
Schlotzky's Corn Chowder	1 cup	284	38	17	73	30	40	35	97	48
Schlotzky's Creamy Turkey Vegetable	1 cup	218	21	14	56	23	31	27	74	37
Schlotzky's French Onion	1 cup	78	9	3	20	8	11	9	27	13
Schlotzky's Minestrone	1 cup	89	17	1	23	9	13	11	30	15
Schlotzky's Wisconsin Cheese Soup	1 cup	319	26	25	82	34	45	39	109	54
Schlotzky's Vegetable Cheese Soup	1 cup	289	24	19	74	31	41	35	98	49
Shoney's Vegetable Beef Soup	6 oz	82	14	2	21	9	12	10	28	14
Shoney's Cheese Florentine Soup	6 oz	110	12	8	28	12	16	13	37	19
Shoney's Clam Chowder	6 oz	94	10	5	24	10	13	11	32	16
Shoney's Potato Soup	6 oz	102	17	3	26	11	14	12	35	17
Shoney's Tomato Soup with Vegetables	6 oz	46	10	0	12	5	7	6	16	8
Sizzler Clam Chowder	4 oz	118	11	6	30	13	17	14	40	20
Sizzler Vegetarian Vegetable Soup	6 oz	50	6	1	13	5	7	6	17	9
Sizzler Vegetable Sirloin Soup	4 oz	60	6	2	15	6	9	7	20	10

FOOD	AMOUNT	CAL	CARBS	FAT	WALK	RUN	BIKE	SWIM	YOGA	DANCE
Subway Chili Con Carne	1 cup	240	23	10	62	26	34	29	82	41
Subway Vegetable Beef Soup	1 cup	90	15	1	23	10	13	11	31	15
Subway Cream of Broccoli	1 cup	130	15	6	34	14	18	16	44	22
Subway Tomato Garden Vegetable with Rotini	1 cup	100	20	1	26	11	14	12	34	17
Subway Roasted Chicken Noodle	1 cup	60	7	2	15	6	9	7	20	10
Wendy's Large Chili	12 oz	310	32	10	80	33	44	38	105	53
Wendy's Small Chili	8 oz	210	21	7	54	22	30	26	71	36
White Castle Chili	12 oz	375	45	15	97	40	53	46	128	64

Dessert

Frozen Yogurt

■ General

FOOD	AMOUNT	CAL	CARBS	FAT	WALK	RUN	BIKE	SWIM	YOGA	DANCE
Frozen yogurt	.5 cup	110	19	3	28	12	16	13	37	19
Vanilla soft-serve frozen yogurt	.5 cup	117	17	4	30	12	17	14	40	20
Chocolate soft-serve frozen yogurt	.5 cup	115	18	4	30	12	16	14	39	20
Chocolate frozen yogurt	.5 cup	110	19	3	28	12	16	13	37	19
Sugar-free chocolate yogurt	.5 cup	100	18	1	26	11	14	12	34	17

■ Baskin Robbins

FOOD	AMOUNT	CAL	CARBS	FAT	WALK	RUN	BIKE	SWIM	YOGA	DANCE
Nonfat Vanilla Frozen Yogurt	.5 cup	150	32	0	39	16	21	18	51	26
Nonfat Vanilla Soft Serve Yogurt	.5 cup	110	23	0	28	12	16	13	37	19
Nonfat Chocolate Soft Serve Yogurt	.5 cup	120	25	0	31	13	17	15	41	20
Nonfat Raspberry Soft Serve Yogurt	.5 cup	110	25	0	28	12	16	13	37	19
Nonfat Peppermint Soft Serve Yogurt	.5 cup	110	24	0	28	12	16	13	37	19
Maui Brownie Madness Low Fat Frozen Yogurt	.5 cup	210	41	4	54	22	30	26	71	36
Perils of Praline Low Fat Frozen Yogurt	.5 cup	190	37	4	49	20	27	23	65	32

■ Ben and Jerry's

FOOD	AMOUNT	CAL	CARBS	FAT	WALK	RUN	BIKE	SWIM	YOGA	DANCE
Ben and Jerry's Cherry Garcia Low Fat Frozen Yogurt	.5 cup	170	32	3	44	18	24	21	58	29

FOOD	AMOUNT	CAL	CARBS	FAT	WALK	RUN	BIKE	SWIM	YOGA	DANCE
Ben and Jerry's Chocolate Fudge Brownie Low Fat Frozen Yogurt	.5 cup	190	35	3	49	20	27	23	65	32
Ben and Jerry's Half Baked Low Fat Frozen Yogurt	.5 cup	190	35	3	49	20	27	23	65	32
Ben and Jerry's Phish Food Frozen Yogurt	.5 cup	220	41	5	57	23	31	27	75	37
■ **Coldstone Creamery**										
Coldstone Creamery Low Fat Chocolate Frozen Yogurt	Gotta have it	530	111	4	137	56	75	64	180	90
Coldstone Creamery Nonfat Cheesecake Frozen Yogurt	Gotta have it	540	113	1	139	58	77	66	184	92
Coldstone Creamery Nonfat Coffee Frozen Yogurt	Gotta have it	510	105	1	131	54	72	62	173	87
Coldstone Creamery Nonfat Sweet Cream Frozen Yogurt	Gotta have it	510	105	1	131	54	72	62	173	87
■ **Dreyer's**										
Dreyer's Vanilla Chocolate Swirl Nonfat Frozen Yogurt	.5 cup	100	17	3	26	11	14	12	34	17
Dreyer's Vanilla Nonfat Frozen Yogurt	.5 cup	90	19	0	23	10	13	11	31	15
■ **Edy's**										
Edy's Fat Free Caramel Praline Crunch Frozen Yogurt	.5 cup	100	23	0	26	11	14	12	34	17
Edy's Fat Free Vanilla Frozen Yogurt	.5 cup	90	19	0	23	10	13	11	31	15
Edy's Fat Free Chocolate Frozen Yogurt	.5 cup	90	19	0	23	10	13	11	31	15
Edy's Fat Free Strawberry Frozen Yogurt	.5 cup	100	22	0	26	11	14	12	34	17
Edy's Black Cherry Vanilla Swirl Frozen Yogurt	.5 cup	90	19	0	23	10	13	11	31	15
■ **Häagen-Dazs**										
Häagen-Dazs Rasberry Sorbet and Vanilla Yogurt	1 bar	90	21	0	23	10	13	11	31	15
Häagen-Dazs Strawberry Frozen Yogurt	.5 cup	140	31	0	36	15	20	17	48	24
Häagen-Dazs Vanilla Low Fat Frozen Yogurt	.5 cup	200	31	5	52	21	28	24	68	34
Häagen-Dazs Vanilla Raspberry Swirl Low Fat Frozen Yogurt	.5 cup	170	32	3	44	18	24	21	58	29

FOOD	AMOUNT	CAL	CARBS	FAT	WALK	RUN	BIKE	SWIM	YOGA	DANCE
Häagen-Dazs Chocolate Fudge Brownie Low Fat Frozen Yogurt	.5 cup	200	35	3	52	21	28	24	68	34
Häagen-Dazs Coffee Low Fat Frozen Yogurt	.5 cup	200	31	5	52	21	28	24	68	34
Häagen-Dazs Dulce de Leche Low Fat Frozen Yogurt	.5 cup	190	35	3	49	20	27	23	65	32
Häagen-Dazs Strawberry Fat Free Frozen Yogurt	.5 cup	140	31	0	36	15	20	17	48	24
■ **TCBY**										
TCBY Low Carb Frozen Yogurt	.5 cup	110	16	7	28	12	16	13	37	19
TCBY Low Fat Frozen Yogurt (any flavor)	.5 cup	140	23	3	36	15	20	17	48	24
TCBY Nonfat Frozen Yogurt	.5 cup	110	23	0	28	12	16	13	37	19
TCBY Nonfat Frozen Yogurt, No Sugar Added (any flavor)	.5 cup	90	20	0	23	10	13	11	31	15
TCBY Butter Pecan Perfection Hand-Scooped Frozen Yogurt	.5 cup	110	14	5	28	12	16	13	37	19
TCBY Chocolate Chocolate Swirl Hand-Scooped Frozen Yogurt	.5 cup	120	19	4	31	13	17	15	41	20
TCBY Chocolate Chunk Cookie Dough Hand-Scooped Frozen Yogurt	.5 cup	160	24	6	41	17	23	19	54	27
TCBY Mint Chocolate Chunk Hand-Scooped Frozen Yogurt	.5 cup	140	22	5	36	15	20	17	48	24
TCBY Cookies and Cream Hand-Scooped Frozen Yogurt	.5 cup	140	22	4	36	15	20	17	48	24
TCBY Cotton Candy Hand-Scooped Frozen Yogurt	.5 cup	120	20	4	31	13	17	15	41	20
TCBY Mocha Almond Hand-Scooped Frozen Yogurt	.5 cup	150	22	5	39	16	21	18	51	26
TCBY Pralines and Cream Hand-Scooped Frozen Yogurt	.5 cup	140	23	5	36	15	20	17	48	24
TCBY Rainbow Cream Hand-Scooped Frozen Yogurt	.5 cup	120	20	4	31	13	17	15	41	20
Syrups and Toppings										
■ **Syrups**										
Heath English Toffee Sundae Syrup	2 tbsp	100	24	0	26	11	14	12	34	17
Hershey's Chocolate Syrup	2 tbsp	100	24	0	26	11	14	12	34	17
Hershey's Dulce de Leche Syrup	2 tbsp	110	28	0	28	12	16	13	37	19

FOOD	AMOUNT	CAL	CARBS	FAT	WALK	RUN	BIKE	SWIM	YOGA	DANCE
Hershey's Sugar Free Syrup	2 tbsp	15	5	0	4	2	2	2	5	3
Hershey's Lite Syrup	2 tbsp	50	12	0	13	5	7	6	17	9
Hershey's Special Dark Syrup	2 tbsp	110	26	0	28	12	16	13	37	19
Hershey's Strawberry Syrup	2 tbsp	100	26	0	26	11	14	12	34	17
Hershey's Double Chocolate Sundae Syrup	2 tbsp	100	24	0	26	11	14	12	34	17
Hershey's Caramel Sundae Syrup	2 tbsp	100	25	0	26	11	14	12	34	17
Whopper's Chocolate Malt Syrup	2 tbsp	100	25	0	26	11	14	12	34	17

■ **Sprinkles**

FOOD	AMOUNT	CAL	CARBS	FAT	WALK	RUN	BIKE	SWIM	YOGA	DANCE
Hershey's Double Chocolate Sprinkles	2 tbsp	90	12	4	23	10	13	11	31	15
Reese's Peanut Butter Sprinkles	2 tbsp	90	12	4	23	10	13	11	31	15

■ **Toppings**

FOOD	AMOUNT	CAL	CARBS	FAT	WALK	RUN	BIKE	SWIM	YOGA	DANCE
Marshmallow topping	1 oz	91	22	0	24	10	13	11	31	16
Nuts in syrup topping	2 tbsp	184	24	9	47	20	26	22	63	31
Pineapple topping	2 tbsp	106	28	0	27	11	15	13	36	18
Hershey's Hot Fudge Topping	2 tbsp	120	20	4	31	13	17	15	41	20
Hershey's Caramel Topping	2 tbsp	110	27	0	28	12	16	13	37	19
Hershey's Butterscotch Topping	2 tbsp	110	27	0	28	12	16	13	37	19
Oreo Crunchies Cookie Crumb Topping	1 serving	52	8	2	13	6	7	6	18	9
Nestlé Crunch Dessert Topping	2 tbsp	125	16	6	32	13	18	15	43	21
Smucker's Marshmallow Topping	2 tbsp	120	29	0	31	13	17	15	41	20
Smucker's Dulce de Leche Topping	2 tbsp	140	25	4	36	15	20	17	48	24
Smucker's Milky Way Topping	2 tbsp	130	23	4	34	14	18	16	44	22
Smucker's Hot Fudge Topping	2 tbsp	140	24	4	36	15	20	17	48	24
Smucker's Light Hot Fudge Topping	2 tbsp	90	23	0	23	10	13	11	31	15
Smucker's Sugar Free Hot Fudge Topping	2 tbsp	90	23	0	23	10	13	11	31	15

■ **Shell Toppings**

FOOD	AMOUNT	CAL	CARBS	FAT	WALK	RUN	BIKE	SWIM	YOGA	DANCE
Heath Shell Topping	2 tbsp	220	17	17	57	23	31	27	75	37
Hershey's Chocolate Shell Topping	2 tbsp	230	16	18	59	24	33	28	78	39

FOOD	AMOUNT	CAL	CARBS	FAT	WALK	RUN	BIKE	SWIM	YOGA	DANCE
Krackel Shell Topping	2 tbsp	190	14	14	49	20	27	23	65	32
Reese's Peanut Butter Shell Topping	2 tbsp	220	17	17	57	23	31	27	75	37
Smucker's Chocolate Magic Shell	2 tbsp	210	16	17	54	22	30	26	71	36
Smucker's Caramel Magic Shell	2 tbsp	220	14	18	57	23	31	27	75	37
Smucker's Chocolate Fudge Magic Shell	2 tbsp	200	19	14	52	21	28	24	68	34
Smucker's Turtle Delight Magic Shell	2 tbsp	210	17	16	54	22	30	26	71	36
Smucker's Twix Magic Shell	2 tbsp	210	18	15	54	22	30	26	71	36
Ice Cream Cones										
Wafer cone	1 cone	17	3	0	4	2	2	2	6	3
Waffle cone	1 large cone	121	23	2	31	13	17	15	41	21
Sugar cone	1 cone	40	8	0	10	4	6	5	14	7
Keebler Sugar Cone	1 cone	50	10	1	13	5	7	6	17	9
Keebler Vanilla Cup Cone	1 cone	15	4	0	4	2	2	2	5	3
Oreo Chocolate Cones	1 cone	60	12	1	15	6	9	7	20	10
Whipped Cream										
Whipped cream (pressurized)	1 cup	154	7	13	40	16	22	19	52	26
Dessert topping (pressurized)	1 cup	185	11	16	48	20	26	22	63	31
Low-fat whipped topping	1 cup	165	18	10	43	18	23	20	56	28
Frozen dessert topping, semi solid	1 cup	239	17	19	61	25	34	29	81	41
Reddi-wip Fat-Free Whipped Topping	2 tbsp	10	2	0	3	1	1	1	3	2
Reddi-wip Original Light Whipped Topping	2 tbsp	15	<1	1	4	2	2	2	5	3
Ice Cream										
■ **General**										
Vanilla ice cream	.5 cup	144	17	8	37	15	20	18	49	25
Rich vanilla ice cream	.5 cup	265	24	17	68	28	38	32	90	45
Light vanilla ice cream	1 serving	125	20	4	32	13	18	15	43	21
Light vanilla soft serve ice cream	1 serving	111	19	2	29	12	16	13	38	19
Light no-sugar-added vanilla ice cream	.5 cup	105	15	5	27	11	15	13	36	18

FOOD	AMOUNT	CAL	CARBS	FAT	WALK	RUN	BIKE	SWIM	YOGA	DANCE
French vanilla soft-serve ice cream	.5 cup	191	19	11	49	20	27	23	65	33
Chocolate ice cream	.5 cup	143	19	7	37	15	20	17	49	24
Rich chocolate ice cream	.5 cup	189	15	13	49	20	27	23	64	32
Light chocolate ice cream	.5 cup	135	20	5	35	14	19	16	46	23
Light no-sugar-added chocolate ice cream	.5 cup	109	18	4	28	12	15	13	37	19
Strawberry ice cream	.5 cup	127	18	6	33	14	18	15	43	22

■ Häagen-Dazs—Regular

FOOD	AMOUNT	CAL	CARBS	FAT	WALK	RUN	BIKE	SWIM	YOGA	DANCE
Banana Split	.5 cup	280	31	16	72	30	40	34	95	48
Bailey's Irish Cream	.5 cup	270	23	17	70	29	38	33	92	46
German Chocolate Cake	.5 cup	300	29	18	77	32	43	36	102	51
Butter Pecan	.5 cup	310	21	23	80	33	44	38	105	53
Caramel Cone	.5 cup	320	32	19	82	34	45	39	109	55
Cherry Vanilla	.5 cup	240	23	15	62	26	34	29	82	41
Chocolate	.5 cup	270	22	18	70	29	38	33	92	46
Chocolate Chip Cookie Dough	.5 cup	310	29	20	80	33	44	38	105	53
Chocolate Chocolate Chip	.5 cup	300	26	20	77	32	43	36	102	51
Chocolate Peanut Butter	.5 cup	360	27	24	93	38	51	44	122	61
Coffee	.5 cup	270	21	18	70	29	38	33	92	46
Cookies & Cream	.5 cup	270	23	17	70	29	38	33	92	46
Crème Brulee	.5 cup	280	23	19	72	30	40	34	95	48
Dulce de Leche	.5 cup	290	28	17	75	31	41	35	99	49
Mango	.5 cup	250	28	14	64	27	35	30	85	43
Mint Chip	.5 cup	300	26	19	77	32	43	36	102	51
Mocha Almond Fudge	.5 cup	340	28	23	88	36	48	41	116	58
Peaches and Cream	.5 cup	240	29	12	62	26	34	29	82	41
Pinapple Coconut	.5 cup	230	25	13	59	24	33	28	78	39
Rocky Road	.5 cup	300	29	18	77	32	43	36	102	51
Pistachio	.5 cup	290	22	20	75	31	41	35	99	49
Rum Raisin	.5 cup	270	22	17	70	29	38	33	92	46
Strawberry	.5 cup	250	23	16	64	27	35	30	85	43
Strawberry Cheesecake	.5 cup	260	27	15	67	28	37	32	88	44
Triple Chocolate	.5 cup	330	31	21	85	35	47	40	112	56
Strawberry shortcake	.5 cup	260	29	14	67	28	37	32	88	44
Vanilla	.5 cup	270	21	18	70	29	38	33	92	46

FOOD	AMOUNT	CAL	CARBS	FAT	WALK	RUN	BIKE	SWIM	YOGA	DANCE
Vanilla Bean	.5 cup	290	26	18	75	31	41	35	99	49
Vanilla Chocolate Chip	.5 cup	310	26	20	80	33	44	38	105	53
Vanilla Fudge	.5 cup	290	26	18	75	31	41	35	99	49
Vanilla Fudge Brownie	.5 cup	300	28	19	77	32	43	36	102	51
Vanilla Swiss Almond	.5 cup	300	24	20	77	32	43	36	102	51
White Chocolate Raspberry Truffle	.5 cup	310	32	18	80	33	44	38	105	53
■ Häagen-Dazs—Light										
Cherry Fudge Truffle	.5 cup	230	37	7	59	24	33	28	78	39
Coffee	.5 cup	210	32	7	54	22	30	26	71	36
Dutch Chocolate	.5 cup	190	33	5	49	20	27	23	65	32
Dulce de Leche	.5 cup	220	33	7	57	23	31	27	75	37
Mint Chip	.5 cup	230	34	8	59	24	33	28	78	39
Smores	.5 cup	240	42	6	62	26	34	29	82	41
Vanilla Bean	.5 cup	200	29	7	52	21	28	24	68	34
■ Ben and Jerry's—Regular										
Brownie Batter	.5 cup	310	32	18	80	33	44	38	105	53
Butter Pecan	.5 cup	280	20	21	72	30	40	34	95	48
Cherry Garcia	.5 cup	250	26	14	64	27	35	30	85	43
Chocolate	.5 cup	260	25	16	67	28	37	32	88	44
Chocolate Chip Cookie Dough	.5 cup	270	32	15	70	29	38	33	92	46
Chocolate Fudge Brownie	.5 cup	260	32	13	67	28	37	32	88	44
Chubby Hubby	.5 cup	330	31	20	85	35	47	40	112	56
Chunky Monkey	.5 cup	300	30	18	77	32	43	36	102	51
Coffee	.5 cup	240	21	15	62	26	34	29	82	41
Coffee Heath Bar Crunch	.5 cup	290	29	18	75	31	41	35	99	49
Dave Matthews Band Magic Brownies	.5 cup	250	29	13	64	27	35	30	85	43
Dublin Mudslide	.5 cup	270	28	16	70	29	38	33	92	46
Everything but the	.5 cup	310	30	19	80	33	44	38	105	53
Fossil Fuel	.5 cup	280	30	17	72	30	40	34	95	48
Fudge Central	.5 cup	300	31	18	77	32	43	36	102	51
Half Baked	.5 cup	280	34	14	72	30	40	34	95	48
In a Crunch	.5 cup	350	30	23	90	37	50	43	119	60
Karamel Sutra	.5 cup	280	32	15	72	30	40	34	95	48
Marsha Marsha Marshmallow	.5 cup	300	33	17	77	32	43	36	102	51

FOOD	AMOUNT	CAL	CARBS	FAT	WALK	RUN	BIKE	SWIM	YOGA	DANCE
Mint Chocolate Cookie	.5 cup	260	26	16	67	28	37	32	88	44
New York Super Fudge Chunk	.5 cup	310	29	20	80	33	44	38	105	53
Oatmeal Cookie Chunk	.5 cup	270	31	15	70	29	38	33	92	46
Peanut Butter Cup	.5 cup	360	27	26	93	38	51	44	122	61
Phish Food	.5 cup	280	37	13	72	30	40	34	95	48
Pistachio, Pistachio	.5 cup	260	21	17	67	28	37	32	88	44
Strawberry	.5 cup	230	26	13	59	24	33	28	78	39
The Gobfather	.5 cup	270	32	14	70	29	38	33	92	46
Uncanny Cashew	.5 cup	290	27	19	75	31	41	35	99	49
Vanilla	.5 cup	240	21	16	62	26	34	29	82	41
Vanilla Caramel Fudge	.5 cup	280	31	15	72	30	40	34	95	48
Vanilla Heath Bar Crunch	.5 cup	290	29	18	75	31	41	35	99	49

■ **Ben and Jerry's—Body and Soul Ice Cream (25% less fat, sugar, and calories)**

Cherry Garcia	.5 cup	170	22	9	44	18	24	21	58	29
Chocolate Chip Cookie Dough	.5 cup	190	26	9	49	20	27	23	65	32
Chocolate Fudge Brownie	.5 cup	180	25	7	46	19	26	22	61	31
Half Baked	.5 cup	190	29	8	49	20	27	23	65	32

■ **Ben and Jerry's—Organic Ice Cream**

Chocolate Fudge Brownie	.5 cup	270	30	13	70	29	38	33	92	46
Strawberry	.5 cup	210	21	12	54	22	30	26	71	36
Sweet Cream and Cookies	.5 cup	250	24	15	64	27	35	30	85	43
Vanilla	.5 cup	220	18	14	57	23	31	27	75	37

■ **TCBY Hand-Dipped Ice Cream**

Butter Pecan	.5 cup	170	14	12	44	18	24	21	58	29
Chunk	.5 cup	150	16	9	39	16	21	18	51	26
Chocolate Chip	.5 cup	160	15	10	41	17	23	19	54	27
Cookie Dough	.5 cup	160	17	9	41	17	23	19	54	27
Chocolate	.5 cup	150	15	9	39	16	21	18	51	26
Mint Chocolate Chip	.5 cup	160	15	10	41	17	23	19	54	27
Pistachio	.5 cup	160	12	10	41	17	23	19	54	27
Pralines and Cream	.5 cup	160	16	9	41	17	23	19	54	27
Rocky Road	.5 cup	170	20	9	44	18	24	21	58	29
Strawberry	.5 cup	140	13	8	36	15	20	17	48	24
Vanilla	.5 cup	150	13	9	39	16	21	18	51	26
White Chocolate Caramel	.5 cup	150	13	9	39	16	21	18	51	26
Arthur's Favorites	.5 cup	150	16	9	39	16	21	18	51	26

FOOD	AMOUNT	CAL	CARBS	FAT	WALK	RUN	BIKE	SWIM	YOGA	DANCE
■ Yarnell's Guilt Free Ice Cream										
Homemade Vanilla	.5 cup	100	20	3	26	11	14	12	34	17
Carb Aware Vanilla	.5 cup	80	15	3	21	9	11	10	27	14
Carb Aware Chocolate	.5 cup	80	15	3	21	9	11	10	27	14
Carb Aware Praline Pecan Crunch	.5 cup	80	14	3	21	9	11	10	27	14
Carb Aware Rocky Road	.5 cup	100	14	5	26	11	14	12	34	17
Carb Aware Butter Pecan	.5 cup	100	15	5	26	11	14	12	34	17
Chocolate Decadence Cup	.5 cup	90	16	3	23	10	13	11	31	15
Strawberry Cheesecake Cup	.5 cup	80	16	3	21	9	11	10	27	14
■ Edy's—Grand Ice Cream										
Andes Cool Mint	.5 cup	170	19	9	44	18	24	21	58	29
Butter Pecan	.5 cup	170	16	10	44	18	24	21	58	29
Cherry Chocolate Chip	.5 cup	160	19	8	41	17	23	19	54	27
Chocolate	.5 cup	150	17	8	39	16	21	18	51	26
Chocolate Caramel Swirl	.5 cup	170	19	9	44	18	24	21	58	29
Chocolate Chips	.5 cup	170	18	9	44	18	24	21	58	29
Chocolate Fudge Mousse	.5 cup	160	20	8	41	17	23	19	54	27
Chocolate Fudge Sundae	.5 cup	170	20	9	44	18	24	21	58	29
Coffee	.5 cup	140	15	8	36	15	20	17	48	24
Cookie Dough	.5 cup	180	21	9	46	19	26	22	61	31
Cookies 'n Cream	.5 cup	160	19	8	41	17	23	19	54	27
Double Fudge Brownie	.5 cup	170	20	9	44	18	24	21	58	29
Double Vanilla	.5 cup	140	16	7	36	15	20	17	48	24
Dulce de Leche	.5 cup	150	20	7	39	16	21	18	51	26
Espresso Chip	.5 cup	150	17	8	39	16	21	18	51	26
French Vanilla	.5 cup	150	16	9	39	16	21	18	51	26
Fudge Tracks	.5 cup	180	18	11	46	19	26	22	61	31
Ice Cream Sandwich	.5 cup	150	19	7	39	16	21	18	51	26
Mint Chocolate Chip	.5 cup	170	18	9	44	18	24	21	58	29
Neapolitan	.5 cup	140	16	7	36	15	20	17	48	24
Nestlé Toll House Cookie Swirl	.5 cup	170	21	9	44	18	24	21	58	29
Peanut Butter Cup	.5 cup	180	19	10	46	19	26	22	61	31
Real Strawberry	.5 cup	130	16	6	34	14	18	16	44	22
Rocky Road	.5 cup	170	19	10	44	18	24	21	58	29
Spumoni	.5 cup	150	16	8	39	16	21	18	51	26

FOOD	AMOUNT	CAL	CARBS	FAT	WALK	RUN	BIKE	SWIM	YOGA	DANCE
Toffee Bar Crunch	.5 cup	170	19	9	44	18	24	21	58	29
Turtle Sundae	.5 cup	160	18	9	41	17	23	19	54	27
Ultimate Caramel Cup	.5 cup	170	22	8	44	18	24	21	58	29
Vanilla	.5 cup	140	15	8	36	15	20	17	48	24
Vanilla Bean	.5 cup	140	15	8	36	15	20	17	48	24
Vanilla Chocolate	.5 cup	150	16	8	39	16	21	18	51	26

■ Edy's—Slow Churned Light Ice Cream

FOOD	AMOUNT	CAL	CARBS	FAT	WALK	RUN	BIKE	SWIM	YOGA	DANCE
Butter Pecan	.5 cup	120	16	5	31	13	17	15	41	20
Caramel Delight	.5 cup	120	19	4	31	13	17	15	41	20
Chocolate	.5 cup	110	16	4	28	12	16	13	37	19
Chocolate Chips	.5 cup	120	17	5	31	13	17	15	41	20
Chocolate Fudge Chunk	.5 cup	120	18	5	31	13	17	15	41	20
Coffee	.5 cup	105	15	4	27	11	15	13	36	18
Cookie Dough	.5 cup	130	20	5	34	14	18	16	44	22
Cookies 'n Cream	.5 cup	120	18	4	31	13	17	15	41	20
French Silk	.5 cup	130	20	5	34	14	18	16	44	22
French Vanilla	.5 cup	100	15	4	26	11	14	12	34	17
Fudge Tracks	.5 cup	120	18	5	31	13	17	15	41	20
Girl Scouts Samoas Cookie	.5 cup	120	19	5	31	13	17	15	41	20
Girl Scouts Thin Mints Cookie	.5 cup	120	18	5	31	13	17	15	41	20
Mint Chocolate Chip	.5 cup	120	17	5	31	13	17	15	41	20
Mocha Almond Fudge	.5 cup	120	16	5	31	13	17	15	41	20
Neapolitan	.5 cup	100	15	3	26	11	14	12	34	17
Rocky Road	.5 cup	120	17	4	31	13	17	15	41	20
Strawberry	.5 cup	110	18	3	28	12	16	13	37	19
Vanilla	.5 cup	100	15	4	26	11	14	12	34	17
Vanilla Bean	.5 cup	100	15	4	26	11	14	12	34	17
Vanilla Chocolate	.5 cup	100	15	4	26	11	14	12	34	17

■ Edy's—Slow Churned No Sugar Added

FOOD	AMOUNT	CAL	CARBS	FAT	WALK	RUN	BIKE	SWIM	YOGA	DANCE
Butter Pecan	.5 cup	120	15	5	31	13	17	15	41	20
Chocolate	.5 cup	95	14	3	24	10	13	12	32	16
Cookie Dough	.5 cup	110	16	4	28	12	16	13	37	19
Fudge Tracks	.5 cup	110	16	4	28	12	16	13	37	19
Mint Chocolate Chip	.5 cup	110	15	5	28	12	16	13	37	19
Neapolitan	.5 cup	95	14	3	24	10	13	12	32	16
Triple Chocolate	.5 cup	110	17	4	28	12	16	13	37	19

FOOD	AMOUNT	CAL	CARBS	FAT	WALK	RUN	BIKE	SWIM	YOGA	DANCE
Vanilla	.5 cup	90	13	3	23	10	13	11	31	15
■ **Edy's—Carb Benefit**										
Butter Pecan	.5 cup	170	13	12	44	18	24	21	58	29
Chocolate	.5 cup	150	13	10	39	16	21	18	51	26
Chocolate Chip	.5 cup	160	14	11	41	17	23	19	54	27
Mint Chocolate Chip	.5 cup	160	14	11	41	17	23	19	54	27
Vanilla Bean	.5 cup	140	13	9	36	15	20	17	48	24
■ **Edy's—Fat Free, No Sugar Added Ice Cream**										
Chocolate Fudge	.5 cup	100	22	0	26	11	14	12	34	17
Raspberry Vanilla Swirl	.5 cup	90	19	0	23	10	13	11	31	15
Vanilla	.5 cup	90	2	0	23	10	13	11	31	15
Vanilla Chocolate Swirl	.5 cup	100	20	0	26	11	14	12	34	17
■ **Breyer's**										
Breyer's All Natural Light Vanilla	.5 cup	110	17	3	28	12	16	13	37	19
Breyer's No Sugar Added Vanilla	.5 cup	99	15	4	26	11	14	12	34	17
Breyer's 98% Fat Free Vanilla	.5 cup	93	21	2	24	10	13	11	32	16
Breyer's No Sugar Added French Vanilla	.5 cup	105	14	5	27	11	15	13	36	18
Breyer's All Natural Light French Vanilla	.5 cup	118	18	4	30	13	17	14	40	20
Breyer's No Sugar Added Vanilla Fudge Twirl	.5 cup	110	18	4	28	12	16	13	37	19
Breyer's All Natural Light Vanilla, Chocolate, Strawberry	.5 cup	109	18	3	28	12	15	13	37	19
Breyer's No Sugar Added Vanilla, Chocolate, Strawberry	.5 cup	97	15	4	25	10	14	12	33	17
Breyer's All Natural Light French Chocolate	.5 cup	137	20	5	35	15	19	17	46	23
Breyer's 98% Fat Free Chocolate	.5 cup	92	21	1	24	10	13	11	31	16
Breyer's Chocolate Caramel No Sugar Added	.5 cup	107	18	4	28	11	15	13	36	18
Breyer's All Natural Light Mint Chocolate Chip	.5 cup	133	19	5	34	14	19	16	45	23
Breyer's No Sugar Added Butter Pecan	1 serving	122	14	7	32	13	17	15	42	21
■ **Healthy Choice—General**										
Brownie Bliss	.5 cup	130	25	2	34	14	18	16	44	22
Butter Pecan	.5 cup	120	20	2	31	13	17	15	41	20

FOOD	AMOUNT	CAL	CARBS	FAT	WALK	RUN	BIKE	SWIM	YOGA	DANCE
Cappuccino Chocolate Chunk	.5 cup	120	20	2	31	13	17	15	41	20
Caramel Fudge Brownie	.5 cup	120	21	2	31	13	17	15	41	20
Chocolate Cherry Mambo	.5 cup	120	21	2	31	13	17	15	41	20
Chocolate Chocolate Chunk	.5 cup	120	21	2	31	13	17	15	41	20
Chocolate Mocha Silk	.5 cup	120	24	2	31	13	17	15	41	20
Cookies 'n Cream	.5 cup	120	21	2	31	13	17	15	41	20
Crazy for Caramel	.5 cup	120	23	2	31	13	17	15	41	20
Double Karma	.5 cup	140	28	2	36	15	20	17	48	24
In the Beginning	.5 cup	110	21	2	28	12	16	13	37	19
Jumpin' Java	.5 cup	130	25	2	34	14	18	16	44	22
Mint Chocolate Chip	.5 cup	120	20	2	31	13	17	15	41	20
Peanut Butter Cup	.5 cup	120	21	2	31	13	17	15	41	20
Praline and Caramel	.5 cup	120	23	2	31	13	17	15	41	20
Rocky Road	.5 cup	130	25	2	34	14	18	16	44	22
So Happy Together	.5 cup	150	29	2	39	16	21	18	51	26
Tin Roof Sundae	.5 cup	120	21	2	31	13	17	15	41	20
Turtle Fudge Cake	.5 cup	130	23	2	34	14	18	16	44	22
Vanilla	.5 cup	110	19	2	28	12	16	13	37	19
■ **Healthy Choice—No Sugar Added**										
Vanilla	.5 cup	100	17	2	26	11	14	12	34	17
Butter Pecan	.5 cup	110	18	3	28	12	16	13	37	19
Chocolate Fudge Brownie	.5 cup	120	21	2	31	13	17	15	41	20
Coffee Almond Fudge	.5 cup	110	20	2	28	12	16	13	37	19
Mint Chocolate Chip	.5 cup	110	18	2	28	12	16	13	37	19
■ **M&M's Ice Cream**										
M&M's Vanilla Fudge	.5 cup	180	20	10	46	19	26	22	61	31
M&M's Mint	.5 cup	170	20	9	44	18	24	21	58	29
Bars and Sandwiches										
■ **Chocolate Bar Ice Cream**										
Chocolate Covered Ice Cream Bar with Nuts	1 bar	171	17	2	44	18	24	21	58	29
Eskimo Pie Bar	1 bar	166	12	12	43	18	24	20	56	28
M&M's Singles Ice Cream Cone	1 cone	250	33	12	64	27	35	30	85	43
M&M's Singles Ice Cream Sandwich	1 sandwich	260	34	12	67	28	37	32	88	44
Snickers Ice Cream Cone	1 cone	280	33	15	72	30	40	34	95	48

FOOD	AMOUNT	CAL	CARBS	FAT	WALK	RUN	BIKE	SWIM	YOGA	DANCE
Snickers Ice Cream Bar	1 large bar	180	18	11	46	19	26	22	61	31
Twix Ice Cream Bar	1 bar	170	19	10	44	18	24	21	58	29
■ Edy's Dibs										
Chocolate with Chocolaty Coating	26 pieces	420	28	32	108	45	60	51	143	72
Mint with Chocolaty Coating	26 pieces	420	29	32	108	45	60	51	143	72
Vanilla with Chocolaty Coating	26 pieces	420	29	32	108	45	60	51	143	72
Vanilla with Nestlé Crunch Coating	26 pieces	380	29	28	98	40	54	46	129	65
Vanilla with Nestlé Drumstick Coating	26 pieces	390	29	29	101	42	55	47	133	66
■ Häagen-Dazs										
Brownie Bar	1 bar	360	30	24	93	38	51	44	122	61
Chocolate and Dark Chocolate	1 bar	300	24	21	77	32	43	36	102	51
Coffee and Almond Crunch	1 bar	310	23	22	80	33	44	38	105	53
Dulce de Leche	1 bar	300	28	19	77	32	43	36	102	51
Vanilla and Almonds	1 bar	320	22	12	82	34	45	39	109	55
Vanilla and Dark Chocolate	1 bar	300	23	21	77	32	43	36	102	51
Vanilla and Milk Chocolate	1 bar	290	22	21	75	31	41	35	99	49
■ Klondike										
Klondike	1 bar	250	22	17	64	27	35	30	85	43
Klondike with Oreo Ice Cream Sandwiches	1 sandwich	230	35	9	59	24	33	28	78	39
Push-Up Pops										
Nestlé Push-Up Rainbow Sherbet	1 tube	90	19	1	23	10	13	11	31	15
Diet Bars and Sandwiches										
Breyer's Carb Smart Fudge Bar	1 bar	100	9	7	26	11	14	12	34	17
Fat-free fudgesicles	1 bar	65	14	0	17	7	9	8	22	11
Healthy Choice Caramel Swirl Ice Cream Sandwich	1 bar	140	27	3	36	15	20	17	48	24
Healthy Choice Fudge Bar	1 bar	80	13	1	21	9	11	10	27	14
Healthy Choice Fudge Swirl Ice Cream Sandwich	1 bar	140	27	3	36	15	20	17	48	24
Healthy Choice Mocha Fudge Swirl Bar	1 bar	90	17	2	23	10	13	11	31	15
Healthy Choice Raspberry Orange Sorbet Swirls	1 bar	90	18	1	23	10	13	11	31	15

FOOD	AMOUNT	CAL	CARBS	FAT	WALK	RUN	BIKE	SWIM	YOGA	DANCE
Healthy Choice Strawberries and Cream Bar	1 bar	80	13	2	21	9	11	10	27	14
Healthy Choice Vanilla Ice Cream Bar with Fudge Coating	1 bar	80	13	1	21	9	11	10	27	14
Healthy Choice Vanilla Ice Cream Sandwich	1 bar	130	24	3	34	14	18	16	44	22
Klondike No Sugar Added Slim-a-Bear Fudge Bar	1 bar	90	22	2	23	10	13	11	31	15
Klondike No Sugar Added Slim-a-Bear Vanilla	1 bar	170	21	9	44	18	24	21	58	29
Klondike Slim-a-Bear Chocolate Cone	1 cone	177	36	3	46	19	25	22	60	30
Klondike Slim-a-Bear Chocolate Sandwich	1 sandwich	136	28	2	35	14	19	17	46	23
Klondike Slim-a-Bear Mint Sandwich	1 sandwich	134	28	2	35	14	19	16	46	23
Klondike Slim-a-Bear Vanilla Cone	1 cone	175	35	3	45	19	25	21	60	30
Klondike Slim-a-Bear Vanilla Sandwich	1 sandwich	135	28	2	35	14	19	16	46	23
No Sugar Added Creamsicle	1 pop	25	6	0	6	3	4	3	9	4
No-sugar-added fudgesicles	2 pops	88	19	1	23	9	12	11	30	15
Skinny Cow Caramel Low Fat Ice Cream Sandwiches	1 sandwich	140	27	3	36	15	20	17	48	24
Skinny Cow Chocolate Peanut Butter Low Fat Ice Cream Sandwiches	1 sandwich	140	27	3	36	15	20	17	48	24
Skinny Cow Coffee Low Fat Ice Cream Sandwiches	1 sandwich	140	28	2	36	15	20	17	48	24
Skinny Cow Cookies 'N Cream Low Fat Ice Cream Sandwiches	1 sandwich	150	31	2	39	16	21	18	51	26
Skinny Cow Fat Free Fudge Bar	1 bar	100	21	0	26	11	14	12	34	17
Skinny Cow Mint Low Fat Ice Cream Sandwiches	1 sandwich	140	30	2	36	15	20	17	48	24
Skinny Cow Mint No Sugar Added Ice Cream Sandwiches	1 sandwich	140	30	2	36	15	20	17	48	24
Skinny Cow Skinny Carb Fudge	1 bar	130	12	8	34	14	18	16	44	22
Skinny Cow Skinny Carb Vanilla Caramel Pecan	1 bar	150	14	9	39	16	21	18	51	26

FOOD	AMOUNT	CAL	CARBS	FAT	WALK	RUN	BIKE	SWIM	YOGA	DANCE
Skinny Cow Strawberry Shortcake Low Fat Ice Cream Sandwiches	1 sandwich	140	28	2	36	15	20	17	48	24
Skinny Cow Vanilla and Chocolate Combo Low Fat Ice Cream Sandwiches	1 sandwich	140	30	2	36	15	20	17	48	24
Skinny Cow Vanilla Low Fat Ice Cream Sandwiches	1 sandwich	140	30	2	36	15	20	17	48	24
Skinny Cow Vanilla No Sugar Added Ice Cream Sandwiches	1 sandwich	140	30	2	36	15	20	17	48	24
Sugar Free Creamsicle	2 pops	39	10	2	10	4	6	5	13	7
Weight Watchers Chocolate Mousse Ice Cream Bar	2 bars	120	28	1	31	13	17	15	41	20
Weight Watchers Frozen Chocolate Éclairs	1 éclair	140	23	4	36	15	20	17	48	24
Weight Watchers Giant Chocolate Fudge Ice Cream Bar	1 bar	110	25	1	28	12	16	13	37	19
Weight Watchers Giant Cookies and Cream Ice Cream Bar	1 bar	140	26	5	36	15	20	17	48	24
Weight Watchers Giant Premium Peanut Butter Fudge Ice Cream Sundae Cone	1 cone	120	29	4	31	13	17	15	41	20
Weight Watchers Vanilla Ice Cream Sandwich	1 sandwich	120	28	2	31	13	17	15	41	20
Yarnell's Carb Aware Deluxe Fudge Bar	1 bar	45	11	0	12	5	6	5	15	8
Yarnell's Guilt Free Ice Cream Sandwich	1 sandwich	140	24	5	36	15	20	17	48	24
Fruit Bars										
Edy's Whole Fruit Creamy Coconut Bars	1 bar	120	21	3	31	13	17	15	41	20
Edy's Whole Fruit Lemon Bars	1 bar	80	20	0	21	9	11	10	27	14
Edy's Whole Fruit Lime Bars	1 bar	80	20	0	21	9	11	10	27	14
Edy's Whole Fruit Low Fat Orange & Cream Bars	1 bar	80	16	2	21	9	11	10	27	14
Edy's Whole Fruit Peach Bars	1 bar	90	23	0	23	10	13	11	31	15
Edy's Whole Fruit Strawberry Bars	1 bar	80	21	0	21	9	11	10	27	14
Edy's Whole Fruit Tangerine Bars	1 bar	80	20	0	21	9	11	10	27	14
Edy's Whole Fruit Tropical Bars	1 bar	100	26	0	26	11	14	12	34	17
Edy's Whole Fruit Wild Berry Bars	1 bar	80	20	0	21	9	11	10	27	14

FOOD	AMOUNT	CAL	CARBS	FAT	WALK	RUN	BIKE	SWIM	YOGA	DANCE
Frozen Fruit and Juice Bar	1 bar (3 oz)	80	19	0	21	9	11	10	27	14
Frozen Fruit Bar, No Sugar Added	1 bar	12	3	0	3	1	2	1	4	2
Orange Juice Bar	1 bar	70	17	0	18	7	10	9	24	12
Yarnell's Guilt Free Fruit Bars	1 bar	45	13	0	12	5	6	5	15	8
Ices										
Lime ice	.5 cup	127	32	0	33	13	18	15	43	22
Italian ice	.5 cup	61	16	0	16	6	9	7	21	10
Sugar-free flavored ice pop	1 pop	12	3	0	3	1	2	1	4	2
Pineapple-coconut ice	.5 cup	112	24	3	29	12	16	14	38	19
Sorbet										
Häagen-Dazs Chocolate	.5 cup	130	28	1	34	14	18	16	44	22
Häagen-Dazs Mango	.5 cup	120	37	0	31	13	17	15	41	20
Häagen-Dazs Orchard Peach	.5 cup	130	33	0	34	14	18	16	44	22
Häagen-Dazs Raspberry	.5 cup	120	30	0	31	13	17	15	41	20
Häagen-Dazs Strawberry	.5 cup	120	30	0	31	13	17	15	41	20
Häagen-Dazs Tropical	.5 cup	150	38	0	39	16	21	18	51	26
Häagen-Dazs Zesty Lemon	.5 cup	110	28	0	28	12	16	13	37	19
Sharon's Coconut Sorbet	.5 cup	160	22	8	41	17	23	19	54	27
Sharon's Fat Free Lemon Sorbet	.5 cup	75	19	0	19	8	11	9	26	13
Sharon's Low Fat Chocolate Sorbet Bars	1 bar	90	20	2	23	10	13	11	31	15
Sharon's Passion Fruit Sorbet	.5 cup	80	20	0	21	9	11	10	27	14
TCBY Nonfat, Nondairy Sorbet	.5 cup	100	24	0	26	11	14	12	34	17
Sherbet										
Orange sherbet	.5 cup	107	23	1	27	11	15	13	36	18
Edy's Berry Rainbow	.5 cup	130	29	2	34	14	18	16	44	22
Edy's Key Lime	.5 cup	130	28	2	34	14	18	16	44	22
Edy's Orange Cream	.5 cup	120	23	2	31	13	17	15	41	20
Edy's Raspberry	.5 cup	130	28	1	34	14	18	16	44	22
Edy's Swiss Orange	.5 cup	150	30	3	39	16	21	18	51	26
Edy's Tropical Rainbow	.5 cup	130	29	1	34	14	18	16	44	22
Gelatin										
Gelatin dessert (prepared with water)	.5 cup	84	19	0	22	9	12	10	29	14

FOOD	AMOUNT	CAL	CARBS	FAT	WALK	RUN	BIKE	SWIM	YOGA	DANCE
Sugar-free gelatin dessert (prepared with water)	.5 cup	23	5	0	6	2	3	3	8	4
Jell-O										
Jell-O Gelatin	.25 package	80	19	0	21	9	11	10	27	14
Sugar Free Jell-O Gelatin Dessert	.25 package	10	0	0	3	1	1	1	3	2
Jell-O Gelatin Snacks	1 snack	70	17	0	18	7	10	9	24	12
Sugar Free Jell-O Gelatin Snacks	1 snack	10	0	0	3	1	1	1	3	2
Jell-O Strawberry Cheesecake Dessert	1 slice	340	52	12	88	36	48	41	116	58
Jell-O Homestyle Cheesecake Dessert	1 slice	360	50	15	93	38	51	44	122	61
Other Gelatin										
Knox Unflavored Gelatin	1 envelope	25	0	0	6	3	4	3	9	4
Royal Gelatin Dessert	.5 cup prepared	70	17	0	18	7	10	9	24	12
Royal Sugar Free Gelatin Dessert	.5 cup prepared	5	0	0	1	1	1	1	2	1
Custard and Flan										
Egg custard (prepared with whole milk)	4 oz	137	20	5	35	15	19	17	47	23
Egg custard (prepared with 2% milk)	4 oz	125	20	3	32	13	18	15	43	21
Flan (prepared with 2% milk)	1 oz	116	21	2	30	12	16	14	39	20
Flan (prepared with whole milk)	4 oz	128	21	3	33	14	18	16	44	22
Pudding										
■ General										
Chocolate pudding	4 oz	157	26	5	40	17	22	19	53	27
Regular chocolate pudding (prepared with whole milk)	.5 cup	169	28	4	44	18	24	21	57	29
Instant chocolate pudding (prepared with whole milk)	.5 cup	163	28	5	42	17	23	20	55	28
Vanilla pudding	4 oz	147	25	4	38	16	21	18	50	25
Fat-free vanilla pudding	4 oz	105	26	0	27	11	15	13	36	18
Regular vanilla pudding (prepared with whole milk)	.5 cup	157	26	5	40	17	22	19	53	27

FOOD	AMOUNT	CAL	CARBS	FAT	WALK	RUN	BIKE	SWIM	YOGA	DANCE
Instant vanilla pudding (prepared with whole milk)	.5 cup	162	28	4	42	17	23	20	55	28
Regular coconut cream pudding (prepared with whole milk)	.5 cup	160	25	5	41	17	23	19	54	27
Regular coconut cream pudding (prepared with 2% milk)	.5 cup	146	25	4	38	16	21	18	50	25
Instant coconut cream pudding (prepared with whole milk)	.5 cup	172	28	5	44	18	24	21	59	29
Instant coconut cream pudding (prepared with 2% milk)	.5 cup	157	28	3	40	17	22	19	53	27
Lemon pudding	4 oz	142	28	3	37	15	20	17	48	24
Instant lemon pudding (prepared with whole milk)	.5 cup	169	30	4	44	18	24	21	57	29
Tapioca pudding	4 oz	134	22	4	35	14	19	16	46	23
Rice pudding	4 oz	185	25	9	48	20	26	23	63	32
Banana pudding	4 oz	144	24	4	37	15	20	18	49	25
■ **Brand Names**										
Hunt's Chocolate Pudding Snack	1 pudding cup	140	22	5	36	15	20	17	48	24
Hunt's Vanilla Pudding Snack	1 pudding cup	130	21	5	34	14	18	16	44	22
Jell-O Chocolate Pudding	.25 package	100	25	0	26	11	14	12	34	17
Jell-O Chocolate Pudding Snack	1 snack	140	27	4	36	15	20	17	48	24
Jell-O Chocolate Vanilla Swirls Pudding Snack	1 snack	140	26	6	36	15	20	17	48	24
Jell-O Fat Free Chocolate Pudding Snack	1 snack	100	23	0	26	11	14	12	34	17
Jell-O Fat Free Chocolate Vanilla Swirl Pudding Snack	1 snack	100	23	0	26	11	14	12	34	17
Jell-O Fat Free Devil's Food Pudding Snack	1 snack	100	22	0	26	11	14	12	34	17
Jell-O Sugar Free Pudding Snack	1 snack	60	14	2	15	6	9	7	20	10
Jell-O Vanilla Pudding	.25 package	90	23	0	23	10	13	11	31	15
Kozy Shack Chocolate Pudding	1 cup	140	24	4	36	15	20	17	48	24
Kozy Shack Rice Pudding	1 cup	130	22	3	34	14	18	16	44	22
Kozy Shack Tapioca Pudding	1 cup	130	23	3	34	14	18	16	44	22

FOOD	AMOUNT	CAL	CARBS	FAT	WALK	RUN	BIKE	SWIM	YOGA	DANCE
Sugar Free Jell-O Chocolate Pudding	.25 package	35	8	0	9	4	5	4	12	6
Sugar Free Jell-O Vanilla Pudding	.25 package	35	6	0	9	4	5	4	12	6
Swiss Miss Chocolate Pudding	1 pudding cup	160	25	5	41	17	23	19	54	27
Swiss Miss Chocolate Vanilla Swirl Pudding	1 pudding cup	160	26	6	41	17	23	19	54	27
Swiss Miss Vanilla Pudding	1 pudding cup	160	24	6	41	17	23	19	54	27

Granola and Nutrition Bars

Granola Bars

■ Hard Granola Bars

FOOD	AMOUNT	CAL	CARBS	FAT	WALK	RUN	BIKE	SWIM	YOGA	DANCE
Plain granola bar	1 bar	118	16	5	30	13	17	14	40	20
Almond granola bar	1 bar	199	15	6	51	21	28	24	68	34
Chocolate chip granola bar	1 bar	105	17	4	27	11	15	13	36	18
Peanut granola bar	1 bar	136	18	6	35	14	19	17	46	23
Peanut butter granola bar	1 bar	116	15	6	30	12	16	14	39	20

■ Soft Granola Bars

FOOD	AMOUNT	CAL	CARBS	FAT	WALK	RUN	BIKE	SWIM	YOGA	DANCE
Plain granola bar	1 bar	124	19	5	32	13	18	15	42	21
Raisin granola bar	1 bar	125	19	5	32	13	18	15	43	21
Nut and raisin granola bar	1 bar	127	18	6	33	14	18	15	43	22
Chocolate chip granola bar	1 bar	118	0	5	30	13	17	14	40	20
Chocolate chip, graham and marshmallow granola bar	1 bar	120	20	4	31	13	17	15	41	20
Peanut butter granola bar	1 bar	119	18	4	31	13	17	14	40	20
Peanut butter chocolate chip granola bar	1 bar	121	17	6	31	13	17	15	41	21
Milk chocolate-coated chocolate chip granola bar	1 bar	130	18	7	34	14	18	16	44	22
Milk chocolate-coated peanut butter granola bar	1 bar	188	20	12	48	20	27	23	64	32

■ Other Granola Bars

FOOD	AMOUNT	CAL	CARBS	FAT	WALK	RUN	BIKE	SWIM	YOGA	DANCE
Nonfat fruit-filled granola bar	1 bar	96	22	0	25	10	14	12	33	16
Chocolate coated-coconut granola bar	1 bar	149	15	9	38	16	21	18	51	25

FOOD	AMOUNT	CAL	CARBS	FAT	WALK	RUN	BIKE	SWIM	YOGA	DANCE
■ Kudos										
Chocolate chip	1 bar	120	20	4	31	13	17	15	41	20
Peanut butter	1 bar	130	18	6	34	14	18	16	44	22
Snickers	1 bar	100	16	3	26	11	14	12	34	17
■ Health Valley										
Low Fat Raspberry Granola Bars	1 bar	150	35	1	39	16	21	18	51	26
Moist & Chewy Peanut Crunch	1 bar	110	19	3	28	12	16	13	37	19
Moist & Chewy Dutch Apple	1 bar	100	22	1	26	11	14	12	34	17
Moist & Chewy Wild Berry	1 bar	100	22	1	26	11	14	12	34	17
Nonfat Raisin Granola Bar	1 bar	140	35	0	36	15	20	17	48	24
Nonfat Strawberry Granola Bar	1 bar	140	35	0	36	15	20	17	48	24
Nonfat Raspberry Granola Bar	1 bar	140	35	0	36	15	20	17	48	24
■ Quaker										
Chewy Chocolate Chip	1 bar	120	21	4	31	13	17	15	41	20
Low Fat Chocolate Chunk	1 bar	110	22	2	28	12	16	13	37	19
■ Nature Valley										
Oat and Honey	2 bars (1 pack)	180	29	6	46	19	26	22	61	31
Peanut Butter	2 bars (1 pack)	180	30	7	46	19	26	22	61	31
Trail Mix Chewy Fruit and Nut	1 bar	140	25	4	36	15	20	17	48	24
■ Sierra Club										
Organic Apple Cinnamon	1 bar	140	25	5	36	15	20	17	48	24
Organic Cranberry Crunch	1 bar	170	18	10	44	18	24	21	58	29
Organic Mixed Nut	1 bar	180	18	11	46	19	26	22	61	31
Breakfast Bars/Tarts										
Breakfast bar	1 bar	200	29	8	52	21	28	24	68	34
Crisped rice bar	1 bar	113	20	4	29	12	16	14	38	19
Rice Krispie treat	1 bar	90	18	2	23	10	13	11	31	15
Cocoa Krispies Milk and Cereal Bars	1 bar	100	17	3	26	11	14	12	34	17
Nutri-Grain Cereal Bars, all flavors	1 bar	140	27	3	36	15	20	17	48	24
■ Pop-Tarts										
Strawberry	1 pastry	200	37	5	52	21	28	24	68	34
Frosted Brown Sugar Cinnamon	1 pastry	210	34	7	54	22	30	26	71	36

FOOD	AMOUNT	CAL	CARBS	FAT	WALK	RUN	BIKE	SWIM	YOGA	DANCE
Frosted Strawberry with Sprinkles	1 pastry	200	38	5	52	21	28	24	68	34
S'mores	1 pastry	200	36	6	52	21	28	24	68	34
Health Valley Fruit Tarts										
Low Fat Baked Apple	1 bar	130	28	2	34	14	18	16	44	22
Low Fat Blueberry	1 bar	130	28	2	34	14	18	16	44	22
Low Fat Raspberry	1 bar	130	28	2	34	14	18	16	44	22
Low Fat Red Cherry	1 bar	130	28	2	34	14	18	16	44	22
Low Fat Strawberry	1 bar	130	28	2	34	14	18	16	44	22
Nutrition Bars										
■ **Hershey's**										
Crunchy Chocolate Peanut Butter Hershey's SmartZone	1 bar (50 g)	200	21	7	52	21	28	24	68	34
Crunchy Chocolate Brownie Hershey's SmartZone	1 bar (50 g)	200	21	7	52	21	28	24	68	34
Crunchy Chocolate Caramel Hershey's SmartZone	1 bar (50 g)	210	23	7	54	22	30	26	71	36
■ **Snickers**										
Snickers Marathon Energy Chewy Chocolate Peanut	1 bar (1.94 oz)	220	27	7	57	23	31	27	75	37
Snickers Marathon Energy Multigrain Crunch	1 bar (1.94 oz)	220	32	7	57	23	31	27	75	37
■ **Clif Bars**										
Apple Cherry	1 bar	250	52	2	64	27	35	30	85	43
Chocolate Almond Fudge	1 bar	250	39	5	64	27	35	30	85	43
Chocolate Chip	1 bar	250	51	3	64	27	35	30	85	43
Chocolate Chip Peanut	1 bar	250	40	6	64	27	35	30	85	43
Cookies 'n Cream	1 bar	250	42	5	64	27	35	30	85	43
Crunchy Peanut Butter	1 bar	250	45	4	64	27	35	30	85	43
Real Berry	1 bar	250	52	2	64	27	35	30	85	43
■ **Power Bar**										
Apple Cinnamon	1 bar	230	45	3	59	24	33	28	78	39
Wild Berry	1 bar	230	45	3	59	24	33	28	78	39
Chocolate	1 bar	230	45	2	59	24	33	28	78	39
Mocha	1 bar	230	45	3	59	24	33	28	78	39
Oatmeal Raisin	1 bar	230	45	3	59	24	33	28	78	39
Peanut Butter	1 bar	230	45	3	59	24	33	28	78	39

FOOD	AMOUNT	CAL	CARBS	FAT	WALK	RUN	BIKE	SWIM	YOGA	DANCE
■ **Power Bar Harvest**										
Cherry Crunch	1 bar	240	45	4	62	26	34	29	82	41
Peanut Butter Chocolate Chip	1 bar	240	45	5	62	26	34	29	82	41
Strawberry	1 bar	240	45	4	62	26	34	29	82	41
■ **Power Bar Essentials**										
Chocolate	1 bar	180	28	4	46	19	26	22	61	31
■ **Power Bar Protein Plus**										
Chocolate	1 bar	290	38	5	75	31	41	35	99	49
Vanilla Yogurt	1 bar	290	38	5	75	31	41	35	99	49
■ **Odwalla**										
Berries Go Mega	1 bar	220	41	5	57	23	31	27	75	37
Cranberry C Monster	1 bar	220	44	3	57	23	31	27	75	37
Organic Carrot Raisin	1 bar	220	43	4	57	23	31	27	75	37
Peanut Crunch	1 bar	240	37	7	62	26	34	29	82	41
Super Protein	1 bar	230	31	5	59	24	33	28	78	39
Superfood	1 bar	230	43	4	59	24	33	28	78	39
■ **Luna**										
Chocolate Pecan Pie	1 bar	180	25	5	46	19	26	22	61	31
Lemonzest	1 bar	180	26	4	46	19	26	22	61	31
Nutz Over Chocolate	1 bar	180	26	4	46	19	26	22	61	31
Toasted Nuts and Cranberry	1 bar	170	26	4	44	18	24	21	58	29
S'mores	1 bar	180	26	5	46	19	26	22	61	31
■ **Kashi**										
GoLean Chocolate Peanut Butter Bar	1 bar	290	48	6	75	31	41	35	99	49

Pantry

Cocoa										
Hershey's Natural Cocoa	1 tbsp	20	3	1	5	2	3	2	7	3
Hershey's Dutch Processed Dark Cocoa	1 tbsp	20	3	1	5	2	3	2	7	3
Sugar										
Brown sugar	1 cup, packed	829	214	0	214	88	118	101	282	141
White sugar	1 cup	774	200	0	199	82	110	94	263	132
Powdered sugar	1 cup	467	0	0	120	50	66	57	159	80

FOOD	AMOUNT	CAL	CARBS	FAT	WALK	RUN	BIKE	SWIM	YOGA	DANCE
Splenda	1 tsp	0	<1	0	0	0	0	0	0	0
Syrups										
Dark corn syrup	2 tbsp	114	31	0	29	12	16	14	39	19
Light corn syrup	2 tbsp	62	17	0	16	7	9	8	21	11
Malt syrup	.25 cup	305	68	0	79	32	43	37	104	52
Maple syrup	.25 cup	210	54	0	54	22	30	26	71	36
Grains										
Couscous	1 cup, cooked	176	36	0	45	19	25	21	60	30
Millet	1 cup	207	41	2	53	22	29	25	70	35
Puffed millet	1 cup	74	17	1	19	8	10	9	25	13
Buckwheat groats	1 cup	155	34	1	40	16	22	19	53	26
Bulgur	1 cup	151	34	0	39	16	21	18	51	26
Pearled barley	1 cup	193	44	1	50	21	27	23	66	33
Cornmeal, white or yellow	1 cup	442	94	4	114	47	63	54	150	75
Yellow canned hominy	1 cup	115	23	1	30	12	16	14	39	20
White canned hominy	1 cup	119	23	1	31	13	17	14	40	20
Rice										
Glutinous white rice, cooked	1 cup	169	37	0	44	18	24	21	57	29
Instant white rice, cooked	1 cup	193	41	1	50	21	27	23	66	33
Long-grain brown rice, cooked	1 cup	216	45	2	56	23	31	26	74	37
Long-grain parboiled white rice, cooked	1 cup	194	41	1	50	21	28	24	66	33
Long-grain white rice, cooked	1 cup	205	45	0	53	22	29	25	70	35
Medium-grain brown rice, cooked	1 cup	218	46	2	56	23	31	27	74	37
Medium-grain white rice, cooked	1 cup	242	53	0	62	26	34	29	82	41
Short-grain white rice, cooked	1 cup	242	53	0	62	26	34	29	82	41
Wild rice, cooked	1 cup	166	35	1	43	18	23	20	56	28
Arrowhead Mills Organic Quinoa	.66 cup	160	30	3	41	17	23	19	54	27
Flour										
Whole-grain wheat flour	1 cup	407	87	2	105	43	58	49	138	69
White flour	1 cup	455	95	1	117	48	65	55	155	78
White self-rising flour	1 cup	443	93	1	114	47	63	54	151	75
White bread flour	1 cup	495	99	2	127	53	70	60	168	84
White cake flour	1 cup	496	107	1	128	53	70	60	169	84

FOOD	AMOUNT	CAL	CARBS	FAT	WALK	RUN	BIKE	SWIM	YOGA	DANCE
Pasta										
Fresh pasta, cooked	2 oz	75	14	1	19	8	11	9	25	13
Fresh spinach pasta, cooked	2 oz	74	14	1	19	8	11	9	25	13
Homemade egg pasta, cooked	2 oz	74	13	1	19	8	11	9	25	13
Homemade pasta, cooked	2 oz	71	14	1	18	8	10	9	24	12
Macaroni, cooked	1 cup	221	43	1	57	24	31	27	75	38
Pasta shells, cooked	1 cup	182	35	1	47	19	26	22	62	31
Pasta spirals, cooked	1 cup	212	41	1	55	23	30	26	72	36
Vegetable pasta, cooked	1 cup	172	36	0	44	18	24	21	59	29
Whole wheat macaroni, cooked	1 cup	174	37	1	45	18	25	21	59	30
Spaghetti, cooked	1 cup	220	43	1	57	23	31	27	75	37
Whole wheat spaghetti, cooked	1 cup	174	37	1	45	18	25	21	59	30
Tortellini with cheese filling	.75 cup	249	38	6	64	26	35	30	85	42
Noodles										
Chinese chow mein noodles	1 cup	237	26	14	61	25	34	29	81	40
Egg noodles, cooked	1 cup	221	40	3	57	24	31	27	75	38
Egg spinach noodles, cooked	1 cup	211	39	3	54	22	30	26	72	36
Rice noodles, cooked	1 cup	192	44	0	49	20	27	23	65	33
Japanese soba noodles, cooked	1 cup	113	24	0	29	12	16	14	38	19
Japanese somen noodles, cooked	1 cup	231	48	0	59	25	33	28	78	39

Candies and Chocolate

Candies										
■ **Miscellaneous**										
Brach's Bridge Mix	16 pieces	190	26	8	49	20	27	23	65	32
Brach's California Raisins	35 pieces	170	28	6	44	18	24	21	58	29
Brach's Cinnamon Imperials	52 pieces	60	15	0	15	6	9	7	20	10
Brach's Lemon Drops	4 pieces	70	17	0	18	7	10	9	24	12
Brach's Maple Nut Goodies	7 pieces	200	30	8	52	21	28	24	68	34
Brach's Peanut Clusters	3 pieces	210	21	13	54	22	30	26	71	36
Charleston Chews	13 pieces	180	32	5	46	19	26	22	61	31
Crème Savers Chocolate and Caramel Crème Hard Candy	3 candies	60	0	2	15	6	9	7	20	10
Crème Savers Soft Candy	7 candies	170	34	4	44	18	24	21	58	29

FOOD	AMOUNT	CAL	CARBS	FAT	WALK	RUN	BIKE	SWIM	YOGA	DANCE
Dots	12 dots	140	35	0	36	15	20	17	48	24
Glo-Worms	13 worms	130	32	0	34	14	18	16	44	22
Gobstopper	9 pieces	50	14	0	13	5	7	6	17	9
Goobers	.25 cup	210	22	14	54	22	30	26	71	36
Good & Plenty	1 box (50 g)	170	43	0	44	18	24	21	58	29
Good & Plenty	33 pieces	130	33	0	34	14	18	16	44	22
Gummy Worms	5 worms	160	37	0	41	17	23	19	54	27
Hot Tamales	20 pieces	150	36	0	39	16	21	18	51	26
Jelly Belly Original Jelly Beans	1 package (45 g)	160	42	0	41	17	23	19	54	27
Jelly Belly Sour Jelly Beans	1 package (45 g)	160	41	0	41	17	23	19	54	27
Farley's Chocolate Double Dipped Peanuts	15 pieces	200	25	11	52	21	28	24	68	34
Jordan Almonds	11 almonds (1.5 oz)	190	35	5	49	20	27	23	65	32
Jujubes	55 pieces	110	28	0	28	12	16	13	37	19
JujyFruits	16 pieces	120	32	0	31	13	17	15	41	20
Halavah	1 oz	131	17	6	34	14	19	16	45	22
Gumdrops	1 cup	721	180	0	186	77	102	88	245	123
Gumdrops with Sorbitol	1 cup	295	160	0	76	31	42	36	100	50
Hard candies	5 candies	118	29	0	30	13	17	14	40	20
Jellybeans	10 small	41	10	0	11	4	6	5	14	7
Marshmallows	10 marsh-mallows	229	59	0	59	24	32	28	78	39
Mini marshmallows	1 cup	159	41	0	41	17	23	19	54	27
Sesame crunch candy	20 pieces	181	18	12	47	19	26	22	62	31
Chocolate hazelnut spread	2 tbsp	200	23	11	52	21	28	24	68	34
Mike and Ike	23 pieces	150	36	0	39	16	21	18	51	26
Milk chocolate-coated peanuts	.5 cup	387	37	25	100	41	55	47	132	66
Milk chocolate-coated raisins	.5 cup	351	61	13	90	37	50	43	119	60
Milk chocolate-coated coffee beans	1 oz	144	17	7	37	15	20	18	49	25
Farley's Gummy Bears	18 pieces	110	27	0	28	12	16	13	37	19
Lifesavers Gummies	1 package (42 g)	140	33	0	36	15	20	17	48	24

FOOD	AMOUNT	CAL	CARBS	FAT	WALK	RUN	BIKE	SWIM	YOGA	DANCE
Lifesavers Gummies	10 pieces	130	30	0	34	14	18	16	44	22
Jolly Rancher Gummies	10 pieces	120	29	0	31	13	17	15	41	20
Laffy Taffy	1 bar	160	34	4	41	17	23	19	54	27
Nerds	1 tbsp	60	14	0	15	6	9	7	20	10
Now and Later	1 package (71 g)	210	50	2	54	22	30	26	71	36
Riesen	4 pieces	170	28	6	44	18	24	21	58	29
Runts	13 pieces	60	14	1	15	6	9	7	20	10
Sathers Candy Corn	23 pieces	150	36	0	39	16	21	18	51	26
Sathers Circus Peanuts	5 pieces	150	37	0	39	16	21	18	51	26
Sathers Spearmint Leaves	3 pieces	130	34	0	34	14	18	16	44	22
Sathers Spice Drops	10 pieces	120	32	0	31	13	17	15	41	20
Farley's Spice Drops	10 pieces	120	32	0	31	13	17	15	41	20
Sathers Vanilla Caramels	6 pieces	160	32	3	41	17	23	19	54	27
Skittles	.25 cup (1.5 oz)	170	39	2	44	18	24	21	58	29
Sour Skittles	.25 cup (1.5 oz)	160	36	2	41	17	23	19	54	27
Sour Patch	16 pieces	140	36	0	36	15	20	17	48	24
Starburst Original Chews	8 pieces	160	33	4	41	17	23	19	54	27
Starburst Sour Fruit Chews	1 pack (2.07 oz)	240	47	5	62	26	34	29	82	41
Sugar Babies	30 pieces	180	41	2	46	19	26	22	61	31
Swedish Fish	19 pieces	160	39	0	41	17	23	19	54	27
Tootsie Roll	1 serving, 6 pieces	155	35	1	40	16	22	19	53	26
Tootsie Roll Bar	1 bar	220	46	5	57	23	31	27	75	37
Werther's Original	3 pieces	60	13	1	15	6	9	7	20	10
Butterscotch candies	3 pieces	63	14	0	16	7	9	8	21	11
Caramel candy	5 caramels	193	39	4	50	21	27	23	66	33
Carob bar	1 bar (3 oz)	470	49	27	121	50	67	57	160	80
Nestlé Bit-O-Honey Chews	6 pieces	160	32	3	41	17	23	19	54	27
■ **Homemade Candy**										
Homemade fondant	1 oz	105	26	0	27	11	15	13	36	18
Homemade fudge	1 oz	115	21	3	30	12	16	14	39	20
Homemade fudge with nuts	1 oz	129	19	5	33	14	18	16	44	22

FOOD	AMOUNT	CAL	CARBS	FAT	WALK	RUN	BIKE	SWIM	YOGA	DANCE
Homemade vanilla fudge	1 oz	108	23	2	28	12	15	13	37	18
Homemade vanilla fudge with nuts	1 oz	122	21	4	31	13	17	15	41	21
Homemade chocolate marshmallow fudge	1 oz	132	19	6	34	14	19	16	45	22
■ **Lollipops**										
Lollipops	1 pop	40	10	0	10	4	6	5	14	7
Blow Pop	1 pop	50	14	0	13	5	7	6	17	9
Dum Dum Pops	2 pops	51	13	0	13	5	7	6	17	9
Tootsie Roll Pops	1 pop	60	15	0	15	6	9	7	20	10
■ **Twizzlers**										
Strawberry Twists	3 pieces	130	30	1	34	14	18	16	44	22
Licorice Twists	4 pieces	120	28	1	31	13	17	15	41	20
Cherry Twists	4 pieces	160	36	1	41	17	23	19	54	27
Chocolate Twists	4 pieces	160	35	2	41	17	23	19	54	27
Cherry Bites	17 pieces	140	32	1	36	15	20	17	48	24
Licorice Bites	18 pieces	130	31	1	34	14	18	16	44	22
Nibs Cherry Bits	1 package (64 g)	220	50	2	57	23	31	27	75	37
Nibs Licorice Bits	1 package (63 g)	210	48	2	54	22	30	26	71	36
Twerpz	1 package (51 g)	190	41	3	49	20	27	23	65	32
Cherry Pull 'n Peel	1 package (62 g)	210	47	1	54	22	30	26	71	36
Twizted Berry Pull 'n Peel	1 package (56 g)	190	43	1	49	20	27	23	65	32
Twizted Paradise Punch Pull 'n Peel	2 pieces	170	40	0	44	18	24	21	58	29
Sourz	33 pieces	140	32	1	36	15	20	17	48	24
■ **Nips**										
Coffee Nips	2 pieces	60	11	2	15	6	9	7	20	10
Dulce de Leche Nips	2 pieces	60	11	2	15	6	9	7	20	10
Chocolate Parfait Nips	2 pieces	60	11	2	15	6	9	7	20	10
Caramel Nips	2 pieces	60	11	2	15	6	9	7	20	10
■ **Mints**										
Breathsavers	1 mint	5	2	0	1	1	1	1	2	1
Ice Breakers Mints	1 mint	0	0	0	0	0	0	0	0	0

FOOD	AMOUNT	CAL	CARBS	FAT	WALK	RUN	BIKE	SWIM	YOGA	DANCE
Ice Breakers Liquid Mints	1 mint	0	0	0	0	0	0	0	0	0
Haviland Thin Mints	6 pieces	160	33	5	41	17	23	19	54	27
Wint o Green Lifesavers	4 mints	60	16	0	15	6	9	7	20	10
Altoids Mints	3 mints	10	2	0	3	1	1	1	3	2
Nestlé After 8 Mints	5 pieces	147	31	6	38	16	21	18	50	25
Junior Mints	16 pieces	170	35	3	44	18	24	21	58	29
■ **Gum**										
Chewing gum	1 stick	7	2	0	2	1	1	1	3	1
Sugarless chewing gum	1 piece	5	2	0	1	1	1	1	2	1
Bubble Bubble Bubble Gum	1 piece	20	5	0	5	2	3	2	7	3
Bubble Yum	1 piece	25	6	0	6	3	4	3	9	4
Sugarless Bubble Yum	1 piece	10	3	0	3	1	1	1	3	2
Ice Breakers Chewing Gum	1 piece	5	2	0	1	1	1	1	2	1
Ice Breakers Gum and Mint Dual Packs	1 mint	0	0	0	0	0	0	0	0	0
■ **Nougat**										
Almond nougat candy	1 piece	56	13	0	14	6	8	7	19	9
Zero	1 bar (52 g)	240	36	9	62	26	34	29	82	41
■ **Nut**										
Zagnut	1 bar (49 g)	230	31	10	59	24	33	28	78	39
Mauna Loa Nut Kona Coffee Bar	7 pieces	210	21	13	54	22	30	26	71	36
Homemade Peanut Brittle	1 oz	136	20	5	35	14	19	17	46	23
Sophie Mae Peanut Brittle	.5 cup	150	26	5	39	16	21	18	51	26
■ **Payday**										
Payday	1 bar (52 g)	250	28	13	64	27	35	30	85	43
King-Size Payday	1 bar (96 g)	480	52	24	124	51	68	58	163	82
Honey Roasted Payday	1 bar (51 g)	240	30	11	62	26	34	29	82	41
Payday Avalanche	1 bar (51 g)	250	29	13	64	27	35	30	85	43
Snack Size Payday	1 bar (19 g)	90	10	5	23	10	13	11	31	15
Payday Pro	1 bar (52 g)	240	19	12	62	26	34	29	82	41

FOOD	AMOUNT	CAL	CARBS	FAT	WALK	RUN	BIKE	SWIM	YOGA	DANCE
■ Reese's										
Peanut Butter Cups	1 package (42 g)	230	23	13	59	24	33	28	78	39
White Chocolate Peanut Butter Cups	1 package (42 g)	230	22	13	59	24	33	28	78	39
Caramel Peanut Butter Cups	1 package (39 g)	190	24	10	49	20	27	23	65	32
Double Chocolate Peanut Butter Cups	1 package (39 g)	210	23	11	54	22	30	26	71	36
Extra Smooth and Creamy Chocolate Peanut Butter Cups	1 package (42 g)	220	22	13	57	23	31	27	75	37
Fudge Peanut Butter Cups	1 package (42 g)	230	22	13	59	24	33	28	78	39
Peanut Butter Lovers Peanut Butter Cups	1 package (42 g)	210	21	14	54	22	30	26	71	36
Chocolate Lovers Peanut Butter Cups	1 package (42 g)	220	24	12	57	23	31	27	75	37
Big Cup Peanut Butter Cup	1 piece (42 g)	230	23	13	59	24	33	28	78	39
White Chocolate Big Cup Peanut Butter Cup	1 piece (42 g)	230	22	13	59	24	33	28	78	39
Reese's Pieces	1 package (43 g)	220	26	11	57	23	31	27	75	37
Reese's Pieces with Peanuts	1 package (45 g)	230	24	12	59	24	33	28	78	39
Fast Break Candy Bar	1 bar (56 g)	270	34	13	70	29	38	33	92	46
Reesesticks Wafer Bars	1 package (42 g)	230	23	13	59	24	33	28	78	39
■ Jolly Rancher										
Fruit Chews	6 chews	150	33	2	39	16	21	18	51	26
Gummies	10 gummies	120	29	0	31	13	17	15	41	20
Hard Candy	3 candies	70	17	0	18	7	10	9	24	12
Sugar Free Hard Candy	4 candies	35	13	0	9	4	5	4	12	6
Rocks	1 container (31 g)	120	30	0	31	13	17	15	41	20
Stix	1 package (18 g)	70	17	0	18	7	10	9	24	12
Paletas Surtido Tropical	1 candy	60	16	0	15	6	9	7	20	10

FOOD	AMOUNT	CAL	CARBS	FAT	WALK	RUN	BIKE	SWIM	YOGA	DANCE
Chocolate										
■ Almond Joy										
Almond Joy	1 package (45 g)	220	27	12	57	23	31	27	75	37
Almond Joy (snack size)	1 snack size bar	91	11	5	23	10	13	11	31	16
Almond Joy Piña Colada	1 bar (45 g)	230	25	13	59	24	33	28	78	39
Almond Joy Chocolate Chocolate	1 bar (45 g)	230	25	13	59	24	33	28	78	39
Almond Joy Key Lime	1 bar (45 g)	230	25	13	59	24	33	28	78	39
Almond Joy Passion Fruit	1 bar (45 g)	230	26	13	59	24	33	28	78	39
■ Hershey's Bites										
Almond Joy	18 pieces	218	23	14	56	23	31	27	74	37
Reese's Peanut Butter	16 pieces	220	23	12	57	23	31	27	75	37
Heath Toffee	15 pieces	210	25	12	54	22	30	26	71	36
Kit Kat Wafers	15 pieces	200	25	10	52	21	28	24	68	34
Mini Rolo	19 pieces	190	26	9	49	20	27	23	65	32
Mr. GoodBar	25 pieces	230	21	14	59	24	33	28	78	39
York Peppermint Pattie	15 pieces	150	33	3	39	16	21	18	51	26
White Chocolate Pretzels	23 pieces	200	25	9	52	21	28	24	68	34
■ Pop'ables										
Pop'ables Snickers	13 pieces	190	24	9	49	20	27	23	65	32
Pop'ables Milky Way	13 pieces	180	28	7	46	19	26	22	61	31
■ Hershey's Kisses										
Milk Chocolate	9 kisses	230	24	13	59	24	33	28	78	39
Dulce de Leche	8 kisses	180	24	8	46	19	26	22	61	31
Hugs	9 kisses	210	23	12	54	22	30	26	71	36
Milk Chocolate with Almonds	9 kisses	230	21	14	59	24	33	28	78	39
Dark Chocolate	9 kisses	230	25	13	59	24	33	28	78	39
Cherry Cordial	9 kisses	200	29	8	52	21	28	24	68	34
Peanut Butter Filled	9 kisses	230	21	14	59	24	33	28	78	39
Kissables	1 package (42 g)	210	28	10	54	22	30	26	71	36
■ Milk Duds										
Milk Duds	13 pieces	180	28	7	46	19	26	22	61	31

FOOD	AMOUNT	CAL	CARBS	FAT	WALK	RUN	BIKE	SWIM	YOGA	DANCE
■ **Cadbury Chocolate**										
Milk Chocolate	10 blocks	220	24	12	57	23	31	27	75	37
Fruit and Nut	10 blocks	200	25	10	52	21	28	24	68	34
Royal Dark	10 blocks	220	24	13	57	23	31	27	75	37
Roast Almond	10 blocks	220	21	13	57	23	31	27	75	37
Caramello	6 blocks	200	27	9	52	21	28	24	68	34
Crème Egg	1 egg	170	28	6	44	18	24	21	58	29
Chocolate Egg	1 egg	180	25	8	46	19	26	22	61	31
Caramel Egg	1 egg	190	24	10	49	20	27	23	65	32
Mini Eggs Candies	12 pieces	190	28	8	49	20	27	23	65	32
■ **Chocolate Bars**										
5th Avenue Bar	1 bar (56 g)	280	35	14	72	30	40	34	95	48
Heath Toffee	1 package (39 g)	220	24	13	57	23	31	27	75	37
Hershey's Milk Chocolate	1 bar (43 g)	230	25	13	59	24	33	28	78	39
Hershey's Milk Chocolate with Almonds	1 bar (41 g)	230	22	14	59	24	33	28	78	39
Hershey's Cookies 'n' Crème	1 bar (43 g)	230	26	12	59	24	33	28	78	39
Hershey's Special Dark	1 bar (41 g)	220	25	12	57	23	31	27	75	37
Hershey's Fudge Crème	1 bar (36 g)	200	21	11	52	21	28	24	68	34
Hershey's Mocha Almond	1 bar (39 g)	220	20	14	57	23	31	27	75	37
Hershey's Extra Creamy Chocolate	1 bar (36 g)	180	22	9	46	19	26	22	61	31
Hershey's 'n' More Caramel	1 bar (25 g)	110	15	5	28	12	16	13	37	19
Hershey's 'n' More Creamy Fudge	1 bar (25 g)	120	16	6	31	13	17	15	41	20
Hershey's 'n' More Marshmallow	1 bar (25 g)	110	15	5	28	12	16	13	37	19
Hershey's Pure Dark Chocolate	3 blocks	210	20	13	54	22	30	26	71	36
Hershey's Cranberries, Blueberries and Almonds Extra Dark Chocolate	3 blocks	200	20	12	52	21	28	24	68	34

FOOD	AMOUNT	CAL	CARBS	FAT	WALK	RUN	BIKE	SWIM	YOGA	DANCE
Hershey's Cranberry Macadamia Extra Dark Chocolate	3 blocks	210	20	13	54	22	30	26	71	36
Krackel	1 bar (41 g)	210	28	10	54	22	30	26	71	36
Mounds	1 package (49 g)	240	29	13	62	26	34	29	82	41
Mr. Goodbar	1 package (49 g)	270	27	16	70	29	38	33	92	46
Rolo	1 package (48 g)	210	31	9	54	22	30	26	71	36
Hershey's S'mores Bar	1 bar (46 g)	230	31	11	59	24	33	28	78	39
Skør	1 bar (39 g)	210	24	12	54	22	30	26	71	36
Symphony	1 bar (42 g)	230	24	13	59	24	33	28	78	39
Symphony with Almonds and Toffee	1 bar (42 g)	230	23	14	59	24	33	28	78	39
Take 5	1 package (42 g)	210	26	10	54	22	30	26	71	36
White Chocolate Take 5	1 package (42 g)	200	25	10	52	21	28	24	68	34
Peanut Butter Take 5	1 package (42 g)	220	23	11	57	23	31	27	75	37
Whatchamacallit	1 package (45 g)	220	28	11	57	23	31	27	75	37
100 Grand	1 package (43 g)	180	29	8	46	19	26	22	61	31
Nestlé Crunch	1 bar	220	30	11	57	23	31	27	75	37
Three Musketeers	1 bar	200	35	6	52	21	28	24	68	34
Toblerone	1 bar	260	31	15	67	28	37	32	88	44
Baby Ruth	1 bar (1 oz)	130	17	7	34	14	18	16	44	22
Chunky	1 bar (1.4 oz)	198	23	12	51	21	28	24	67	34
Mars Almond	1 bar (1.76 oz)	234	31	12	60	25	33	28	79	40
Oh! Henry	1 bar	120	17	6	31	13	17	15	41	20
Sweet Escapes Triple Chocolate Wafer Bars	1 bar	82	14	3	21	9	12	10	28	14

FOOD	AMOUNT	CAL	CARBS	FAT	WALK	RUN	BIKE	SWIM	YOGA	DANCE
■ Whoppers										
Whoppers	1 pouch (21 g)	100	16	4	26	11	14	12	34	17
Mini Robin Eggs	24 pieces	170	31	5	44	18	24	21	58	29
■ York Peppermint Patties										
Peppermint Patties	1 pattie	160	32	3	41	17	23	19	54	27
Mini Peppermint Patties	3 patties	160	33	3	41	17	23	19	54	27
Chocolate Truffle Mint Patties	1 pattie	170	29	6	44	18	24	21	58	29
Pink Pattie	1 pattie	150	31	3	39	16	21	18	51	26
■ Hershey's Swoops										
Milk Chocolate	1 cup	190	20	11	49	20	27	23	65	32
Almond Joy	1 cup	200	21	12	52	21	28	24	68	34
Reese's Peanut Butter	1 cup	190	17	11	49	20	27	23	65	32
York Peppermint Pattie	1 cup	190	21	11	49	20	27	23	65	32
White Chocolate Peppermint	1 cup	190	21	10	49	20	27	23	65	32
White Chocolate Reese's	1 cup	190	20	11	49	20	27	23	65	32
Toffee and Almond	1 cup	190	20	11	49	20	27	23	65	32
Special Dark with Almonds	1 cup	190	19	12	49	20	27	23	65	32
Strawberries 'n' Crème	1 cup	190	21	10	49	20	27	23	65	32
■ Hershey's Miniatures and Nuggets										
Hershey's Assorted Miniatures	5 pieces	230	26	13	59	24	33	28	78	39
Hershey's Assorted Nut Lovers Miniatures	5 pieces	230	24	13	59	24	33	28	78	39
Hershey's Milk Chocolate Nuggets	4 pieces	230	24	13	59	24	33	28	78	39
Hershey's Extra Creamy Milk Chocolate with Raisins and Almonds Nuggets	4 pieces	200	23	11	52	21	28	24	68	34
Hershey's Extra Creamy Milk Chocolate with Toffee and Almonds Nuggets	4 pieces	210	21	13	54	22	30	26	71	36
Hershey's Milk Chocolate with Almonds Nuggets	4 pieces	210	20	13	54	22	30	26	71	36
Hershey's Special Dark with Almonds Nuggets	4 pieces	220	20	14	57	23	31	27	75	37
Hershey's Cookies 'n' Mint Nuggets	4 pieces	200	22	11	52	21	28	24	68	34
Hershey's Dark Chocolate Raspberry Nuggets	4 pieces	220	24	13	57	23	31	27	75	37

FOOD	AMOUNT	CAL	CARBS	FAT	WALK	RUN	BIKE	SWIM	YOGA	DANCE
Hershey's Strawberries and Cookies Nuggets	4 pieces	200	22	11	52	21	28	24	68	34
Hershey's Extra Creamy Milk Chocolate with Macadamia Nuts Nuggets	4 pieces	220	20	14	57	23	31	27	75	37
Hershey's Extra Creamy Milk Chocolate with Toasted Coconut and Macadamia Nuts Nuggets	4 pieces	220	21	14	57	23	31	27	75	37
■ **Dove**										
Dove Smooth Milk Chocolate with Caramel	5 pieces	200	24	11	52	21	28	24	68	34
Dove Rich Dark Chocolate	5 pieces	210	24	13	54	22	30	26	71	36
Dove Smooth Milk Chocolate	5 pieces	220	24	13	57	23	31	27	75	37
■ **Kit Kat**										
Milk Chocolate	1 4-piece bar	220	27	11	57	23	31	27	75	37
White Chocolate	1 4-piece bar	220	26	12	57	23	31	27	75	37
Coffee	1 4-piece bar	220	27	11	57	23	31	27	75	37
Milkshake	1 4-piece bar	220	26	12	57	23	31	27	75	37
Orange Creme	1 4-piece bar	220	26	12	57	23	31	27	75	37
■ **M&M'S**										
M&M's	.25 cup (1.5 oz)	210	30	9	54	22	30	26	71	36
Peanut M&M's	.25 cup (1.5 oz)	220	26	11	57	23	31	27	75	37
Almond M&M's	1.31 oz	200	21	11	52	21	28	24	68	34
Peanut Butter M&M's	1.63 oz	240	26	14	62	26	34	29	82	41
Crispy M&M's	1.65 oz	200	31	8	52	21	28	24	68	34
M&M's Minis	1.08 oz	150	21	7	39	16	21	18	51	26
■ **Snickers**										
Snickers	1 bar (2.07 oz)	280	35	14	72	30	40	34	95	48
Snickers, King Size	1 bar	510	63	24	131	54	72	62	173	87
Snickers Crunchier	1 bar (1.56 oz)	230	25	13	59	24	33	28	78	39
Snickers Almond	1 bar (1.76 oz)	240	32	11	62	26	34	29	82	41

FOOD	AMOUNT	CAL	CARBS	FAT	WALK	RUN	BIKE	SWIM	YOGA	DANCE
Snickers Almond, King Size	1 bar	460	58	22	119	49	65	56	156	78
Snickers Minis Mix	4 pieces	170	23	9	44	18	24	21	58	29
■ **Milky Way**										
Milky Way	1 bar (2.05 oz)	260	41	10	67	28	37	32	88	44
Milky Way, King Size	1 bar	450	72	18	116	48	64	55	153	77
Milky Way Midnight	1 bar (1.76 oz)	220	36	8	57	23	31	27	75	37
Milky Way Chocolate Covered Caramels	5 pieces	200	30	8	52	21	28	24	68	34
■ **Twix**										
Twix	2 cookies	280	37	14	72	30	40	34	95	48
Peanut Butter Twix	2 cookies	280	28	17	72	30	40	34	95	48
■ **Butterfinger**										
Butterfinger	1 bar	270	43	11	70	29	38	33	92	46
Butterfinge, King Size	1 bar	480	78	18	124	51	68	58	163	82
Butterfinger Crisp	1 bar	250	33	13	64	27	35	30	85	43
Butterfinger Fun Size	1 bar	100	15	4	26	11	14	12	34	17
■ **Hershey's Cookies**										
Almond Joy Cookies	2 cookies	150	17	9	39	16	21	18	51	26
Hershey's with Almonds Cookies	2 cookies	150	16	9	39	16	21	18	51	26
Hershey's Cookies 'n' Creme Cookies	1 package (56 g)	300	33	17	77	32	43	36	102	51
Hershey's Caramel Cookies	1 package (56 g)	270	12	38	70	29	38	33	92	46
Hershey's Miniature Chocolate Cookie Mix	6 pieces	220	25	12	57	23	31	27	75	37
Mauna Loa Chocolate Chip Cookies	4 cookies	150	16	9	39	16	21	18	51	26
Mauna Loa White Chocolate Chip Cookies	4 cookies	150	16	9	39	16	21	18	51	26
Mauna Loa Toffee Crunch Cookies	4 cookies	150	16	9	39	16	21	18	51	26
Reese's Cookies	2 cookies	150	17	8	39	16	21	18	51	26
York Peppermint Pattie Cookies	2 cookies	160	17	9	41	17	23	19	54	27
■ **Low-Carb Chocolate**										
Hershey's 1 Gram Sugar Chocolate Carb Bar	1 bar (31 g)	130	18	11	34	14	18	16	44	22

FOOD	AMOUNT	CAL	CARBS	FAT	WALK	RUN	BIKE	SWIM	YOGA	DANCE
Hershey's 1 Gram Sugar Chocolate with Soy Crisps Carb Bar	1 bar (31 g)	120	16	10	31	13	17	15	41	20
Hershey's 1 Gram Sugar Chocolate with Almonds Carb Bar	1 bar (31 g)	140	16	12	36	15	20	17	48	24
Hershey's 1 Gram Sugar Dark Chocolatey Carb Bar	1 bar (31 g)	140	17	12	36	15	20	17	48	24
Reese's 1 Gram Sugar Carb Peanut Butter Cups	1 bar (34 g)	160	17	12	41	17	23	19	54	27
Russell Stover Net Carb Peanut Butter Cups	4 pieces	180	18	14	46	19	26	22	61	31
Russell Stover Net Carb Toffee Squares	3 pieces	170	22	11	44	18	24	21	58	29
Russell Stover Net Carb Truffle Cups	4 pieces	170	23	11	44	18	24	21	58	29
Sugar Free										
Hershey's Sugar Free Chocolate Candy	5 pieces	170	25	13	44	18	24	21	58	29
Hershey's Sugar Free Chocolate with Almonds Candy	5 pieces	180	23	14	46	19	26	22	61	31
Hershey's Sugar Free Dark Chocolate Candy	5 pieces	190	23	15	49	20	27	23	65	32
Russell Stover Sugar Free Toffee Squares	3 pieces	160	21	11	41	17	23	19	54	27
Russell Stover Sugar Free Peanut Butter Cups	4 pieces	180	17	13	46	19	26	22	61	31
Sugar Free Jolly Ranchers	4 pieces	35	13	0	9	4	5	4	12	6
Sugar Free Reese's Peanut Butter Cups	5 pieces	170	24	12	44	18	24	21	58	29
Sugar Free York Peppermint Patties	3 pieces	110	28	5	28	12	16	13	37	19
Sugar Free Twizzlers	6 pieces	130	33	1	34	14	18	16	44	22
Sugar Free White Reese's	5 pieces	180	21	13	46	19	26	22	61	31
Sugar Free Nestlé Turtles	3 pieces	160	19	11	41	17	23	19	54	27
Sugar Free Go Lightly Crème Doublers	7 pieces	150	33	6	39	16	21	18	51	26
Sugar Free Go Lightly Vanilla Caramels	5 pieces	150	31	6	39	16	21	18	51	26
Sugar Free Go Lightly Fruit Chews	7 pieces	120	34	3	31	13	17	15	41	20
Sugar Free Lifesavers	4 candies	30	14	0	8	3	4	4	10	5

FOOD	AMOUNT	CAL	CARBS	FAT	WALK	RUN	BIKE	SWIM	YOGA	DANCE
Sugar Free Nestlé Crunch	1 bar	140	18	11	36	15	20	17	48	24
Boxed Chocolates										
Ferroro Rocher Fine Hazelnut Chocolate	3 pieces	220	17	15	57	23	31	27	75	37
Ghiradelli Milk Chocolate with Caramelized Almond Squares	4 squares	220	24	14	57	23	31	27	75	37
Ghiradelli Milk Chocolate Squares with Caramel Filling	3 squares	220	27	12	57	23	31	27	75	37
Guylian Original Praline	4 pieces	195	17	13	50	21	28	24	66	33
Hershey's Pot of Gold Nut Assortment	1.5 oz	240	21	16	62	26	34	29	82	41
Hershey's Pot of Gold Almond Caramel Clusters	3 pieces	240	24	14	62	26	34	29	82	41
Hershey's Pot of Gold Caramel Assortment	1.5 oz	200	27	9	52	21	28	24	68	34
Hershey's Pot of Gold Chocolate Assortment	1 box (30 g)	130	21	5	34	14	18	16	44	22
Hershey's Pot of Gold Creme Assortment	1.5 oz	170	32	4	44	18	24	21	58	29
Hershey's Pot of Gold Mint Assortment	1.5 oz	200	26	10	52	21	28	24	68	34
Hershey's Pot of Gold Pecan Caramel Clusters	3 pieces	250	24	16	64	27	35	30	85	43
Hershey's Pot of Gold Premium Assortment	1.5 oz	220	26	11	57	23	31	27	75	37
Hershey's Pot of Gold Sugar Free Assortment	1.5 oz	180	22	16	46	19	26	22	61	31
Hershey's Pot of Gold Truffle Assortment	1.5 oz	200	27	9	52	21	28	24	68	34
Lindt Milk Chocolate Truffles	3 balls	220	16	17	57	23	31	27	75	37
Lindt Dark Chocolate Truffles	3 balls	220	15	18	57	23	31	27	75	37
Lindt White Chocolate Truffles	3 balls	230	14	19	59	24	33	28	78	39
Mauna Loa Mountains	4 pieces	230	18	16	59	24	33	28	78	39
Nestlé Turtles	4 pieces	210	25	12	54	22	30	26	71	36
Whitman's Milk Chocolate Sampler	3 pieces	180	22	9	46	19	26	22	61	31
Whitman's Sugar Free Chocolate Sampler	3 pieces	150	22	11	39	16	21	18	51	26
Baking Chocolate										
Unsweetened baking chocolate	1 square	145	9	15	37	15	21	18	49	25

FOOD	AMOUNT	CAL	CARBS	FAT	WALK	RUN	BIKE	SWIM	YOGA	DANCE
Semi-sweet chocolate chips	1 cup	805	106	50	207	86	114	98	274	137
Milk chocolate chips	1 cup	899	100	50	232	96	127	109	306	153
Mexican baking chocolate	1 tablet	85	15	3	22	9	12	10	29	15
Hershey's Bake Shoppe Unsweetened Chocolate	.5 bar (14 g)	90	4	7	23	10	13	11	31	15
Hershey's Bake Shoppe Semi-Sweet Chocolate	.5 bar (14 g)	70	9	4	18	7	10	9	24	12
Hershey's Bake Shoppe Semi-Sweet Chocolate Chips	1 tbsp	80	10	5	21	9	11	10	27	14
Hershey's Bake Shoppe Butterscotch Chips	1 tbsp	80	10	4	21	9	11	10	27	14
Hershey's Bake Shoppe Cinnamon Chips	1 tbsp	80	9	4	21	9	11	10	27	14
Hershey's Bake Shoppe Milk Chocolate Chips	1 tbsp	80	9	5	21	9	11	10	27	14
Hershey's Bake Shoppe Mini Chips Semi-Sweet Chocolates	1 tbsp	80	9	5	21	9	11	10	27	14
Hershey's Bake Shoppe Mini Milk Chocolate Kisses	11 pieces	80	9	5	21	9	11	10	27	14
Hershey's Bake Shoppe Mini Mint Chocolate Kisses	1 tbsp	80	10	4	21	9	11	10	27	14
Hershey's Bake Shoppe Premier White Chips	1 tbsp	80	9	4	21	9	11	10	27	14
Hershey's Bake Shoppe Raspberry Chips	1 tbsp	80	10	4	21	9	11	10	27	14
Hershey's Bake Shoppe Special Dark Chocolate Chips	1 tbsp	80	9	5	21	9	11	10	27	14
Hershey's Bake Shoppe Unwrapped Kisses	9 pieces	230	24	13	59	24	33	28	78	39
Hershey's Milk Chocolate Filled with Caramel Baking Pieces	1 tbsp	70	10	4	18	7	10	9	24	12
Hershey's Dark Chocolate Filled with Raspberry Creme Baking Pieces	1 tbsp	80	10	5	21	9	11	10	27	14
Hershey's Special Dark Chips with Macadamia Nuts	1 tbsp	90	7	7	23	10	13	11	31	15
Hershey's White Chips with Macadamia Nuts	1 tbsp	90	7	6	23	10	13	11	31	15
Hershey's Sugar Free Baking Chunks	1 tbsp	70	9	5	18	7	10	9	24	12
M&M's Chocolate Mini Baking Bits	1 tbsp	70	10	4	18	7	10	9	24	12

FOOD	AMOUNT	CAL	CARBS	FAT	WALK	RUN	BIKE	SWIM	YOGA	DANCE
M&M's Semi-Sweet Chocolate Mini Baking Bits	1 tbsp	70	9	4	18	7	10	9	24	12
Reese's Milk Chocolate Filled with Peanut Butter Creme Baking Pieces	1 tbsp	80	9	5	21	9	11	10	27	14
Reese's Peanut Butter Chips	1 tbsp	80	8	4	21	9	11	10	27	14

Snack Food

Beef Jerky										
Beef jerky	1 piece	82	2	5	21	9	12	10	28	14
Jack Link's Jumbo Kippered Beef Teriyaki Steak	2 oz	160	10	2	41	17	23	19	54	27
Slim Jim Twin Pack Spicy Smoked Snack	1 package (55 g)	290	4	26	75	31	41	35	99	49
Slim Jim Beef Jerky	1 package (19 g)	80	2	5	21	9	11	10	27	14
Smoked Beef Sticks	1 stick	110	1	10	28	12	16	13	37	19
Potato Chips										
■ **General**										
Potato chips	1 oz	155	14	11	40	17	22	19	53	26
Barbecue potato chips	1 oz	139	15	9	36	15	20	17	47	24
Reduced-fat potato chips	1 oz	136	0	6	35	14	19	17	46	23
Fat-free potato chips	1 oz	107	24	0	28	11	15	13	36	18
Fat-free potato chips made with Olestra	1 oz	75	17	0	19	8	11	9	26	13
Cheese-flavored potato chips	1 oz	141	16	8	36	15	20	17	48	24
Sour cream and onion potato chips	1 oz	151	15	10	39	16	21	18	51	26
■ **Lay's**										
Classic Lay's	1 oz	150	15	10	39	16	21	18	51	26
Lay's Deli Style Potato Chips	1 oz	150	16	10	39	16	21	18	51	26
Baked Lay's	1 oz	110	23	2	28	12	16	13	37	19
KC Masterpiece BBQ Baked Lay's Potato Chips	1 oz	120	22	3	31	13	17	15	41	20
Sour Cream and Onion Baked Lay's Potato Chips	1 oz	120	21	3	31	13	17	15	41	20
Chile Limon Lay's	1 oz	150	14	10	39	16	21	18	51	26
Pickle Flavored Lay's	1 oz	160	13	10	41	17	23	19	54	27

FOOD	AMOUNT	CAL	CARBS	FAT	WALK	RUN	BIKE	SWIM	YOGA	DANCE
Flamin' Hot Lay's	1 oz	160	15	10	41	17	23	19	54	27
KC Masterpiece BBQ Lay's Potato Chips	1 oz	150	15	10	39	16	21	18	51	26
Kettle Cooked Original Lay's	1 oz	150	18	8	39	16	21	18	51	26
Kettle Cooked Jalapeño Lay's	1 oz	140	16	8	36	15	20	17	48	24
Kettle Cooked Mesquite BBQ Lay's	1 oz	140	16	8	36	15	20	17	48	24
Kettle Cooked Sea Salt and Vinegar Lay's	1 oz	140	17	7	36	15	20	17	48	24
Limon Lay's	1 oz	150	15	10	39	16	21	18	51	26
Salt and Vinegar Lay's	1 oz	150	15	10	39	16	21	18	51	26
Sour Cream and Onion Lay's	1 oz	160	15	10	41	17	23	19	54	27
Lay's Stax	1 oz	160	15	10	41	17	23	19	54	27
Wavy Lay's	1 oz	150	15	10	39	16	21	18	51	26
Au Gratin Wavy Lay's	1 oz	150	14	10	39	16	21	18	51	26
Hickory Barbecue Wavy Lay's	1 oz	150	16	9	39	16	21	18	51	26
Hidden Vally Ranch Wavy Lay's	1 oz	150	16	10	39	16	21	18	51	26
■ Ruffles										
Original Ruffles	1 oz	160	14	10	41	17	23	19	54	27
KC Masterpiece Mesquite Barbecue Ruffles	1 oz	160	15	10	41	17	23	19	54	27
Cheddar and Sour Cream Ruffles	1 oz	160	14	10	41	17	23	19	54	27
Sour Cream and Onion Ruffles	1 oz	160	14	10	41	17	23	19	54	27
Baked Ruffles	1 oz	120	21	3	31	13	17	15	41	20
■ Munchos										
Munchos Potato Chips	1 oz	160	16	10	41	17	23	19	54	27
■ Pringles										
Original	1 oz	160	14	11	41	17	23	19	54	27
Salt and Vinegar	1 oz	150	14	10	39	16	21	18	51	26
Ranch	1 oz	150	14	10	39	16	21	18	51	26
Pizza-licious	1 oz	160	14	11	41	17	23	19	54	27
Sour Cream and Onion	1 oz	150	14	10	39	16	21	18	51	26
Spicy Cajun	1 oz	160	14	11	41	17	23	19	54	27
Reduced Fat Original	1 oz	140	19	7	36	15	20	17	48	24
Reduced Fat Sour Cream and Onion	1 oz	140	18	7	36	15	20	17	48	24
White Cheddar	1 oz	160	15	10	41	17	23	19	54	27

FOOD	AMOUNT	CAL	CARBS	FAT	WALK	RUN	BIKE	SWIM	YOGA	DANCE
Chili Cheese	1 oz	160	15	11	41	17	23	19	54	27
Cheezums	1 oz	150	15	10	39	16	21	18	51	26

Tortilla Chips

■ General

FOOD	AMOUNT	CAL	CARBS	FAT	WALK	RUN	BIKE	SWIM	YOGA	DANCE
White corn tortilla chips	1 oz	138	19	7	36	15	20	17	47	24
Low-fat tortilla chips	1 oz	116	22	2	30	12	16	14	39	20
Nacho-flavored tortilla chips	1 oz	141	18	7	36	15	20	17	48	24
Ranch-flavored tortilla chips	1 oz	142	18	7	37	15	20	17	48	24
Taco-flavored tortilla chips	1 oz	136	18	7	35	14	19	17	46	23
Low-fat baked tortilla chips	1 oz	116	22	2	30	12	16	14	39	20
Reduced-fat nacho-flavored tortilla chips	1 oz	126	20	4	32	13	18	15	43	21
Low-fat nacho cheese tortilla chips made with Olestra	1 oz	91	18	1	23	10	13	11	31	16
Light tortilla chips	1 oz	130	21	4	34	14	18	16	44	22

■ Doritos

FOOD	AMOUNT	CAL	CARBS	FAT	WALK	RUN	BIKE	SWIM	YOGA	DANCE
Baked Cooler Ranch Doritos	1 oz	120	21	4	31	13	17	15	41	20
Baked Nacho Cheese Doritos	1 oz	120	21	4	31	13	17	15	41	20
Black PepperJack Doritos	1 oz	150	18	7	39	16	21	18	51	26
Cool Ranch Doritos	1 oz	140	18	7	36	15	20	17	48	24
Cooler Ranch Doritos	1 oz	140	18	7	36	15	20	17	48	24
Guacamole Flavored Doritos	1 oz	150	16	8	39	16	21	18	51	26
Mini Cooler Ranch Doritos	1 oz	140	18	7	36	15	20	17	48	24
Mini Nacho Cheese Doritos	1 oz	150	17	9	39	16	21	18	51	26
Nacho Cheesier Doritos	1 oz	140	17	7	36	15	20	17	48	24
Ranchero Doritos	1 oz	150	17	8	39	16	21	18	51	26
Cooler Ranch Rollitos	1 oz	140	17	8	36	15	20	17	48	24
Nacho Cheesier Rollitos	1 oz	150	17	8	39	16	21	18	51	26
Zesty Taco Rollitos	1 oz	150	17	8	39	16	21	18	51	26
Salsa Verde Doritos	1 oz	140	19	7	36	15	20	17	48	24
Spicier Nacho Doritos	1 oz	140	18	7	36	15	20	17	48	24
Taco Flavored Doritos	1 oz	140	18	7	36	15	20	17	48	24
Toasted Corn Doritos	1 oz	140	18	7	36	15	20	17	48	24

■ Tostitos

FOOD	AMOUNT	CAL	CARBS	FAT	WALK	RUN	BIKE	SWIM	YOGA	DANCE
Baked Bite-Size Tostitos	1 oz	110	24	1	28	12	16	13	37	19
Bite-Size Tostitos	1 oz	140	17	8	36	15	20	17	48	24

FOOD	AMOUNT	CAL	CARBS	FAT	WALK	RUN	BIKE	SWIM	YOGA	DANCE
Crispy Rounds Tostitos	1 oz	140	18	7	36	15	20	17	48	24
Gold Tostitos	1 oz	140	19	7	36	15	20	17	48	24
Natural Blue Corn Restaurant Style Tostitos	1 oz	140	19	6	36	15	20	17	48	24
Natural Yellow Corn Restaurant Style Tostitos	1 oz	140	19	6	36	15	20	17	48	24
Restaurant Style Tostitos	1 oz	140	19	7	36	15	20	17	48	24
Restaurant Style Hint of Lime Tostitos	1 oz	140	19	6	36	15	20	17	48	24
Santa Fe Yellow Corn Round Tostitos	1 oz	140	20	6	36	15	20	17	48	24
Tostitos Scoops	1 oz	140	18	7	36	15	20	17	48	24
■ Santitas										
White Corn Santitas	1 oz	130	19	6	34	14	18	16	44	22
Yellow Corn Santitas	1 oz	130	19	6	34	14	18	16	44	22
Chips										
■ Chester's										
Chester's Flamin' Hot Fries	1 oz	150	17	8	39	16	21	18	51	26
■ French's										
Potato Sticks	.5 cup	94	10	6	24	10	13	11	32	16
French's Potato Sticks	.75 cup	180	16	12	46	19	26	22	61	31
■ Taro Chips										
Taro Chips	1 oz	141	19	7	36	15	20	17	48	24
■ Plantain Chips										
El Isleno Plantain Chips	1 oz	150	17	9	39	16	21	18	51	26
Top Banana Plantain Chips	1 oz	150	19	8	39	16	21	18	51	26
■ Shrimp Chips										
Maui Shrimp Chips	1 oz	140	19	8	36	15	20	17	48	24
■ Banana Chips										
Banana chips	1 oz	147	17	1	38	16	21	18	50	25
■ Corn Chips										
Corn chips	1 oz	147	18	8	38	16	21	18	50	25
Barbecue corn chips	1 oz	148	16	9	38	16	21	18	50	25
Onion-flavored corn chips	1 oz	142	18	6	37	15	20	17	48	24
Corn cones	1 oz	145	18	8	37	15	21	18	49	25
Nacho-flavored corn cones	1 oz	152	16	9	39	16	22	18	52	26
Corn cheese twists or puffs	1 oz	157	15	10	40	17	22	19	53	27

FOOD	AMOUNT	CAL	CARBS	FAT	WALK	RUN	BIKE	SWIM	YOGA	DANCE
■ **Fritos**										
Fritos	1 oz	160	15	10	41	17	23	19	54	27
Barbecue Fritos	1 oz	150	16	10	39	16	21	18	51	26
Chili Cheese Fritos	1 oz	160	15	10	41	17	23	19	54	27
Flamin Hot Fritos	1 oz	160	15	10	41	17	23	19	54	27
Fritos Cheddar Ranch Flavor Twists	1 oz	150	17	9	39	16	21	18	51	26
Fritos Honey BBQ Flavor Twists	1 oz	160	16	10	41	17	23	19	54	27
Fritos King Size	1 oz	160	16	10	41	17	23	19	54	27
Fritos Scoops	1 oz	160	16	10	41	17	23	19	54	27
■ **Cheetos**										
Cheetos Puffs	1 oz	160	13	10	41	17	23	19	54	27
Cheetos White Cheddar Puffs	1 oz	150	16	9	39	16	21	18	51	26
Crunchy Cheetos	1 oz	160	15	10	41	17	23	19	54	27
Baked Cheetos	1 oz	130	19	5	34	14	18	16	44	22
Baked Flamin' Hot Cheetos	1 package	200	29	8	52	21	28	24	68	34
Asteroids	1 oz	160	15	10	41	17	23	19	54	27
Flamin' Hot Asteroids	1 cup	160	13	11	41	17	23	19	54	27
Flamin' Hot Crunchy Cheetos	1 oz	170	14	11	44	18	24	21	58	29
Flamin' Hot Limon Crunchy Cheetos	1 oz	160	15	11	41	17	23	19	54	27
Twisted Cheetos Puffs	1 oz	160	13	10	41	17	23	19	54	27
■ **Bugles**										
Original Bugles	1.333 cups	160	18	9	41	17	23	19	54	27
Smokin' Barbecue Bugles	1.333 cups	150	18	8	39	16	21	18	51	26
Salsa Bugles	1.333 cups	160	18	9	41	17	23	19	54	27
Chili Cheese Bugles	1.333 cups	160	18	9	41	17	23	19	54	27
Nacho Cheese Bugles	1.333 cups	160	18	9	41	17	23	19	54	27
Southwest Ranch Bugles	1.333 cups	170	18	10	44	18	24	21	58	29
Corn Nuts										
Corn nuts	1 oz	126	20	4	33	13	18	15	43	22

FOOD	AMOUNT	CAL	CARBS	FAT	WALK	RUN	BIKE	SWIM	YOGA	DANCE
Nacho-flavored corn nuts	1 oz	124	20	4	32	13	18	15	42	21
Barbecue-flavored corn nuts	1 oz	124	20	4	32	13	18	15	42	21
Fruit Leather										
Fruit Leather Bars	1 bar	81	18	1	21	9	11	10	27	14
Fruit Leather Pieces	1 packet (.75 oz)	75	17	1	19	8	11	9	26	13
Fruit Leather Rolls	1 large	78	18	1	20	8	11	9	27	13
Fruit Roll-Ups	2 rolls	104	24	1	27	11	15	13	36	18
Farley Fruit Snacks	1 pouch	89	21	0	23	9	13	11	30	15
Sunkist Fruit Roll	1 roll	72	17	0	19	8	10	9	24	12
Stretch Island 100% Fruit Snack	1 bar	45	12	0	12	5	6	5	15	8
Onion Rings										
Funyuns Onion Flavored Rings	1 oz	140	18	7	36	15	20	17	48	24
Funyuns Mini Onion Flavored Rings	1 package	260	30	4	67	28	37	32	88	44
Rice Cake										
Rice cake	1 cake	35	7	0	9	4	5	4	12	6
Plain brown rice cake	1 cake	35	7	0	9	4	5	4	12	6
Sesame brown rice cake	1 cake	35	7	0	9	4	5	4	12	6
Rye brown rice cake	1 cake	35	7	0	9	4	5	4	12	6
Multigrain brown rice cake	1 cake	35	7	0	9	4	5	4	12	6
Corn brown rice cake	1 cake	35	7	0	9	4	5	4	12	6
Buckwheat brown rice cake	1 cake	34	7	0	9	4	5	4	12	6
Hain Mini Munchies Ranch Rice Snacks	9 mini cakes	80	10	4	21	9	11	10	27	14
Hain Mini Munchies Plain Rice Snacks	14 mini cakes	60	13	1	15	6	9	7	20	10
Hain Mini Munchies Peanut Butter Rice Snacks	9 mini cakes	70	12	2	18	7	10	9	24	12
Hain Mini Munchies Honey Nut Rice Snacks	9 mini cakes	60	14	1	15	6	9	7	20	10
Hain Honey Nut Rice Cake	1 cake	50	11	0	13	5	7	6	17	9
Hain Mini Munchies Apple Cinnamon Rice Snacks	9 mini cakes	60	14	1	15	6	9	7	20	10
Lundberg Nutra-Farm Brown Rice Cake	1 cake	70	15	0	18	7	10	9	24	12
Lundberg Nutra-Farm Salt Free Brown Rice Cake	1 cake	70	15	0	18	7	10	9	24	12

FOOD	AMOUNT	CAL	CARBS	FAT	WALK	RUN	BIKE	SWIM	YOGA	DANCE
Lundberg Organic Sesame Tamari Rice Cake	1 cake	70	16	1	18	7	10	9	24	12
Lundberg Organic Tamari Seaweed Rice Cake	1 cake	70	15	0	18	7	10	9	24	12
Weightwise Plain Rice Cake	1 cake	30	5	0	8	3	4	4	10	5
Corn Cakes										
Popcorn cakes	2 cakes	77	16	1	20	8	11	9	26	13
Hain Caramel Popped Corn Cakes	1 cake	50	11	0	13	5	7	6	17	9
Hain Organic White Cheddar Popped Corn Snacks	6 mini cakes	60	11	1	15	6	9	7	20	10
Hain Organic Mild Cheddar Popped Corn Snacks	6 mini cakes	50	10	1	13	5	7	6	17	9
Snack Mix										
Cheez-It Party Mix	.5 cup	120	21	5	31	13	17	15	41	20
Cheez-It Double Cheese Baked Snack Mix	.75 cup	140	20	5	36	15	20	17	48	24
Doo Dads Snack Mix	1 cup	260	37	11	67	28	37	32	88	44
Gardetto's Snack Mix	.5 cup	150	20	6	39	16	21	18	51	26
Oriental Mix	1 oz	143	15	7	37	15	20	17	49	24
Chex Mix										
Traditional Chex Mix	.66 cup	130	22	4	34	14	18	16	44	22
Cheddar Chex Mix	.66 cup	130	22	4	34	14	18	16	44	22
Sweet 'n Salty Chex Mix	.5 cup	140	22	5	36	15	20	17	48	24
Chocolate Peanut Butter Chex Mix	.66 cup	150	23	5	39	16	21	18	51	26
Chocolate Turtle Chex Mix	.66 cup	150	23	5	39	16	21	18	51	26
Munchies										
Munchies Traditional Mix	1 serving	130	19	5	34	14	18	16	44	22
Munchies Classic Mix	1 serving	140	18	7	36	15	20	17	48	24
Munchies Cooler Ranch Mix	1 serving	140	19	8	36	15	20	17	48	24
Munchies Kids Mix	1 serving	130	20	4	34	14	18	16	44	22
Munchies Ultimate Cheddar Mix	1 serving	130	19	5	34	14	18	16	44	22
Popcorn										
Air-popped popcorn	1 cup	31	6	0	8	3	4	4	10	5
Oil-popped popcorn	1 cup	55	6	3	14	6	8	7	19	9
Low-fat oil-popped popcorn	1 cup	45	8	1	12	5	6	5	15	8

FOOD	AMOUNT	CAL	CARBS	FAT	WALK	RUN	BIKE	SWIM	YOGA	DANCE
Microwave oil-popped popcorn	1 cup	60	6	4	15	6	9	7	20	10
Low fat microwave popcorn	1 cup	45	8	1	12	5	6	5	15	8
Sugar-free caramel popcorn	2 oz	213	50	1	55	23	30	26	72	36
Caramel popcorn with peanuts	2 oz	228	46	4	59	24	32	28	78	39
Caramel popcorn	2 oz	244	45	7	63	26	35	30	83	42
Cheese-flavored popcorn	1 cup	58	6	4	15	6	8	7	20	10
■ **SmartFood**										
White Cheddar Cheese Flavored Popcorn	1 single-serving bag	160	14	10	41	17	23	19	54	27
Reduced Fat White Cheddar Cheese Flavored Popcorn	3 cups	140	19	6	36	15	20	17	48	24
■ **Chester's**										
Chester's Butter Flavored Popcorn	3 cups	170	16	12	44	18	24	21	58	29
Chester's Cheddar Flavored Popcorn	3 cups	200	17	3	52	21	28	24	68	34
Chester's Butter Puffcorn	1 oz	160	12	11	41	17	23	19	54	27
Chester's Cheese Flavored Puffcorn	1 oz	160	12	11	41	17	23	19	54	27
■ **Cracker Jack**										
Cracker Jack	.5 cup	120	23	2	31	13	17	15	41	20
Cracker Jack Butter Toffee Clusters	.75 cup	140	22	4	36	15	20	17	48	24
■ **Poppycock**										
Poppycock Original Popcorn and Nut Clusters	.5 cup	160	20	8	41	17	23	19	54	27
Poppycock Pecan Delight	.5 cup	150	20	7	39	16	21	18	51	26
Poppycock Cashew Lovers	.5 cup	140	21	6	36	15	20	17	48	24
■ **Microwave Popcorn—Orville Redenbacher's**										
Smart Pop	1 cup popped	15	4	0	4	2	2	2	5	3
Movie Theater	1 cup popped	35	4	3	9	4	5	4	12	6
Butter	1 cup popped	35	4	2	9	4	5	4	12	6
Kettle Korn	1 cup popped	35	4	3	9	4	5	4	12	6

FOOD	AMOUNT	CAL	CARBS	FAT	WALK	RUN	BIKE	SWIM	YOGA	DANCE
■ **Microwave Popcorn—Act II**										
Light Butter	1 cup popped	25	5	1	6	3	4	3	9	4
Butter Lover's	1 cup popped	35	4	3	9	4	5	4	12	6
Buttery Kettle Korn	1 cup popped	30	3	2	8	3	4	4	10	5
Butter	1 cup popped	30	4	2	8	3	4	4	10	5
Pretzels										
■ **General**										
Hard pretzels	1 oz	108	23	1	28	12	15	13	37	18
Hard whole-wheat pretzels	1 oz	103	23	1	27	11	15	13	35	18
Soft pretzel	1 large	483	99	4	124	51	69	59	164	82
■ **Combos**										
Combos Cheddar Cheese Pretzels	1 oz	130	19	5	34	14	18	16	44	22
Combos Pizzeria Pretzels	1 oz	130	19	5	34	14	18	16	44	22
Combos Nacho Cheese Pretzels	1 oz	130	19	5	34	14	18	16	44	22
■ **Snyder**										
Snyder's Cheddar Pretzels	1 oz	130	18	6	34	14	18	16	44	22
Snyder's Honey Mustard and Onion Pretzels	1 oz	140	18	7	36	15	20	17	48	24
Snyder's Mini Unsalted Pretzels	20 pretzels	110	25	0	28	12	16	13	37	19
Snyder's Organic Honey Wheat Sticks	15 pretzels	130	24	2	34	14	18	16	44	22
Snyder's Organic Oat Bran Sticks	18 pretzels	120	25	0	31	13	17	15	41	20
Snyder's Organic Pumpernickel and Onion Sticks	14 pretzels	120	24	2	31	13	17	15	41	20
Snyder's Snaps	24 pretzels	120	25	1	31	13	17	15	41	20
Snyder's Sourdough Nibblers	16 pretzels	120	25	0	31	13	17	15	41	20
Snyder's Sticks Lunch Packs	1 pack (42.5 g)	160	33	2	41	17	23	19	54	27
■ **Rold Gold**										
Cheddar Tiny Twists	1 oz	110	22	1	28	12	16	13	37	19

FOOD	AMOUNT	CAL	CARBS	FAT	WALK	RUN	BIKE	SWIM	YOGA	DANCE
Pretzel Sticks	1 oz	100	23	0	26	11	14	12	34	17
Pretzel Thins	1 oz	110	23	1	28	12	16	13	37	19
Braided Pretzel Twists	1 oz	110	22	1	28	12	16	13	37	19
Pretzel Rods	1 oz	110	22	1	28	12	16	13	37	19
Tiny Twists	1 oz	110	23	1	28	12	16	13	37	19
Hard Sourdough Pretzels	1 oz	100	21	1	26	11	14	12	34	17
Honey Mustard Tiny Twists	1 oz	110	23	1	28	12	16	13	37	19
Honey Wheat Braided Twists	1 oz	110	22	1	28	12	16	13	37	19
Land O' Lakes Butter Flavored Checkers	1 oz	110	22	2	28	12	16	13	37	19
■ **Chocolate-Covered Pretzels**										
Chocolate-covered pretzels	1 oz	130	20	5	33	14	18	16	44	22
Flipz White Chocolate Covered Pretzels	1 oz	130	20	5	34	14	18	16	44	22
Sierra Club Organic Milk Chocolate Covered Pretzels	4 pieces	50	9	2	13	5	7	6	17	9
■ **Auntie Anne's Pretzels**										
Almond Pretzel	1 pretzel	400	72	8	103	43	57	49	136	68
Almond Pretzel Without Butter	1 pretzel	350	72	2	90	37	50	43	119	60
Cinnamon Sugar Pretzel	1 pretzel	450	83	9	116	48	64	55	153	77
Cinnamon Sugar Pretzel Without Butter	1 pretzel	350	74	2	90	37	50	43	119	60
Garlic Pretzel	1 pretzel	350	68	5	90	37	50	43	119	60
Garlic Pretzel Without Butter	1 pretzel	320	66	1	82	34	45	39	109	55
Glazin' Raisin Pretzel	1 pretzel	510	107	4	131	54	72	62	173	87
Glazin' Raisin Pretzel Without Butter	1 pretzel	470	104	1	121	50	67	57	160	80
Jalapeño Pretzel	1 pretzel	310	59	5	80	33	44	38	105	53
Jalapeño Pretzel Without Butter	1 pretzel	270	58	1	70	29	38	33	92	46
Original Pretzel	1 pretzel	370	72	4	95	39	52	45	126	63
Original Pretzel Without Butter	1 pretzel	340	72	1	88	36	48	41	116	58
Pretzel Dog	1 pretzel	290	25	16	75	31	41	35	99	49
Sesame Pretzel	1 pretzel	410	64	12	106	44	58	50	139	70
Sesame Pretzel Without Butter	1 pretzel	350	63	6	90	37	50	43	119	60
Sour Cream & Onion Pretzel	1 pretzel	340	66	5	88	36	48	41	116	58
Sour Cream and Onion Pretzel Without Butter	1 pretzel	310	66	1	80	33	44	38	105	53
Stix	4 sticks	247	48	3	64	26	35	30	84	42

FOOD	AMOUNT	CAL	CARBS	FAT	WALK	RUN	BIKE	SWIM	YOGA	DANCE
Stix Without Butter	4 sticks	227	48	1	59	24	32	28	77	39
Whole Wheat Pretzel	1 pretzel	370	72	5	95	39	52	45	126	63
Whole Wheat Pretzel Without Butter	1 pretzel	350	72	2	90	37	50	43	119	60
Puffed Wheat Snacks										
Chile and Lime Sabritones	1 oz	150	13	10	39	16	21	18	51	26
Original Sun Chips	1 oz	140	19	6	36	15	20	17	48	24
Harvest Cheddar Sun Chips	1 oz	140	19	6	36	15	20	17	48	24
French Onion Sun Chips	1 oz	140	18	6	36	15	20	17	48	24
Dips										
Fritos Bean Dip	2 tbsp	40	5	1	10	4	6	5	14	7
Fritos Chili Cheese Dip	2 tbsp	45	3	3	12	5	6	5	15	8
Fritos Hot Bean Dip with Jalapeño Peppers	2 tbsp	40	5	1	10	4	6	5	14	7
Fritos Mild Cheddar Cheese Dip	2 tbsp	60	3	4	15	6	9	7	20	10
Ruffles French Onion Dip	4 tbsp	200	9	15	52	21	28	24	68	34
Ruffles Ranch Dip	2 tbsp	60	1	5	15	6	9	7	20	10
■ **Auntie Anne's Dips**										
Light Cream Cheese	1.25 oz	70	1	6	18	7	10	9	24	12
Strawberry Cream Cheese	1.25 oz	110	4	10	28	12	16	13	37	19
Caramel Dip	1.5 oz	135	27	3	35	14	19	16	46	23
Cheese Sauce	1.25 oz	100	4	8	26	11	14	12	34	17
Chocolate Flavored Dip	1.25 oz	130	24	4	34	14	18	16	44	22
Marinara Sauce	1.25 oz	10	4	0	3	1	1	1	3	2
Sweet Mustard	1.25 oz	60	8	2	15	6	9	7	20	10
Hot Salsa Cheese	1.25 oz	100	4	8	26	11	14	12	34	17
Salsa										
Salsa	2 tbsp	9	2	0	2	1	1	1	3	2
Breakstone's Nonfat Creamy Salsa	2 tbsp	20	3	0	5	2	3	2	7	3
Guiltless Gourmet Roasted Red Pepper Salsa	2 tbsp	10	2	0	3	1	1	1	3	2
Guiltless Gourmet Tomatillo Salsa	2 tbsp	10	2	0	3	1	1	1	3	2
Kraft Nonfat Salsa Dip	2 tbsp	20	3	0	5	2	3	2	7	3
La Victoria Hot Salsa Brava	2 tbsp	4	1	0	1	0	1	0	1	1
La Victoria Hot Salsa Victoria	2 tbsp	7	1	0	2	1	1	1	2	1

FOOD	AMOUNT	CAL	CARBS	FAT	WALK	RUN	BIKE	SWIM	YOGA	DANCE
La Victoria Hot Salsa Ranchera	2 tbsp	9	2	0	2	1	1	1	3	2
La Victoria Mild or Medium Salsa Picante	2 tbsp	8	1	0	2	1	1	1	3	1
La Victoria Mild Salsa Suprema	2 tbsp	8	2	0	2	1	1	1	3	1
La Victoria Medium Salsa Suprema	2 tbsp	8	1	0	2	1	1	1	3	1
La Victoria Mild Green Chile Salsa	2 tbsp	8	1	0	2	1	1	1	3	1
La Victoria Mild, Medium or Hot Thick 'n Chunky Salsa	2 tbsp	8	1	0	2	1	1	1	3	1
La Victoria Green Salsa Jalapeña	2 tbsp	10	1	0	2	1	1	1	3	2
La Victoria Red Salsa Jalapeña	2 tbsp	12	2	0	3	1	2	1	4	2
Old El Paso Cheese and Salsa Dip	2 tbsp	40	3	3	10	4	6	5	14	7
Old El Paso Hot Taco Salsa, Hot, Medium, Mild	2 tbsp	10	2	0	3	1	1	1	3	2
Old El Paso Green Chili Salsa	2 tbsp	10	2	0	3	1	1	1	3	2
Old El Paso Picante Salsa	2 tbsp	10	2	0	3	1	1	1	3	2
Ortega Thick and Chunky Salsa	2 tbsp	8	2	0	2	1	1	1	3	1
Pace Medium Chunky Salsa	2 tbsp	4	1	1	1	0	1	0	1	1
Pace Mild Chunky Salsa	2 tbsp	4	1	1	1	0	1	0	1	1
Tostitos Salsa Con Queso	2 tbsp	80	10	5	21	9	11	10	27	14
Tostitos Fire Roasted Tomato Salsa	2 tbsp	30	4	0	8	3	4	4	10	5
Tostitos Restaurant Style or Mild, Medium or Hot Salsa	4 tbsp	30	6	0	8	3	4	4	10	5
Tostitos Monterey Jack Queso Party Bowl	2 tbsp	40	4	3	10	4	6	5	14	7
Santa Barbara Black Bean and Corn Salsa	2 tbsp	20	4	0	5	2	3	2	7	3
Santa Barbara Artichoke Salsa	2 tbsp	15	2	1	4	2	2	2	5	3
Santa Barbara Fire-Roasted Chili Salsa	2 tbsp	10	2	0	3	1	1	1	3	2
Cheese Sauce										
Cheez Whiz Original Cheese Dip	2 tbsp	90	4	7	23	10	13	11	31	15
Cheez Whiz Light	2 tbsp	80	6	4	21	9	11	10	27	14
Cheez Whiz Cheezin 'n Squeezin	2 tbsp	100	4	8	26	11	14	12	34	17
Velveeta Spread	1 oz	85	3	6	22	9	12	10	29	14

FOOD	AMOUNT	CAL	CARBS	FAT	WALK	RUN	BIKE	SWIM	YOGA	DANCE
Velveeta Reduced Fat	1 oz	62	3	3	16	7	9	8	21	11
La Victoria Cheddar Cheese Sauce	.25 cup	105	6	8	27	11	15	13	36	18
La Victoria Medium Nacho Cheese Sauce with Jalapeño Pepper	.25 cup	122	7	10	31	13	17	15	41	21
Ortega Mild Nacho Cheese Sauce	1 cup	476	10	41	123	51	68	58	162	81
Ortega Nacho Cheese Sauce	1 cup	512	16	40	132	54	73	62	174	87
Pork Skins										
Plain pork skins	1 oz	155	0	9	40	17	22	19	53	26
Barbecue-flavored pork skins	1 oz	153	0	9	39	16	22	19	52	26
Baken-ets Fried Pork Skins	9 pieces	80	0	5	21	9	11	10	27	14
Baken-ets Hot 'n Spicy Fried Pork Skins	9 pieces	80	<1	5	21	9	11	10	27	14
Baken-ets Chili Limon Fried Pork Skins	9 pieces	70	0	5	18	7	10	9	24	12
Baken-ets Sweet 'n Tangy BBQ Fried Pork Skins	9 pieces	80	1	5	21	9	11	10	27	14
Baken-ets Pork Cracklins	8 pieces	90	<1	6	23	10	13	11	31	15
Baken-ets Hot 'n Spicy Pork Cracklins	8 pieces	80	<1	5	21	9	11	10	27	14

Fats, Oils, and Dressings

Fats										
Fat, beef tallow	1 tbsp	115	0	13	30	12	16	14	39	20
Lard	1 tbsp	115	0	13	30	12	16	14	39	20
Household shortening	1 tbsp	113	0	13	29	12	16	14	38	19
Crisco Shortening	1 tbsp	110	0	12	28	12	16	13	37	19
Crisco Butter Flavor	1 tbsp	110	0	12	28	12	16	13	37	19
Wesson Shortening	1 tbsp	109	0	12	28	12	15	13	37	19
chicken fat	1 tbsp	115	0	13	30	12	16	14	39	20
bacon grease	1 tsp	39	0	4	10	4	6	5	13	7
goose fat	1 tbsp	115	0	13	30	12	16	14	39	20
duck fat	1 tbsp	115	0	13	30	12	16	14	39	20
turkey fat	1 tbsp	115	0	13	30	12	16	14	39	20
meat drippings	1 oz	249	0	28	64	27	35	30	85	42

FOOD	AMOUNT	CAL	CARBS	FAT	WALK	RUN	BIKE	SWIM	YOGA	DANCE
■ **Fat Substitute**										
Prune puree	1 oz	72	18	0	19	8	10	9	24	12
Oils										
■ **General**										
Avocado oil	1 tbsp	120	0	14	31	13	17	15	41	20
Canola oil (rapeseed)	1 tbsp	124	0	14	32	13	18	15	42	21
Cocoa butter oil	1 tbsp	120	0	14	31	13	17	15	41	20
Coconut oil	1 tbsp	120	0	14	31	13	17	15	41	20
Coconut vegetable oil	1 tbsp	117	0	14	30	12	17	14	40	20
Corn oil	1 tbsp	120	0	14	31	13	17	15	41	20
Cottonseed oil	1 tbsp	120	0	14	31	13	17	15	41	20
Grapeseed oil	1 tbsp	120	0	14	31	13	17	15	41	20
Hazelnut (filbert) oil	1 tbsp	120	0	14	31	13	17	15	41	20
Herring oil	1 tbsp	123	0	14	32	13	17	15	42	21
Hydrogenated soybean oil	1 tbsp	120	0	14	31	13	17	15	41	20
Mustard oil	1 tbsp	124	0	14	32	13	18	15	42	21
Olive oil	1 tbsp	119	0	14	31	13	17	14	40	20
Palm kernel oil	1 tbsp	117	0	14	30	12	17	14	40	20
Palm oil	1 tbsp	120	0	14	31	13	17	15	41	20
Peanut oil	1 tbsp	119	0	14	31	13	17	14	40	20
Rice bran oil	1 tbsp	120	0	14	31	13	17	15	41	20
Safflower oil (linoleic)	1 tbsp	120	0	14	31	13	17	15	41	20
Safflower oil (oleic)	1 tbsp	120	0	14	31	13	17	15	41	20
Salmon oil	1 tbsp	123	0	14	32	13	17	15	42	21
Sardine oil	1 tbsp	123	0	14	32	13	17	15	42	21
Soybean and canola oil	1 tbsp	120	0	14	31	13	17	15	41	20
Soybean and Cottonseed oil	1 tbsp	120	0	14	31	13	17	15	41	20
Soybean oil	1 tbsp	120	0	14	31	13	17	15	41	20
Sunflower oil	1 tbsp	120	0	14	31	13	17	15	41	20
Vegetable corn oil	1 tbsp	120	0	14	31	13	17	15	41	20
Wheat germ oil	1 tbsp	120	0	14	31	13	17	15	41	20
White truffle oil	1 tbsp	120	0	14	31	13	17	15	41	20
Cod Liver Oil										
Cod liver oil	100 g	902	0	100	232	96	128	110	307	154
Cod liver oil concentrate	100 g	883	0	100	228	94	125	107	300	150
Cod liver oil pellet	1 pellet	2	0	0	1	0	0	0	1	0

FOOD	AMOUNT	CAL	CARBS	FAT	WALK	RUN	BIKE	SWIM	YOGA	DANCE
Brand Name Oils										
Bertolli Olive Oil	1 tbsp	120	0	14	31	13	17	15	41	20
Crisco Canola and Corn Oil blend	1 tbsp	120	0	14	31	13	17	15	41	20
Crisco Soybean Oil	1 tbsp	120	0	14	31	13	17	15	41	20
Eden Foods Toasted Sesame Oil	1 tbsp	120	0	14	31	13	17	15	41	20
Hain Cod Liver Oil	1 tbsp	120	0	14	31	13	17	15	41	20
Hain Garlic and Oil	1 tbsp	120	0	14	31	13	17	15	41	20
Hain Peanut Oil	1 tbsp	120	0	14	31	13	17	15	41	20
Hain Soybean Oil	1 tbsp	120	0	14	31	13	17	15	41	20
Hain Vegetable Oil	1 tbsp	120	0	14	31	13	17	15	41	20
Mazola Right Blend Canola and Corn Oil	1 tbsp	120	0	14	31	13	17	15	41	20
Orville Redenbacher Popcorn and Topping Oil	1 tbsp	120	0	14	31	13	17	15	41	20
Planters 100% Peanut Oil	1 tbsp	120	0	14	31	13	17	15	41	20
Planters Popcorn Oil	1 tbsp	120	0	14	31	13	17	15	41	20
Progresso Extra Virgin Olive Oil	1 tbsp (15 mL)	120	0	14	31	13	17	15	41	20
Smart Beat Canola Oil	1 tbsp	117	0	14	30	12	17	14	40	20
Wesson Best Blend Canola and Vegetable Oil	1 tbsp	120	0	14	31	13	17	15	41	20
Wesson Butter Flavor Oil	1 tbsp	122	0	14	31	13	17	15	41	21
Wesson Butter Flavor Popcorn Oil	1 tbsp	120	0	14	31	13	17	15	41	20
Wesson Canola Oil	1 tbsp	122	0	14	31	13	17	15	41	21
Wesson Cottonseed Oil	1 tbsp	122	0	14	31	13	17	15	41	21
Wesson Olive Oil	1 tbsp	122	0	14	31	13	17	15	41	21
Wesson Peanut Oil	1 tbsp	122	0	14	31	13	17	15	41	21
Cooking Sprays										
Pam Cooking Spray	1 serving	0	0	0	0	0	0	0	0	0
Pam Butter Cooking Spray	1 serving	0	0	0	0	0	0	0	0	0
Pam Olive Oil Cooking Spray	1 serving	0	0	0	0	0	0	0	0	0
Mazola Corn Oil Spray	1 tsp	2	0	0	0	0	0	0	1	0
Weight Watchers Canola Oil Spray	.33 g	2	0	1	1	0	0	0	1	0
Wesson Light Cooking Oil Spray	.27 g	1	0	1	0	0	0	0	0	0

FOOD	AMOUNT	CAL	CARBS	FAT	WALK	RUN	BIKE	SWIM	YOGA	DANCE
Wesson No-Stick Cooking Oil Spray	.25 g	2	0	0	1	0	0	0	1	0
Salad Dressings										
■ Blue Cheese Dressing										
Blue cheese dressing	1 tbsp	76	1	8	20	8	11	9	26	13
Low-calorie blue cheese dressing	1 tbsp	15	0	1	4	2	2	2	5	3
Fat-free blue cheese dressing	1 tbsp	20	4	0	5	2	3	2	7	3
Walden Farms Calorie-Free Bleu Cheese	2 tbsp	0	0	0	0	0	0	0	0	0
■ Creamy Dressings										
Fat free creamy dressing	1 tbsp	18	3	1	5	2	3	2	6	3
Reduced-calorie creamy dressing	1 tbsp	24	1	2	6	3	3	3	8	4
Kraft Onion and Chives Creamy Dressing	1 tbsp	70	1	7	18	7	10	9	24	12
■ Coleslaw Dressing										
Coleslaw dressing	1 tbsp	62	4	5	16	7	9	8	21	11
Reduced-fat coleslaw dressing	1 tbsp	56	7	3	14	6	8	7	19	10
■ Russian Dressing										
Russian	1 tbsp	53	5	4	14	6	8	6	18	9
Low-calorie Russian	1 tbsp	23	4	1	6	2	3	3	8	4
■ Thousand Island Dressing										
Thousand Island	1 tbsp	59	2	6	15	6	8	7	20	10
Reduced-calorie Thousand Island	1 tbsp	31	3	2	8	3	4	4	11	5
Fat-free Thousand Island	1 tbsp	21	5	0	5	2	3	3	7	4
Kraft Nonfat Thousand Island	2 tbsp	40	9	0	10	4	6	5	14	7
■ French Dressing										
French	1 tbsp	73	2	7	19	8	10	9	25	12
Reduced-fat French	1 tbsp	37	5	2	10	4	5	5	13	6
Fat-free French	1 tbsp	21	5	0	5	2	3	3	7	4
■ Italian Dressing										
Italian	1 tbsp	43	2	4	11	5	6	5	15	7
Reduced-fat Italian	1 tbsp	11	1	1	3	1	2	1	4	2
Reduced-calorie Italian	1 tbsp	28	1	3	7	3	4	3	10	5
Fat-free Italian	1 tbsp	7	1	0	2	1	1	1	2	1

FOOD	AMOUNT	CAL	CARBS	FAT	WALK	RUN	BIKE	SWIM	YOGA	DANCE
Good Seasons Cheese Italian Lite Mix	1 tbsp	25	1	3	6	3	4	3	9	4
Good Seasons Nonfat Italian Mix	1 serving	80	24	0	21	9	11	10	27	14
Good Seasons Italian Mix	1 serving	40	8	0	10	4	6	5	14	7
Good Seasons Cheese Italian Lite Mix (prepared)	1 tbsp	70	1	8	18	7	10	9	24	12
Kraft House Italian	1 tbsp	60	1	6	15	6	9	7	20	10
Kraft House Italian, Reduced Calorie	1 tbsp	30	1	2	8	3	4	4	10	5
Kraft Italian Deliciously Light	1 tbsp	35	1	3	9	4	5	4	12	6
Newman's Own Family Recipe Italian	1 tbsp	60	1	7	15	6	9	7	20	10
Wish-Bone Just 2 Good Light Italian	1 tbsp	18	2	1	5	2	2	2	6	3
Wish-Bone Light Italian	1 tbsp	7	1	0	2	1	1	1	2	1
■ **Ranch Dressing**										
Ranch	1 tbsp	73	1	8	19	8	10	9	25	12
Reduced-fat ranch	1 tbsp	33	2	3	9	4	5	4	11	6
Fat-free ranch	1 tbsp	17	4	0	4	2	2	2	6	3
Good Seasons Ranch Mix	1 serving	80	16	0	21	9	11	10	27	14
Good Seasons Lower Calorie Ranch Mix	1 serving	160	32	0	41	17	23	20	55	27
Kraft Ranch	1 tbsp	74	1	8	19	8	10	9	25	13
Kraft Nonfat Ranch	2 tbsp	50	11	0	13	5	7	6	17	9
Kraft Light Done Right Ranch	1 tbsp	38	2	3	10	4	5	5	13	6
Kraft Ranch Mix	1.33 tbsp	130	1	13	34	14	18	16	44	22
Litehouse Lite Ranch	1 tbsp	35	1	3	9	4	5	4	12	6
Litehouse Ranch	1 tbsp	59	1	6	15	6	8	7	20	10
Newman's Own Ranch	1 tbsp	70	1	8	18	7	10	9	24	12
T Marzetti Peppercorn Ranch	1 tbsp	85	1	9	22	9	12	10	29	14
Wish-Bone Ranch	1 tbsp	80	1	9	21	9	11	10	27	14
■ **Caesar Dressing**										
Caesar dressing	1 tbsp	78	0	8	20	8	11	9	27	13
Reduced-calorie caesar	1 cup	16	3	1	4	2	2	2	5	3
Emiril's Caesar Dressing	1 tbsp	65	1	7	17	7	9	8	22	11
Good Seasons Caesar Mix (prepared)	1 tbsp	75	2	8	19	8	11	9	26	13

FOOD	AMOUNT	CAL	CARBS	FAT	WALK	RUN	BIKE	SWIM	YOGA	DANCE
Newman's Own Caesar	1 tbsp	75	1	8	19	8	11	9	26	13
Newman's Own Creamy Caesar	1 tbsp	85	1	9	22	9	12	10	29	14
Walden Farms Calorie-Free Caesar	2 tbsp	0	0	0	0	0	0	0	0	0
■ **Vinaigrettes**										
Hain Garden Canola Tomato Vinaigrette	1 tbsp	60	1	6	15	6	9	7	20	10
Hain Natural Classics Creamy Dijon Vinaigrette	2 tbsp	130	3	13	34	14	18	16	44	22
Kraft Nonfat Honey Dijon	2 tbsp	45	10	0	12	5	6	5	15	8
Newman's Own Olive Oil and Vinegar	1 tbsp	75	1	8	19	8	11	9	26	13
Seven Seas Red Wine Vinegar and Oil	1 tbsp	70	1	7	18	7	10	9	24	12
Simply Delicious Lime Cilantro Vinaigrette Undressing	1 tbsp	41	1	4	11	4	6	5	14	7
Simply Delicious Pink Peppercorn Vinaigrette Undressing	1 tbsp	40	1	4	10	4	6	5	14	7
Walden Farms Diet Raspberry	2 tbsp	0	0	0	0	0	0	0	0	0
Walden Farms Honey Dijon Vinaigrette	2 tbsp	0	0	0	0	0	0	0	0	0
Wish-Bone Salad Spritzers Red Wine Mist Cabernet Vinaigrette Dressing	10 sprays	10	1	1	3	1	1	1	3	2
Wish-Bone Salad Spritzers Italian Vinaigrette Dressing	10 sprays	10	1	1	3	1	1	1	3	2
Wish-Bone Salad Spritzers Balsamic Breeze Vinaigrette Dressing	10 sprays	10	1	1	3	1	1	1	3	2
■ **Other Dressings**										
Bacon and tomato salad dressing	1 tbsp	49	0	5	13	5	7	6	17	8
Sesame seed	1 tbsp	66	1	7	17	7	9	8	22	11
Sweet and sour dressing	1 tbsp	2	1	0	1	0	0	0	1	0
Peppercorn dressing	1 tbsp	76	0	8	19	8	11	9	26	13
Cardini's Pesto with Basil	1 tbsp	70	0	7	18	7	10	9	24	12
Mayonnaise										
Mayonnaise	1 tbsp	103	0	12	27	11	15	13	35	18
Reduced-calorie mayonnaise	1 tbsp	49	1	5	13	5	7	6	17	8

FOOD	AMOUNT	CAL	CARBS	FAT	WALK	RUN	BIKE	SWIM	YOGA	DANCE
Diet mayonnaise	1 tbsp	32	2	3	8	3	5	4	11	5
Hellman's Real Mayonnaise	1 tbsp	90	0	10	23	10	13	11	31	15
Hellman's Mayonnaise with Lime Juice	1 tbsp	90	0	10	23	10	13	11	31	15
Hellman's Light Mayonnaise	1 tbsp	45	<1	5	12	5	6	5	15	8
Hellman's Reduced Fat Mayonnaise	1 tbsp	20	2	2	5	2	3	2	7	3
Kraft Light Mayo	1 tbsp	40	2	4	10	4	6	5	14	7
Kraft Miracle Whip	1 tbsp	40	2	4	10	4	6	5	14	7
Kraft Miracle Whip Light	1 tbsp	30	3	2	8	3	4	4	10	5
Kraft Fat Free Mayo Dressing	1 tbsp	10	2	0	3	1	1	1	3	2
Kraft Miracle Whip Free	1 tbsp	15	2	0	4	2	2	2	5	3

Nuts, Seeds, Legumes, and Beans

Nuts

■ General

FOOD	AMOUNT	CAL	CARBS	FAT	WALK	RUN	BIKE	SWIM	YOGA	DANCE
Brazil nuts	1 oz (6–8 kernels)	186	3	19	48	20	26	23	63	32
Pistachio nuts	1 oz (49 kernels)	162	8	13	42	17	23	20	55	28
Honey-roasted almonds	1 oz	168	8	14	43	18	24	20	57	29
Almonds	1 oz	172	5	16	44	18	24	21	59	29
Cashews	1 oz (18 kernels)	164	8	14	42	17	23	20	56	28
Mixed nuts	1 oz	174	6	16	45	19	25	21	59	30
Pecans	1 oz	203	4	21	52	22	29	25	69	35
Pine nuts	1 oz (167 kernels)	191	4	19	49	20	27	23	65	33
Chestnuts	1 oz	68	15	0	17	7	10	8	23	12
Hazelnuts (filberts)	1 oz (21 kernels)	183	5	18	47	20	26	22	62	31
Macadamia nuts	1 oz (10-12 kernels)	204	0	22	53	22	29	25	69	35
Walnuts	1 oz (14 kernels)	185	4	18	48	20	26	23	63	32
Peanuts	1 oz (32 nuts)	165	5	14	43	18	23	20	56	28

FOOD	AMOUNT	CAL	CARBS	FAT	WALK	RUN	BIKE	SWIM	YOGA	DANCE
■ Frito-Lay										
Frito-Lay Salted Peanuts	3 tbsp	160	5	14	41	17	23	19	54	27
Frito-Lay Honey Roasted Peanuts	3 tbsp	170	7	13	44	18	24	21	58	29
Frito-Lay In-Shell Pistachios	1 package (25 g)	150	7	13	39	16	21	18	51	26
Frito-Lay Smoked Almonds	1 package	300	15	22	77	32	43	36	102	51
Frito-Lay Cashews	3 tbsp	160	8	13	41	17	23	19	54	27
Frito-Lay Mixed Nuts	.25 cup	170	6	16	44	18	24	21	58	29
■ Planter's										
Planter's Mixed Nuts	1 oz	170	6	15	44	18	24	21	58	29
■ Mauna Loa										
Mauna Loa Honey Roasted Macadamia Nuts	.25 cup	180	8	16	46	19	26	22	61	31
Mauna Loa Butter Candy Macadamia Nuts	.25 cup	160	10	13	41	17	23	19	54	27
Mauna Loa Kona Coffee Macadamia Nuts	.25 cup	150	11	12	39	16	21	18	51	26
Mauna Loa Maui Onion and Garlic Macadamia Nuts	.25 cup	200	4	20	52	21	28	24	68	34
Mauna Loa Island Nut and Fruit Mix	.25 cup	160	17	9	41	17	23	19	54	27
■ Hershey's										
Hershey's Really Nuts Roasted Peanuts	1 package (70 g)	440	13	35	113	47	62	54	150	75
Hershey's Cocoa Peanuts	1 package (70 g)	390	34	24	101	42	55	47	133	66
Hershey's Cashew Nuts	1 package (42 g)	260	12	20	67	28	37	32	88	44
■ Trail Mix										
Trail mix	1 oz	110	19	4	28	12	16	13	37	19
Raisin and nut trail mix	1 oz	130	13	7	34	14	18	16	44	22
Trail mix with chocolate chips	1 oz	137	13	9	35	15	19	17	47	23
Cranberry-nut trail mix	1 oz	120	15	6	31	13	17	15	41	20
Frito-Lay Original Trail Mix	3 tbsp	160	25	9	41	17	23	19	54	27
Hershey's Trail Mix	1 package (51 g)	280	21	18	72	30	40	34	95	48
Mauna Loa Trail Mix	1 package (48 g)	260	23	17	67	28	37	32	88	44

FOOD	AMOUNT	CAL	CARBS	FAT	WALK	RUN	BIKE	SWIM	YOGA	DANCE
Reese's Trail Mix	1 package (51 g)	300	18	20	77	32	43	36	102	51
Seeds										
Pumpkin and squash seeds	1 oz	148	4	12	38	16	21	18	50	25
Sesame seeds	1 oz	160	7	14	41	17	23	19	54	27
Sunflower seeds	1 cup	168	6	15	43	18	24	20	57	29
Dried acorns	1 oz	144	15	9	37	15	20	18	49	25
Flaxseeds	1 tbsp, ground	37	2	3	10	4	5	5	13	6
Frito-Lay Sunflower Seeds	3 tbsp	180	4	14	46	19	26	22	61	31
Frito-Lay Flamin' Hot Sunflower Seeds	1 package (31 g)	180	6	17	46	19	26	22	61	31
Frito-Lay BBQ Sunflower Seeds	1 oz	140	17	8	36	15	20	17	48	24
Coconut										
Raw coconut	.5 cup, shredded	283	12	27	73	30	40	34	96	48
Raw coconut milk	1 cup	552	13	57	142	59	78	67	188	94
Canned coconut cream	1 cup	568	25	52	146	61	81	69	193	97
Canned coconut milk	1 cup	445	6	48	115	47	63	54	151	76
Dried sweetened coconut flakes	1 cup	351	35	24	90	37	50	43	119	60
Mounds Sweetened Coconut Flakes	2 tbsp	70	6	5	18	7	10	9	24	12
Butters and Spreads										
Sunflower seed butter	1 tbsp	93	4	8	24	10	13	11	32	16
Tahini (sesame butter)	1 tbsp	89	3	8	23	10	13	11	30	15
Almond butter	1 tbsp	101	3	9	26	11	14	12	34	17
Almond paste (marzipan)	1 cup, firmly packed	1040	109	63	268	111	147	126	354	177
Cashew butter	1 tbsp	94	4	8	24	10	13	11	32	16
Chunky peanut butter	2 tbsp	188	6	16	48	20	27	23	64	32
Smooth peanut butter	2 tbsp	188	7	16	48	20	27	23	64	32
Chocolate hazelnut spread	2 tbsp	200	23	11	52	21	28	24	68	34
Halavah	1 oz	131	17	6	34	14	19	16	45	22
Jif/Skippy Peanut Butter	2 tbsp	190	7	16	49	20	27	23	65	32
Jif/Skippy Reduced Fat Peanut Butter	2 tbsp	190	15	12	49	20	27	23	65	32

FOOD	AMOUNT	CAL	CARBS	FAT	WALK	RUN	BIKE	SWIM	YOGA	DANCE
Nutella Chocolate Hazelnut Spread	2 tbsp	200	23	11	52	21	28	24	68	34
Reese's Creamy Peanut Butter	2 tbsp	200	8	15	52	21	28	24	68	34
Reese's Crunchy Peanut Butter	2 tbsp	200	7	15	52	21	28	24	68	34
Candied Nuts										
Sesame crunch candy	20 pieces	181	18	12	47	19	26	22	62	31
Milk chocolate-coated peanuts	.5 cup	387	37	25	100	41	55	47	132	66
Sugar-coated almonds	1 oz	132	19	5	34	14	19	16	45	22
Blue Diamond Jordan Almonds	13 pieces	140	21	5	36	15	20	17	48	24
Blue Diamond Lime 'n Chili Almonds	1 oz	170	5	16	44	18	24	21	58	29
Emerald Glazed Walnuts	1 oz	140	12	10	36	15	20	17	48	24
Emerald Glazed Pecans	1 oz	150	12	11	39	16	21	18	51	26
Farley's Chocolate Double Dipped Peanuts	15 pieces	200	25	11	52	21	28	24	68	34
Fisher Praline Glazed Cashews	.25 cup	170	11	12	44	18	24	21	58	29
Fisher Nut 'N Crunchies Honey Crunch Mix	.25 cup	140	17	6	36	15	20	17	48	24
Goobers	1 package (1.375 oz)	200	19	13	52	21	28	24	68	34
Hershey's Honey Glazed Peanuts	1 package (70 g)	400	31	25	103	43	57	49	136	68
Mauna Loa Milk Chocolate Toffee Macadamia Nuts	7 pieces	210	21	13	54	22	30	26	71	36
Mauna Loa Dark Chocolate Macadamia Nuts	9 pieces	220	19	15	57	23	31	27	75	37
Mauna Loa Chocolate Trio Macadamia Nuts	9 pieces	220	18	15	57	23	31	27	75	37
Mauna Loa Sugar Free Dark Chocolate Macadamia Nuts	6 pieces	200	19	17	52	21	28	24	68	34
Mauna Loa Candy Coated Macadamia Nuts	13 pieces	210	22	13	54	22	30	26	71	36
Mauno Loa Milk Chocolate Macadamia Nuts	9 pieces	220	18	15	57	23	31	27	75	37
Crackers Made from Nuts										
Blue Diamond Nut Thins	16 crackers	130	23	3	34	14	18	16	44	22

FOOD	AMOUNT	CAL	CARBS	FAT	WALK	RUN	BIKE	SWIM	YOGA	DANCE
Legumes and Beans										
■ Fresh										
Raw green snap beans	1 cup	34	8	0	9	4	5	4	12	6
■ Cooked										
Cooked baby lima beans	1 cup	229	42	1	59	24	33	28	78	39
Cooked black beans	1 cup	227	41	1	59	24	32	28	77	39
Cooked black turtle soup beans	1 cup	240	45	1	62	26	34	29	82	41
Cooked California red kidney beans	1 cup	219	40	0	57	23	31	27	75	37
Cooked chickpeas	1 cup	269	45	4	69	29	38	33	91	46
Cooked cowpeas	1 cup	200	36	1	51	21	28	24	68	34
Cooked fava beans	1 cup	187	33	1	48	20	27	23	64	32
Cooked French beans	1 cup	228	43	1	59	24	32	28	78	39
Cooked great northern beans	1 cup	209	37	1	54	22	30	25	71	36
Cooked green snap beans	1 cup	44	10	0	11	5	6	5	15	7
Cooked kidney beans	1 cup	225	40	1	58	24	32	27	76	38
Cooked lentils	1 cup	230	40	1	59	24	33	28	78	39
Cooked lima beans	1 cup	209	40	1	54	22	30	25	71	36
Cooked mungo beans	1 cup	189	33	1	49	20	27	23	64	32
Cooked navy beans	1 cup	255	47	1	66	27	36	31	87	43
Cooked pink beans	1 cup	252	47	1	65	27	36	31	86	43
Cooked pinto beans	1 cup	245	45	1	63	26	35	30	83	42
Cooked red kidney beans	1 cup	225	40	1	58	24	32	27	76	38
Cooked royal red kidney beans	1 cup	218	39	0	56	23	31	26	74	37
Cooked small white beans	1 cup	254	46	1	66	27	36	31	86	43
Cooked split peas	1 cup	231	41	1	60	25	33	28	79	39
Cooked white beans	1 cup	249	45	1	64	26	35	30	85	42
Cooked yellow beans	1 cup	255	45	2	66	27	36	31	87	43
■ Canned										
Canned black turtle soup beans	1 cup	218	40	1	56	23	31	27	74	37
Canned chickpeas	1 cup	286	54	3	74	30	41	35	97	49
Canned fava beans	1 cup	182	32	1	47	19	26	22	62	31
Canned great northern beans	1 cup	299	55	1	77	32	42	36	102	51
Canned green snap beans	.5 cup	18	4	0	5	2	3	2	6	3
Canned kidney beans	1 cup	210	37	2	54	22	30	26	71	36
Canned lima beans	.5 cup	88	17	0	23	9	12	11	30	15

FOOD	AMOUNT	CAL	CARBS	FAT	WALK	RUN	BIKE	SWIM	YOGA	DANCE
Canned navy beans	1 cup	296	54	1	76	32	42	36	101	50
Canned pinto beans	1 cup	206	37	2	53	22	29	25	70	35
Canned red kidney beans	1 cup	218	40	1	56	23	31	26	74	37
Canned white beans	1 cup	307	57	1	79	33	43	37	104	52
Canned cowpeas	1 cup	185	33	1	48	20	26	22	63	31
Canned cowpeas with pork	1 cup	199	40	4	51	21	28	24	68	34
Campbell's Pork and Beans in Tomato Sauce	.5 cup	130	24	2	34	14	18	16	44	22
Goya Black Beans	.5 cup	90	19	1	23	10	13	11	31	15
Goya Cannellini Beans	.5 cup	80	18	0	21	9	11	10	27	14
Goya Chick Peas	.5 cup	100	20	2	26	11	14	12	34	17
Goya Kidney Beans	.5 cup	90	19	1	23	10	13	11	31	15
Goya Pink Beans	.5 cup	80	16	1	21	9	11	10	27	14
Goya Red Beans	.5 cup	90	18	1	23	10	13	11	31	15
Westbrae Organic Red Beans	.5 cup	100	19	0	26	11	14	12	34	17
Westbrae Organic Garbanzo Beans	.5 cup	110	18	2	28	12	16	13	37	19
Westbrae Organic Salad Beans	.5 cup	100	19	1	26	11	14	12	34	17
Westbrae Organic Great Northern Beans	.5 cup	100	19	0	26	11	14	12	34	17
Westbrae Vegetarian Organic Kidney Beans	.5 cup	100	18	0	26	11	14	12	34	17
Westbrae Vegetarian Organic Lentils	.5 cup	100	17	0	26	11	14	12	34	17
Westbrae Vegetarian Organic Pinto Beans	.5 cup	100	19	0	26	11	14	12	34	17
■ **Frozen**										
Frozen lima beans	.5 cup	85	16	0	22	9	12	10	29	14
Frozen baby lima beans	.5 cup	108	21	0	28	12	15	13	37	18
Frozen pinto beans	1 package (10 oz)	483	92	1	124	51	68	59	164	82
Frozen green snap beans	1 cup	41	9	0	11	4	6	5	14	7
Frozen cowpeas	1 cup	222	40	1	57	24	32	27	76	38
■ **Baked Beans**										
Homemade baked beans	1 cup	382	54	13	98	41	54	46	130	65
Canned vegetarian baked beans	1 cup	239	54	1	62	25	34	29	81	41
Canned baked beans with beef	1 cup	322	45	9	83	34	46	39	109	55
Canned baked beans with franks	1 cup	368	40	17	95	39	52	45	125	63

FOOD	AMOUNT	CAL	CARBS	FAT	WALK	RUN	BIKE	SWIM	YOGA	DANCE
Canned baked beans with pork	1 cup	268	51	4	69	29	38	33	91	46
Canned baked beans with pork and sweet sauce	1 cup	283	53	4	73	30	40	34	96	48
Canned baked beans with pork and tomato sauce	1 cup	238	47	2	61	25	34	29	81	41
Amy's Organic Vegetarian Baked Beans	1 cup	240	48	1	62	26	34	29	82	41
Bush's Best Original Baked Beans	1 cup	300	58	2	77	32	43	36	102	51
Bush's Best Vegetarian Baked Beans	1 cup	260	48	0	67	28	37	32	88	44
Heinz Vegetarian Baked Beans	1 cup	280	54	1	72	30	40	34	95	48
■ **Refried Beans**										
Refried beans	1 cup	237	39	3	61	25	34	29	81	40
Amy's Organic Refried Beans with Green Chilies	1 cup	260	40	6	67	28	37	32	88	44
Amy's Organic Traditional Refried Beans	1 cup	280	42	6	72	30	40	34	95	48
Amy's Organic Vegetarian Refried Black Beans	1 cup	280	40	6	72	30	40	34	95	48
Bearitos Fat Free Vegetarian Refried Beans	1 cup	220	40	0	57	23	31	27	75	37
Old El Paso Refried Beans	1 cup	200	34	1	52	21	28	24	68	34
■ **Bean Products—Sauces and Spreads**										
Hummus	1 tbsp	27	3	1	7	3	4	3	9	5
Lee Kum Kee Black Bean Garlic Sauce	1 tbsp	30	3	1	8	3	4	4	10	5
Tribe of Two Sheiks Roasted Garlic Hummus	2 tbsp	50	4	3	13	5	7	6	17	9
Tribe of Two Sheiks Roasted Red Pepper Hummus	2 tbsp	50	4	3	13	5	7	6	17	9
■ **Indian-Style Bean Dishes**										
Kohinoor Pindi Chana Masala	⅓ package	179	20	9	46	19	25	22	61	30
Kohinoor Amritsari Cholle	⅓ package	173	26	6	45	18	25	21	59	29
Kohinoor Dal Palak	⅓ package	107	17	3	28	11	15	13	36	18
Kohinoor Kashmiri Rajma	⅓ package	165	18	7	43	18	23	20	56	28

FOOD	AMOUNT	CAL	CARBS	FAT	WALK	RUN	BIKE	SWIM	YOGA	DANCE
Kohinoor Peshwari Dal Makhani	⅓ package	153	14	8	39	16	22	19	52	26
■ **Bean Salad**										
Black bean salad	4 oz	130	19	4	34	14	18	16	44	22
Four bean salad	4 oz	120	26	1	31	13	17	15	41	20
■ **Bean Chips**										
Garden of Eatin' Black Bean Chili Corn Chips	1 oz	140	17	7	36	15	20	17	48	24
Garden of Eatin' Black Bean Corn Chips	1 oz	140	18	7	36	15	20	17	48	24
■ **Rice and Beans**										
Goya Rice and Black Beans	.25 cup	160	34	0	41	17	23	19	54	27
Goya Rice and Pinto Beans	.25 cup	160	34	0	41	17	23	19	54	27
Goya Rice and Red Beans	.25 cup	160	35	0	41	17	23	19	54	27
Weight Watchers Smart Ones Santa Fe Style Rice and Beans	1 package (283 g)	300	49	8	77	32	43	36	102	51
■ **Chili**										
Canned chili with beans	1 cup	287	30	14	74	31	41	35	98	49
Amy's Organic Medium Chili	1 cup	190	26	6	49	20	27	23	65	32
Amy's Organic Black Bean Chili	1 cup	200	31	2	52	21	28	24	68	34
Amy's Organic Medium Chili with Vegetables	1 cup	190	29	6	49	20	27	23	65	32
Amy's Organic Spicy Chili	1 cup	190	26	6	49	20	27	23	65	32
■ **Other Bean Products**										
Homemade falafel	1 patty (2 ¼" diameter)	57	5	3	15	6	8	7	19	10

Soybeans and Soy Products

Fake Meat and Poultry Products										
Meat extender	1 cup	275	34	3	71	29	39	34	94	47
Meatless bacon	3 strips	46	1	4	12	5	7	6	16	8
Meatless bacon bits	1 tbsp	33	2	2	9	4	5	4	11	6
Meatless chicken	3 oz	190	3	11	49	20	27	23	65	32
Meatless chicken, breaded and fried	3 oz	199	7	11	51	21	28	24	68	34

FOOD	AMOUNT	CAL	CARBS	FAT	WALK	RUN	BIKE	SWIM	YOGA	DANCE
Meatless fish sticks	3 sticks (3 oz)	244	8	15	63	26	35	30	83	42
Meatless frankfurters	1 frank (70 g)	163	5	10	42	17	23	20	55	28
Meatless luncheon slices	3 thin slices (42 g)	79	2	5	20	8	11	10	27	13
Meatless meatballs	3 oz	167	7	8	43	18	24	20	57	28
Meatless sausage	1 link	64	0	5	17	7	9	8	22	11
Soybeans										
Cooked soybeans	1 cup	298	17	15	77	32	42	36	101	51
Dry-roasted soybeans	1 cup	776	56	37	200	83	110	94	264	132
Seapoint Farms Ready-to-Eat Soybeans	.5 cup	100	9	3	26	11	14	12	34	17
Cascadian Farms Frozen Soybeans	.667 cup	120	9	5	31	13	17	15	41	20
Other Soy Products										
Soy nuts	.25 cup	113	8	5	29	12	16	14	38	19
Miso	1 cup	547	73	17	141	58	78	67	186	93
Natto	1 cup	371	25	19	96	40	53	45	126	63
Tempeh	1 cup	320	16	18	83	34	45	39	109	55
Tofu yogurt	1 cup	246	42	5	63	26	35	30	84	42
■ Soy Sauce										
La Choy Mandarin Soy Sauce	.25 cup	35	8	0	9	4	5	4	12	6
La Choy Soy Sauce	1 tbsp	11	1	0	3	1	1	1	4	2
La Choy Light Soy Sauce	1 tbsp	15	2	0	4	2	2	2	5	3
Lum Kum Kee Soy Sauce	1 tbsp	10	1	0	3	1	1	1	3	2
Kikkoman Soy Sauce	1 tbsp	10	0	0	3	1	1	1	3	2
Shoyu Soy Sauce	1 tbsp	8	1	1	2	1	1	1	3	1
Tamari Soy Sauce	1 tbsp	11	1	0	3	1	2	1	4	2
■ Tofu										
Regular tofu (raw)	.5 cup	94	2	6	24	10	13	11	32	16
Firm tofu (prepared with nigari)	.5 cup	88	2	5	23	9	13	11	30	15
Firm tofu (raw)	.5 cup	183	5	11	47	19	26	22	62	31
Extra firm tofu (prepared with nigari)	3 oz	77	2	5	20	8	11	9	26	13
Hard tofu (prepared with nigari)	3 oz	124	4	8	32	13	18	15	42	21

FOOD	AMOUNT	CAL	CARBS	FAT	WALK	RUN	BIKE	SWIM	YOGA	DANCE
Soft tofu (prepared with nigari)	.5 cup	76	2	5	20	8	11	9	26	13
Salted and fermented tofu (fuyu)	3 oz	99	4	7	26	11	14	12	34	17
Fried tofu	3 oz	230	9	17	59	24	33	28	78	39
Mori-Nu Silken Firm Tofu	1 slice (3 oz)	50	2	3	13	5	7	6	17	9
Mori-Nu Enriched Silken Firm Tofu	1 slice (3 oz)	70	6	3	18	7	10	9	24	12
Mori-Nu Organic Silken Firm Tofu	1 slice (3 oz)	60	2	3	15	6	9	7	20	10
Mori-Nu Silken Lite Firm Tofu	1 slice (3 oz)	30	1	1	8	3	4	4	10	5
Mori-Nu Silken Extra Firm Tofu	1 slice (3 oz)	45	2	2	12	5	6	5	15	8
Mori-Nu Silken Lite Extra Firm Tofu	1 slice (3 oz)	35	1	1	9	4	5	4	12	6
Nasoya Super Firm Cubed Tofu	2.8 oz (⅓ package)	100	3	5	26	11	14	12	34	17
Mori-Nu Silken Soft Tofu	1 slice (3 oz)	45	2	3	12	5	6	5	15	8
Mori-Nu Chinese Spice Seasoned Tofu	1 slice (3 oz)	50	3	2	13	5	7	6	17	9
Mori-Nu Japanese Miso Seasoned Tofu	1 slice (3 oz)	60	3	3	15	6	9	7	20	10
Nasoya Firm Tofu	.20 package (79 g)	70	2	3	18	7	10	9	24	12
Nasoya Lite Firm Tofu	.20 package (79 g)	40	0	2	10	4	6	5	14	7
Nasoya Extra Firm Tofu	.20 package (79 g)	80	2	4	21	9	11	10	27	14
Nasoya Silken Tofu	.20 package (91 g)	45	2	3	12	5	6	5	15	8
Nasoya Soft Tofu	.20 package (79 g)	60	1	3	15	6	9	7	20	10
Nasoya Lite Silken Tofu	.20 package (91 g)	30	0	1	8	3	4	4	10	5

FOOD	AMOUNT	CAL	CARBS	FAT	WALK	RUN	BIKE	SWIM	YOGA	DANCE
Nasoya Garlic and Onion Tofu	.25 package (85 g)	90	3	5	23	10	13	11	31	15
Nasoya Chinese Spice Tofu	.25 package (85 g)	90	3	5	23	10	13	11	31	15

■ Soy Milk

FOOD	AMOUNT	CAL	CARBS	FAT	WALK	RUN	BIKE	SWIM	YOGA	DANCE
Soy milk	1 cup	127	12	5	33	14	18	15	43	22
Chocolate soy milk	1 cup	120	14	5	31	13	17	15	41	20
Calcium-fortified soy milk	1 cup	98	8	4	25	10	14	12	33	17
Silk Vanilla Soy Milk	1 cup	100	10	4	26	11	14	12	34	17
Silk Chocolate Soy Milk	1 cup	140	23	4	36	15	20	17	48	24
WestSoy Nonfat Soy Beverage	1 cup	80	15	0	21	9	11	10	27	14
WestSoy Low Fat Vanilla Soy Drink	1 cup	120	21	2	31	13	17	15	41	20
WestSoy Vanilla Soy Shake	1 cup	170	28	3	44	18	24	21	58	29

Beverages

Carbonated Beverages/Soda

FOOD	AMOUNT	CAL	CARBS	FAT	WALK	RUN	BIKE	SWIM	YOGA	DANCE
Club soda	12 fl oz	0	0	0	0	0	0	0	0	0
Cream soda	12 fl oz	189	49	0	49	20	27	23	64	32
Ginger ale	12 fl oz	124	32	0	32	13	18	15	42	21
Cola	12 fl oz	136	35	0	35	14	19	17	46	23
Grape soda	12 fl oz	160	42	0	41	17	23	19	54	27
Lemon-lime soda	12 fl oz	151	38	0	39	16	21	18	51	26
Low-calorie cola	12 fl oz	7	1	0	2	1	1	1	2	1
Orange soda	12 fl oz	179	46	0	46	19	25	22	61	30
Tonic water	12 fl oz	124	32	0	32	13	18	15	42	21
Coca Cola Classic	8 fl oz	100	27	0	26	11	14	12	34	17
Coca Cola Classic	12 fl oz	140	39	0	36	15	20	17	48	24
Cherry Coke	12 fl oz	150	0	0	39	16	21	18	51	26
Diet Coke	8 fl oz	0	0	0	0	0	0	0	0	0
Diet Coke with Lime	8 fl oz	0	0	0	0	0	0	0	0	0
Dr. Brown's Cream Soda	12 fl oz	180	44	0	46	19	26	22	61	31
Dr. Brown's Diet Cream Soda	12 fl oz	0	0	0	0	0	0	0	0	0
Dr Pepper	8 fl oz	100	27	0	26	11	14	12	34	17

FOOD	AMOUNT	CAL	CARBS	FAT	WALK	RUN	BIKE	SWIM	YOGA	DANCE
Fresca	8 fl oz	0	0	0	0	0	0	0	0	0
Canada Dry Ginger Ale	12 fl oz	140	36	0	36	15	20	17	48	24
Canada Dry Diet Ginger Ale	12 fl oz	0	0	0	0	0	0	0	0	0
Mountain Dew	8 fl oz	110	31	0	28	12	16	13	37	19
Diet Mountain Dew	8 fl oz	0	0	0	0	0	0	0	0	0
Minute Maid Orange Soda	8 fl oz	120	32	0	31	13	17	15	41	20
Sierra Mist	12 fl oz	150	39	0	39	16	21	18	51	26
Pepsi	8 fl oz	100	27	0	26	11	14	12	34	17
Pepsi	12 fl oz	150	41	0	39	16	21	18	51	26
Pepsi One	8 fl oz	1	0	0	0	0	0	0	0	0
Diet Pepsi	8 fl oz	0	0	0	0	0	0	0	0	0
Pepsi Twist	12 fl oz	150	42	0	39	16	21	18	51	26
Diet Pepsi Twist	12 fl oz	0	0	0	0	0	0	0	0	0
A&W Root Beer	8 fl oz	120	31	0	31	13	17	15	41	20
A&W Diet Root Beer	8 fl oz	0	0	0	0	0	0	0	0	0
Barq's Root Beer	8 fl oz	110	30	0	28	12	16	13	37	19
Bacardi Margarita Mixer (10% frozen juice concntrate)	8 fl oz	110	29	0	28	12	16	13	37	19
Mug Root Beer	8 fl oz	110	29	0	28	12	16	13	37	19
Mug Diet Root Beer	8 fl oz	0	0	0	0	0	0	0	0	0
Sunkist Orange Soda	8 fl oz	130	35	0	34	14	18	16	44	22
7-Up	12 fl oz	140	39	0	36	15	20	17	48	24
Cherry 7-Up	8 fl oz	150	39	0	39	16	21	18	51	26
Diet 7-Up	8 fl oz	0	0	0	0	0	0	0	0	0
Diet Cherry 7-Up	8 fl oz	0	0	0	0	0	0	0	0	0
Sprite	12 fl oz	140	38	0	36	15	20	17	48	24
Diet Sprite	12 fl oz	0	0	0	0	0	0	0	0	0
Chocolate Drinks										
Chocolate syrup	2 tbsp	109	25	0	28	12	15	13	37	19
Whole chocolate milk prepared with chocolate syrup	1 cup	254	36	8	65	27	36	31	86	43
Chocolate fudge syrup	2 tbsp	133	24	3	34	14	19	16	45	23
Thick chocolate milk shake	16 fl oz	541	96	12	139	58	77	66	184	92
Au Bon Pain Choco Bon Loco: Chocolate	6 oz	220	27	12	57	23	31	27	75	37
Carnation Hot Cocoa with Marshmallows	1 envelope	112	24	1	29	12	16	14	38	19

FOOD	AMOUNT	CAL	CARBS	FAT	WALK	RUN	BIKE	SWIM	YOGA	DANCE
Carnation Rich Chocolate Hot Cocoa Mix	1 serving	112	24	1	29	12	16	14	38	19
Carnation No Sugar Hot Cocoa Mix	1 envelope	55	8	0	14	6	8	7	19	9
Carnation Milk Chocolate Instant Breakfast	1 envelope	130	27	1	34	14	18	16	44	22
Dunkin' Donuts Hot Chocolate	10 fl oz	220	38	8	57	23	31	27	75	37
Hershey's Chocolate Syrup	2 tbsp	100	24	0	26	11	14	12	34	17
Hershey's Sugar Free Syrup	2 tbsp	15	5	0	4	2	2	2	5	3
Hershey's Lite Syrup	2 tbsp	50	12	0	13	5	7	6	17	9
Hershey's Special Dark Syrup	2 tbsp	110	26	0	28	12	16	13	37	19
Hershey's Chocolate Drink	1 box (8 oz)	130	28	1	34	14	18	16	44	22
Hershey's Chocolate Milk Drink Mix	3 tbsp	90	23	0	23	10	13	11	31	15
Hershey's Rich Chocolate Hot Cocoa Mix	1 envelope	110	23	2	28	12	16	13	37	19
Hershey's Chocolate Raspberry Hot Cocoa Mix	1 envelope	140	29	2	36	15	20	17	48	24
Hershey's Dutch Chocolate Hot Cocoa Mix	1 envelope	200	41	3	52	21	28	24	68	34
Hershey's French Vanilla Hot Cocoa Mix	1 envelope	140	28	2	36	15	20	17	48	24
Hershey's Goodnight Hugs Hot Cocoa Mix	1 envelope	140	27	3	36	15	20	17	48	24
Hershey's Goodnight Kisses Hot Cocoa Mix	1 envelope	150	27	3	39	16	21	18	51	26
Hershey's Rich Chocolate with Marshmallows Hot Cocoa Mix	1 envelope	110	23	2	28	12	16	13	37	19
Nestlé Nesquik Chocolate Milk Powder	2 tbsp	90	19	1	23	10	13	11	31	15
Nestlé Nesquik Chocolate Milk	1 cup	230	31	8	59	24	33	28	78	39
Nestlé No Sugar Added Hot Cocoa Mix	1 envelope	50	10	0	13	5	7	6	17	9
Nestlé Rich Chocolate Flavored Hot Cocoa Mix	1 envelope	80	15	3	21	9	11	10	27	14
Ovaltine Chocolate Malt Milk Powder	4 tbsp	80	18	0	21	9	11	10	27	14
Starbucks Hot Chocolate	16 fl oz	350	47	14	90	37	50	43	119	60
Starbucks Hot Chocolate with Whip	16 fl oz	450	49	24	116	48	64	55	153	77

FOOD	AMOUNT	CAL	CARBS	FAT	WALK	RUN	BIKE	SWIM	YOGA	DANCE
Starbucks White Hot Chocolate	16 fl oz	480	63	18	124	51	68	58	163	82
Starbucks White Hot Chocolate with Whip	16 fl oz	580	65	28	149	62	82	71	197	99
Starbucks Chocolate Milk	16 fl oz	340	42	15	88	36	48	41	116	58
Starbucks Chantico Drinking Chocolate	6 fl oz	390	51	21	101	42	55	47	133	66
Swiss Miss Hot Cocoa Mix	1 envelope	120	22	3	31	13	17	15	41	20
Swiss Miss Hot Cocoa Mix with Mini-Marshmallows	1 envelope	120	23	3	31	13	17	15	41	20
Swiss Miss Diet Hot Cocoa Mix	1 envelope	25	4	0	6	3	4	3	9	4
Weight Watchers Chocolate Fudge Shake	1 serving	80	12	1	21	9	11	10	27	14
Yoohoo Chocolate Drink	1 box (6.5 oz)	130	29	1	34	14	18	16	44	22
Coffee and Coffee Substitutes										
Black coffee, brewed	1 cup	2	0	0	1	0	0	0	1	0
Decaf black coffee	1 cup	0	0	0	0	0	0	0	0	0
Espresso	1 fl oz	1	0	0	0	0	0	0	0	0
Decaf espresso	1 fl oz	0	0	0	0	0	0	0	0	0
Instant black coffee	1 cup	5	81	0	1	1	1	1	2	1
Decaf instant black coffee	1 cup	5	1	0	1	1	1	1	2	1
Coffee substitute made from grains, prepared with water	1 cup	14	3	0	4	1	2	2	5	2
■ Brand Names										
Café Westbrae Mocha	1 cup	130	24	3	34	14	18	16	44	22
General Foods Hazelnut Belgian Café Instant Coffee Powder	1.33 tbsp	70	12	2	18	7	10	9	24	12
General Foods Italian Cappuccino Powder	1.33 tbsp	50	10	2	13	5	7	6	17	9
General Foods Kahlua Café Instant Coffee Powder	1.33 tbsp	60	10	2	15	6	9	7	20	10
General Foods Sugar Free Café Vienna Coffee (prepared)	1.33 tbsp	30	3	2	8	3	4	4	10	5
General Foods Sugar Free French Vanilla Coffee (prepared)	8 fl oz	25	5	0	6	3	4	3	9	4
General Foods Sugar Free Suisse Mocha Instant Coffee Powder	1.33 tbsp	30	4	2	8	3	4	4	10	5
General Foods Viennese Chocolate Instant Coffee Powder	1.33 tbsp	60	10	2	15	6	9	7	20	10

FOOD	AMOUNT	CAL	CARBS	FAT	WALK	RUN	BIKE	SWIM	YOGA	DANCE
Kaffree Roma Coffee Substitute	8 fl oz	6	1	0	2	1	1	1	2	1
Nescafé Instant Coffee	8 fl oz	4	1	1	1	0	1	0	1	1
Ultra Slim-Fast Coffee Shake	1 shake	220	38	3	57	23	31	27	75	37
■ **Dunkin' Donuts—Regular and Iced Coffee**										
Black	10 fl oz	15	3	0	4	2	2	2	5	3
With sugar	10 fl oz	60	15	0	15	6	9	7	20	10
Any flavored coffee	10 fl oz	20	4	0	5	2	3	2	7	3
With cream	10 fl oz	70	3	6	18	7	10	9	24	12
With cream and sugar	10 fl oz	120	15	6	31	13	17	15	41	20
With milk	10 fl oz	35	4	1	9	4	5	4	12	6
With milk and sugar	10 fl oz	80	16	1	21	9	11	10	27	14
With skim milk	10 fl oz	25	4	0	6	3	4	3	9	4
With skim milk and sugar	10 fl oz	70	16	0	18	7	10	9	24	12
■ **Dunkin' Donuts—Latte**										
Dunkin' Donuts Latte	10 fl oz	120	10	6	31	13	17	15	41	20
Dunkin' Donuts Latte with Sugar	10 fl oz	160	22	6	41	17	23	19	54	27
Dunkin' Donuts Latte with Soy Milk and Sugar	10 fl oz	150	22	4	39	16	21	18	51	26
Dunkin' Donuts Caramel Swirl Latte	10 fl oz	230	36	6	59	24	33	28	78	39
Dunkin' Donuts Mocha Swirl Latte	10 fl oz	230	37	7	59	24	33	28	78	39
Dunkin' Donuts Caramel Swirl Latte with Soy Milk	10 fl oz	210	34	4	54	22	30	26	71	36
Dunkin' Donuts Mocha Swirl Latte with Soy Milk	10 fl oz	210	35	5	54	22	30	26	71	36
Dunkin' Donuts Caramel Crème Hot Latte	10 fl oz	260	40	9	67	28	37	32	88	44
Dunkin' Donuts Mocha Almond Hot Latte	10 fl oz	290	46	10	75	31	41	35	99	49
Dunkin' Donuts Hot Latte Lite	10 fl oz	70	10	0	18	7	10	9	24	12
Iced Espresso Drinks										
Dunkin' Donuts Caramel Creme Iced Latte	16 fl oz	260	40	9	67	28	37	32	88	44
Dunkin' Donuts Iced Caramel Swirl Latte	16 fl oz	240	37	7	62	26	34	29	82	41
Dunkin' Donuts Iced Caramel Swirl Latte with Skim Milk	16 fl oz	180	36	0	46	19	26	22	61	31

FOOD	AMOUNT	CAL	CARBS	FAT	WALK	RUN	BIKE	SWIM	YOGA	DANCE
Dunkin' Donuts Iced Latte	16 fl oz	120	11	7	31	13	17	15	41	20
Dunkin' Donuts Iced Latte Lite	16 fl oz	80	13	0	21	9	11	10	27	14
Dunkin' Donuts Iced Latte with Skim Milk	16 fl oz	70	11	0	18	7	10	9	24	12
Dunkin' Donuts Iced Latte with Skim Milk and Sugar	16 fl oz	120	23	0	31	13	17	15	41	20
Dunkin' Donuts Iced Latte with Sugar	16 fl oz	170	23	7	44	18	24	21	58	29
Dunkin' Donuts Iced Mocha Swirl Latte	16 fl oz	240	38	8	62	26	34	29	82	41
Dunkin' Donuts Iced Mocha Swirl Latte with Skim Milk	16 fl oz	180	37	1	46	19	26	22	61	31
Dunkin' Donuts Mocha Almond Iced Latte	16 fl oz	290	46	10	75	31	41	35	99	49
Dunkin' Donuts Turbo Ice	16 fl oz	120	14	7	31	13	17	15	41	20
Cappuccino										
Dunkin' Donuts Cappuccino	10 fl oz	80	7	5	21	9	11	10	27	14
Dunkin' Donuts Cappuccino with Soy Milk	10 fl oz	70	6	3	18	7	10	9	24	12
Dunkin' Donuts Cappuccino with Sugar	10 fl oz	130	21	5	34	14	18	16	44	22
Dunkaccino	10 fl oz	230	35	10	59	24	33	28	78	39

■ Dunkin' Donuts—Espresso

FOOD	AMOUNT	CAL	CARBS	FAT	WALK	RUN	BIKE	SWIM	YOGA	DANCE
Dunkin' Donuts Espresso	2 oz	0	1	0	0	0	0	0	0	0
Dunkin' Donuts Espresso with Sugar	2 oz	30	7	0	8	3	4	4	10	5

■ Dunkin' Donuts—Coffee Coolatta

FOOD	AMOUNT	CAL	CARBS	FAT	WALK	RUN	BIKE	SWIM	YOGA	DANCE
With 2% milk	16 fl oz	190	41	2	49	20	27	23	65	32
With cream	16 fl oz	350	40	22	90	37	50	43	119	60
With milk	16 fl oz	210	42	4	54	22	30	26	71	36
With skim milk	16 fl oz	170	41	0	44	18	24	21	58	29

■ Starbucks Coffee—Regular and Iced Coffee

FOOD	AMOUNT	CAL	CARBS	FAT	WALK	RUN	BIKE	SWIM	YOGA	DANCE
Tall	12 fl oz	5	1	0	1	1	1	1	2	1
Grande	16 fl oz	10	2	0	3	1	1	1	3	2
Venti	20 fl oz	15	3	0	4	2	2	2	5	3

■ Starbucks Coffee—Espresso, Hot

FOOD	AMOUNT	CAL	CARBS	FAT	WALK	RUN	BIKE	SWIM	YOGA	DANCE
Caffe Americano	16 fl oz	15	3	0	4	2	2	2	5	3
Caffe Latte with Skim Milk	16 fl oz	160	24	0	41	17	23	19	54	27
Caffe Latte with Whole Milk	16 fl oz	260	21	14	67	28	37	32	88	44

FOOD	AMOUNT	CAL	CARBS	FAT	WALK	RUN	BIKE	SWIM	YOGA	DANCE
Caffe Latte with Soy Milk	16 fl oz	210	28	6	54	22	30	26	71	36
Café Au Lait with Skim Milk	16 fl oz	90	13	0	23	10	13	11	31	15
Café Au Lait with Whole Milk	16 fl oz	140	11	8	36	15	20	17	48	24
Café Au Lait with Soy Milk	16 fl oz	110	15	3	28	12	16	13	37	19
Caffe Mocha with Skim Milk	16 fl oz	220	42	2	57	23	31	27	75	37
Caffe Mocha with Whole Milk	16 fl oz	300	40	12	77	32	43	36	102	51
Caffe Mocha with Soy Milk	16 fl oz	260	46	6	67	28	37	32	88	44
Cappuccino with Skim Milk	16 fl oz	100	14	0	26	11	14	12	34	17
Cappuccino with Whole Milk	16 fl oz	150	13	8	39	16	21	18	51	26
Cappuccino with Soy Milk	16 fl oz	120	17	3	31	13	17	15	41	20
Caramel Macchiato with Skim Milk	16 fl oz	220	40	1	57	23	31	27	75	37
Caramel Macchiato with Whole Milk	16 fl oz	310	37	12	80	33	44	38	105	53
Caramel Macchiato with Soy Milk	16 fl oz	270	44	6	70	29	38	33	92	46
Espresso	2 fl oz	10	2	0	3	1	1	1	3	2
Espresso Con Panna	2 fl oz	110	4	9	28	12	16	13	37	19
Espresso Macchiato	2 fl oz	15	2	0	4	2	2	2	5	3
Toffee Nut Latte with Skim Milk	16 fl oz	230	43	0	59	24	33	28	78	39
Toffee Nut Latte with Whole Milk	16 fl oz	330	41	13	85	35	47	40	112	56
Toffee Nut Latte with Soy Milk	16 fl oz	280	47	6	72	30	40	34	95	48
Vanilla Latte with Skim Milk	16 fl oz	230	42	0	59	24	33	28	78	39
Vanilla Latte with Whole Milk	16 fl oz	320	39	12	82	34	45	39	109	55
Vanilla Latte with Soy Milk	16 fl oz	270	46	5	70	29	38	33	92	46
White Chocolate Mocha with Skim Milk	16 fl oz	340	58	5	88	36	48	41	116	58
White Chocolate Mocha with Whole Milk	16 fl oz	410	56	15	106	44	58	50	139	70
White Chocolate Mocha with Soy Milk	16 fl oz	370	62	9	95	39	52	45	126	63

■ **Starbucks Coffee—Espresso, Iced**

FOOD	AMOUNT	CAL	CARBS	FAT	WALK	RUN	BIKE	SWIM	YOGA	DANCE
Caffe Americano	16 fl oz	20	3	0	5	2	3	2	7	3
Caffe Latte with Skim Milk	16 fl oz	100	14	0	26	11	14	12	34	17
Caffe Latte with Soy Milk	16 fl oz	120	17	4	31	13	17	15	41	20
Caffe Latte with Whole Milk	16 fl oz	160	13	8	41	17	23	19	54	27
Caffe Mocha with Skim Milk	16 fl oz	180	36	2	46	19	26	22	61	31

OOD	AMOUNT	CAL	CARBS	FAT	WALK	RUN	BIKE	SWIM	YOGA	DANCE
Caffe Mocha with Soy Milk	16 fl oz	200	38	5	52	21	28	24	68	34
Caffe Mocha with Whole Milk	16 fl oz	220	35	8	57	23	31	27	75	37
Caramel Macchiato with Skim Milk	16 fl oz	200	36	1	52	21	28	24	68	34
Caramel Macchiato with Soy Milk	16 fl oz	230	39	5	59	24	33	28	78	39
Caramel Macchiato with Whole Milk	16 fl oz	270	34	10	70	29	38	33	92	46
Caramel Mocha with Skim Milk	16 fl oz	260	55	3	67	28	37	32	88	44
Caramel Mocha with Soy Milk	16 fl oz	280	57	5	72	30	40	34	95	48
Caramel Mocha with Whole Milk	16 fl oz	290	54	7	75	31	41	35	99	49
Vanilla Latte with Skim Milk	16 fl oz	160	32	0	41	17	23	19	54	27
Vanilla Latte with Whole Milk	16 fl oz	210	31	7	54	22	30	26	71	36
Vanilla Latte with Soy Milk	16 fl oz	190	34	3	49	20	27	23	65	32
White Chocolate Mocha with Skim Milk	16 fl oz	320	57	6	82	34	45	39	109	55
White Chocolate Mocha with Whole Milk	16 fl oz	360	56	11	93	38	51	44	122	61
White Chocolate Mocha with Soy Milk	16 fl oz	340	59	8	88	36	48	41	116	58

■ Starbucks Coffee—Frappuccino Blended Coffee

FOOD	AMOUNT	CAL	CARBS	FAT	WALK	RUN	BIKE	SWIM	YOGA	DANCE
Coffee Frappuccino	16 fl oz	260	52	4	67	28	37	32	88	44
Mocha Frappuccino	16 fl oz	290	58	4	75	31	41	35	99	49
Mocha Frappuccino with Whip	16 fl oz	420	61	16	108	45	60	51	143	72
White Chocolate Mocha Frappuccino	16 fl oz	320	62	5	82	34	45	39	109	55
White Chocolate Mocha Frappuccino with Whip	16 fl oz	450	65	17	116	48	64	55	153	77
Java Chip Frappuccino	16 fl oz	370	69	9	95	39	52	45	126	63
Java Chip Frappuccino with Whip	16 fl oz	510	73	22	131	54	72	62	173	87
Espresso Frappuccino	16 fl oz	230	46	3	59	24	33	28	78	39

■ Starbucks Coffee—Frappuccino Light Blended Coffee

FOOD	AMOUNT	CAL	CARBS	FAT	WALK	RUN	BIKE	SWIM	YOGA	DANCE
Coffee Frappuccino Light	16 fl oz	150	30	1	39	16	21	18	51	26
Coffee Frappuccino Light with Whip	16 fl oz	280	32	13	72	30	40	34	95	48
Mocha Frappuccino Light	16 fl oz	180	36	2	46	19	26	22	61	31
Mocha Frappuccino Light with Whip	16 fl oz	310	38	14	80	33	44	38	105	53

FOOD	AMOUNT	CAL	CARBS	FAT	WALK	RUN	BIKE	SWIM	YOGA	DANCE
White Chocolate Mocha Frappuccino Light	16 fl oz	200	40	3	52	21	28	24	68	34
White Chocolate Mocha Frappuccino Light with Whip	16 fl oz	340	42	15	88	36	48	41	116	58
Java Chip Frappuccino Light	16 fl oz	260	46	7	67	28	37	32	88	44
Java Chip Frappuccino Light with Whip	16 fl oz	400	50	19	103	43	57	49	136	68
Espresso Frappuccino Light	16 fl oz	140	27	1	36	15	20	17	48	24
Espresso Frappuccino Light with Whip	16 fl oz	270	29	13	70	29	38	33	92	46
■ **Starbucks Coffee—Frappuccino Blended Crème**										
Double Chocolate Chip	16 fl oz	460	79	12	119	49	65	56	156	78
Double Chocolate Chip with Whip	16 fl oz	590	83	24	152	63	84	72	201	101
Strawberries and Crème	16 fl oz	450	90	5	116	48	64	55	153	77
Strawberries and Crème with Whip	16 fl oz	580	92	17	149	62	82	71	197	99
Tazo Chai Crème	16 fl oz	380	72	5	98	40	54	46	129	65
Tazo Chai Crème with Whip	16 fl oz	510	74	17	131	54	72	62	173	87
Vanilla Bean	16 fl oz	370	70	5	95	39	52	45	126	63
Vanilla Bean with Whip	16 fl oz	500	72	17	129	53	71	61	170	85
■ **Starbucks Coffee—Ready-to-Drink Frappuccino**										
Regular	1 bottle (9.5 oz)	200	37	3	52	21	28	24	68	34
Mocha	1 bottle (9.5 oz)	180	33	3	46	19	26	22	61	31
Vanilla	1 bottle (9.5 oz)	200	37	3	52	21	28	24	68	34
■ **Krispy Kreme**										
Frozen Latte Blend	16 fl oz	610	92	22	157	65	87	74	207	104
Frozen Original Kreme with Coffee Blend	16 fl oz	600	95	21	155	64	85	73	204	102
Frozen Double Chocolate with Coffee Blend	16 fl oz	600	93	22	155	64	85	73	204	102
Reduced Calorie Latte Blend (no whipped cream)	12 fl oz	99	34	1	26	11	14	12	34	17
■ **Au Bon Pain—Specialty Coffee Drinks**										
Café Au Lait	16 fl oz	120	12	5	31	13	17	15	41	20
Caffe Latte	16 fl oz	160	17	6	41	17	23	19	54	27
Frozen Mocha Blast	16 fl oz	320	57	13	82	34	45	39	109	55

FOOD	AMOUNT	CAL	CARBS	FAT	WALK	RUN	BIKE	SWIM	YOGA	DANCE
Hot Cappuccino	16 fl oz	120	12	5	31	13	17	15	41	20
Hot Mocha Blast	16 fl oz	360	54	11	93	38	51	44	122	61
Iced Cappuccino	16 fl oz	220	22	8	57	23	31	27	75	37
■ Roaster's Cove Beverage Program										
Gourmet French Vanilla Cappuccino	1 serving	160	28	5	41	17	23	19	54	27
Chocolate Supreme Hot Chocolate	1 serving	180	36	3	46	19	26	22	61	31
English Toffee Cappuccino	1 serving	160	27	5	41	17	23	19	54	27
French Vanilla Cappuccino	1 serving	160	27	5	41	17	23	19	54	27
Caramel Pecan Cappuccino	1 serving	160	28	5	41	17	23	19	54	27
Dutch Cocoa	1 serving	160	40	1	41	17	23	19	54	27
Irish Crème Cappuccino	1 serving	160	28	5	41	17	23	19	54	27
White Chocolate Caramel Cappuccino	1 serving	160	28	5	41	17	23	19	54	27
Tea										
■ General										
Tea, brewed (regular and decaf)	1 cup	2	1	0	1	0	0	0	1	0
Unsweetened instant tea	1 cup	2	0	0	1	0	0	0	1	0
Sugar-free instant lemon-flavored tea	1 cup	5	1	0	1	1	1	1	2	1
Sweetened lemon-flavored instant tea	1 cup	91	22	0	23	10	13	11	31	16
Brewed herbal tea	1 cup	2	0	0	1	0	0	0	1	0
■ Nestea										
Nestea Cool Sweetened Lemon Iced Tea Can	12 fl oz	120	33	0	31	13	17	15	41	20
■ Tazo										
Tazo Giant Peach Bottled Tea	16 fl oz	180	42	0	46	19	26	22	61	31
Tazo Tazoberry Bottled Tea	16 fl oz	160	38	0	41	17	23	19	54	27
Tazo Chai Tea Latte	4 fl oz	70	17	0	18	7	10	9	24	12
Tazo Lemon Ginger Herbal Tea	16 fl oz	140	36	0	36	15	20	17	48	24
■ Au Bon Pain										
Au Bon Pain Peach Iced Tea	22 fl oz	120	30	0	31	13	17	15	41	20
■ Dunkin' Donuts										
Any plain tea (regular, green, Earl Grey, English Breakfast)	10 fl oz	0	1	0	0	0	0	0	0	0
Tea with milk and sugar	10 fl oz	70	14	1	18	7	10	9	24	12

FOOD	AMOUNT	CAL	CARBS	FAT	WALK	RUN	BIKE	SWIM	YOGA	DANC
Tea with skim milk and sugar	10 fl oz	60	14	0	15	6	9	7	20	10
Vanilla Chai	10 fl oz	230	40	8	59	24	33	28	78	39
Tea with milk	10 fl oz	25	2	1	6	3	4	3	9	4
Tea with skim milk	10 fl oz	25	4	0	6	3	4	3	9	4
Tea with sugar	10 fl oz	50	13	0	13	5	7	6	17	9
■ Starbucks—Tazo										
Tazo Iced Tea (green, black, or passion)	16 fl oz	80	21	0	21	9	11	10	27	14
Tazo Tea Lemonade (green, black, or passion)	16 fl oz	120	30	0	31	13	17	15	41	20
Tazo Chai Tea Latte with Skim Milk	16 fl oz	230	51	0	59	24	33	28	78	39
Tazo Chai Tea Latte with Whole Milk	16 fl oz	290	50	7	75	31	41	35	99	49
Tazo Chai Tea Latte with Soy Milk	16 fl oz	260	53	3	67	28	37	32	88	44
Tazo Chai Iced Tea Latte with Skim Milk	16 fl oz	230	50	0	59	24	33	28	78	39
Tazo Chai Iced Tea Latte with Whole Milk	16 fl oz	270	48	7	70	29	38	33	92	46
Tazo Chai Iced Tea Latte with Soy Milk	16 fl oz	250	52	3	64	27	35	30	85	43
■ Snapple										
Lime Green or Lemon Tea	1 bottle (16 oz)	200	50	0	52	21	28	24	68	34
Unsweetened Iced Tea	1 bottle (16 oz)	0	0	0	0	0	0	0	0	0
Mint Tea	1 bottle (16 oz)	220	54	0	57	23	31	27	75	37
Peach, Kiwi, or Raspberry Tea	1 bottle (16 oz)	200	52	0	52	21	28	24	68	34
Lemonade Iced Tea	1 bottle (16 oz)	220	56	0	57	23	31	27	75	37
Diet Lime Green, Peach, Lemon, or Raspberry Tea	1 bottle (16 oz)	0	2	0	0	0	0	0	0	0
Diet Lemonade Iced Tea	1 bottle (16 oz)	20	4	0	5	2	3	2	7	3
Drink Mixes										
■ Kool-Aid										
Kool-Aid Splash Ready-to-Drink Grape Berry Punch	1 serving	90	24	0	23	10	13	11	31	15

FOOD	AMOUNT	CAL	CARBS	FAT	WALK	RUN	BIKE	SWIM	YOGA	DANCE
Kool-Aid Tropical Punch Mix	1 serving	64	16	0	16	7	9	8	22	11
Sugar Free Kool-Aid, all flavors	8 fl oz	4	0	0	1	0	1	0	1	1
Unsweetened Kool-Aid, all flavors	8 fl oz	2	0	0	1	0	0	0	1	0

■ Crystal Light

FOOD	AMOUNT	CAL	CARBS	FAT	WALK	RUN	BIKE	SWIM	YOGA	DANCE
Crystal Light Iced Tea or Lemonade Powder (prepared with water)	1 cup	5	0	0	1	0	1	1	2	1

■ Country Time

FOOD	AMOUNT	CAL	CARBS	FAT	WALK	RUN	BIKE	SWIM	YOGA	DANCE
Country Time Lemonade	1 cup	64	18	0	16	7	9	8	22	11
Sugar Free Country Time Pink Lemonade	1 portion	5	2	0	1	1	1	1	2	1

Shakes and Malteds

■ General

FOOD	AMOUNT	CAL	CARBS	FAT	WALK	RUN	BIKE	SWIM	YOGA	DANCE
Strawberry shake	16 fl oz	425	71	11	110	45	60	52	145	72
Chocolate shake	16 fl oz	478	77	14	123	51	68	58	163	81
Vanilla shake	16 fl oz	556	74	25	143	59	79	68	189	95
Chocolate malted drink (prepared from mix with whole milk)	1 cup	223	29	9	57	24	32	27	76	38
Malted drink (prepared from mix with whole milk)	1 cup	228	28	9	59	24	32	28	78	39
Thick chocolate milk shake	16 fl oz	541	96	12	139	58	77	66	184	92
Thick vanilla milk shake	16 fl oz	509	81	14	131	54	72	62	173	87
Strawberry-flavored drink (prepared from mix with whole milk)	1 cup	234	33	8	60	25	33	28	80	40

■ Dunkin' Donuts

FOOD	AMOUNT	CAL	CARBS	FAT	WALK	RUN	BIKE	SWIM	YOGA	DANCE
Dunkin' Donuts Tropicana Orange Coolatta	16 fl oz	370	92	0	95	39	52	45	126	63
Dunkin' Donuts Strawberry Fruit Coolatta	16 fl oz	290	72	0	75	31	41	35	99	49
Dunkin' Donuts Vanilla Bean Coolatta	16 fl oz	440	70	17	113	47	62	54	150	75
Dunkin' Donuts Lemonade Coolatta	16 fl oz	240	59	0	62	26	34	29	82	41

■ Wendy's

FOOD	AMOUNT	CAL	CARBS	FAT	WALK	RUN	BIKE	SWIM	YOGA	DANCE
Wendy's Junior Frosty	1 drink (113 g)	160	28	4	41	17	23	19	54	27

FOOD	AMOUNT	CAL	CARBS	FAT	WALK	RUN	BIKE	SWIM	YOGA	DANCE
Wendy's Small Frosty	1 drink (227 g)	330	56	8	85	35	47	40	112	56
Wendy's Medium Frosty	1 drink (298 g)	430	74	11	111	46	61	52	146	73
Wendy's Fix 'n Mix Frosty	1 drink (117 g)	170	29	4	44	18	24	21	58	29
■ **Krispy Kreme**										
Frozen Double Chocolate Blend	16 fl oz	610	93	22	157	65	87	74	207	104
Reduced Calorie Double Chocolate Blend (no whipped cream)	12 fl oz	99	38	1	26	11	14	12	34	17
Frozen Raspberry Blend	16 fl oz	590	99	19	152	63	84	72	201	101
Frozen Original Kreme Blend	16 fl oz	600	95	21	155	64	85	73	204	102
Specialty Drinks										
■ **Au Bon Pain**										
Passion Fruit Piña Colada	16 fl oz	170	27	9	44	18	24	21	58	29
Mango Blast	16 fl oz	360	66	10	93	38	51	44	122	61
Strawberry Banana Blast	18 fl oz	400	78	10	103	43	57	49	136	68
Strawberry Blast	16 fl oz	350	73	7	90	37	50	43	119	60
Wildberry Blast	16 fl oz	360	66	10	93	38	51	44	122	61
Homestyle Lemonade	16 fl oz	50	14	0	13	5	7	6	17	9
Tomato Juice	8 fl oz	45	9	0	12	5	6	5	15	8
Water and Flavored Water										
Water	1 cup	0	0	0	0	0	0	0	0	0
Fruit 2 0	1 cup	0	0	0	0	0	0	0	0	0
Vitaminwater	1 cup	50	13	0	13	5	7	6	17	9
Energy Drinks										
Gatorade Sports Drink	1 cup	50	14	0	13	5	7	6	17	9
Red Bull Energy Drink	1 cup	110	28	0	28	12	16	13	37	19
Red Bull Sugar Free Energy Drink	1 cup	10	3	0	3	1	1	1	3	2
Vitaminwater	1 cup	50	13	0	13	5	7	6	17	9
Smoothies										
■ **Dunkin' Donuts**										
Strawberry Banana Smoothie	16 fl oz	360	79	3	93	38	51	44	122	61
Wildberry Smoothie	16 fl oz	360	79	3	93	38	51	44	122	61
Mango Passion Fruit Smoothie	16 fl oz	360	79	3	93	38	51	44	122	61

OOD	AMOUNT	CAL	CARBS	FAT	WALK	RUN	BIKE	SWIM	YOGA	DANCE
■ TCBY—Fruithead Smoothies with Yogurt										
Berry Slim	20 oz	410	95	3	106	44	58	50	139	70
Raspberry Delite	20 oz	360	85	3	93	38	51	44	122	61
Peachy Lean	20 oz	470	116	3	121	50	67	57	160	80
Tropical Replenisher	20 oz	370	87	3	95	39	52	45	126	63
Raspberry Revitalizer	20 oz	370	84	3	95	39	52	45	126	63
Workout Whey	20 oz	460	112	3	119	49	65	56	156	78
Holy Cal	20 oz	470	114	3	121	50	67	57	160	80
A Lotta Coloda	20 oz	550	99	17	142	59	78	67	187	94
Healthy Balance	20 oz	410	95	3	106	44	58	50	139	70
Berry Slim	32 oz	600	143	4	155	64	85	73	204	102
Raspberry Delite	32 oz	510	116	5	131	54	72	62	173	87
Peachy Lean	32 oz	620	151	4	160	66	88	75	211	106
Tropical Replenisher	32 oz	520	121	4	134	55	74	63	177	89
Raspberry Revitalizer	32 oz	530	124	4	137	56	75	64	180	90
Workout Whey	32 oz	600	145	5	155	64	85	73	204	102
Holy Cal	32 oz	610	149	4	157	65	87	74	207	104
A Lotta Coloda	32 oz	710	142	17	183	76	101	86	241	121
Healthy Balance	32 oz	590	138	4	152	63	84	72	201	101
■ TCBY—Fruithead Smoothies without Yogurt										
Berry Slim	20 oz	300	75	0	77	32	43	36	102	51
Raspberry Delite	20 oz	240	59	0	62	26	34	29	82	41
Peachy Lean	20 oz	360	96	0	93	38	51	44	122	61
Tropical Replenisher	20 oz	240	61	0	62	26	34	29	82	41
Raspberry Revitalizer	20 oz	300	79	0	77	32	43	36	102	51
Workout Whey	20 oz	340	92	0	88	36	48	41	116	58
Holy Cal	20 oz	360	94	0	93	38	51	44	122	61
A Lotta Coloda	20 oz	380	69	12	98	40	54	46	129	65
Healthy Balance	20 oz	300	75	0	77	32	43	36	102	51
Berry Slim	32 oz	450	116	1	116	48	64	55	153	77
Raspberry Delite	32 oz	300	74	0	77	32	43	36	102	51
Peachy Lean	32 oz	470	124	0	121	50	67	57	160	80
Tropical Replenisher	32 oz	350	92	0	90	37	50	43	119	60
Raspberry Revitalizer	32 oz	470	118	1	121	50	67	57	160	80
Workout Whey	32 oz	450	119	1	116	48	64	55	153	77
Holy Cal	32 oz	450	118	0	116	48	64	55	153	77

FOOD	AMOUNT	CAL	CARBS	FAT	WALK	RUN	BIKE	SWIM	YOGA	DANCE
A Lotta Coloda	32 oz	620	122	15	160	66	88	75	211	106
Healthy Balance	32 oz	450	116	1	116	48	64	55	153	77

Juice

Fruit Juice

■ Apple Juice

FOOD	AMOUNT	CAL	CARBS	FAT	WALK	RUN	BIKE	SWIM	YOGA	DANCE
Unsweetened apple juice	1 cup	117	29	0	30	12	17	14	40	20
Apple juice made from frozen unsweetened concentrate	1 cup	112	28	0	29	12	16	14	38	19

■ Cranberry Juice

FOOD	AMOUNT	CAL	CARBS	FAT	WALK	RUN	BIKE	SWIM	YOGA	DANCE
Cranberry juice cocktail	1 cup	137	34	0	35	15	19	17	47	23
Cranberry-apple juice drink	1 cup	154	39	0	40	16	22	19	52	26
Cranberry-grape juice drink	1 cup	137	34	0	35	15	19	17	47	23
Cranberry juice cocktail (prepared from frozen concentrate)	1 cup	138	0	0	35	15	20	17	47	23

■ Berry Juice

FOOD	AMOUNT	CAL	CARBS	FAT	WALK	RUN	BIKE	SWIM	YOGA	DANCE
Canned blackberry juice	1 cup	86	18	1	22	9	12	10	29	15

■ Grape Juice

FOOD	AMOUNT	CAL	CARBS	FAT	WALK	RUN	BIKE	SWIM	YOGA	DANCE
Unsweetened grape juice	1 cup	154	38	0	40	16	22	19	52	26
Sweetened grape juice from frozen concentrate	1 cup	128	32	0	33	14	18	16	43	22
Grape juice drink	1 cup	142	36	0	37	15	20	17	48	24

■ Lemon Juice and Lemonade

FOOD	AMOUNT	CAL	CARBS	FAT	WALK	RUN	BIKE	SWIM	YOGA	DANCE
Fresh lemon juice	1 cup	61	21	0	16	6	9	7	21	10
Lemon juice (bottled or canned)	1 cup	51	16	1	13	5	7	6	17	9
Frozen unsweetened lemon juice	1 cup	54	16	1	14	6	8	7	18	9
Lemonade (prepared from frozen concentrate)	1 cup	131	34	0	34	14	19	16	45	22
Lemonade (prepared from mix)	1 cup	103	27	0	27	11	15	13	35	18
Lemonade-flavored drink (prepared from mix)	1 cup	112	29	0	29	12	16	14	38	19
Low-calorie lemonade (prepared from mix)	1 cup	5	1	0	1	1	1	1	2	1
Pink lemonade (prepared from frozen concentrate)	1 cup	99	26	0	26	11	14	12	34	17

FOOD	AMOUNT	CAL	CARBS	FAT	WALK	RUN	BIKE	SWIM	YOGA	DANCE
■ Lime Juice										
Fresh lime juice	1 cup	62	21	0	16	7	9	7	21	10
Lime juice (canned or bottled)	1 cup	52	16	1	13	6	7	6	18	9
Limeade (prepared from frozen concentrate)	1 cup	104	26	0	27	11	15	13	35	18
■ Citrus Juice										
Citrus-flavored juice drink (prepared from frozen concentrate)	1 cup	124	30	0	32	13	18	15	42	21
■ Orange Juice										
Fresh orange juice	1 cup	112	26	1	29	12	16	14	38	19
Unsweetened orange juice	1 cup	105	25	0	27	11	15	13	36	18
Orange juice (from frozen unsweetened concentrate)	1 cup	112	27	0	29	12	16	14	38	19
Orange-grapefruit juice	1 cup	106	25	0	27	11	15	13	36	18
Low-calorie orange-flavored breakfast drink (prepared from mix)	1 cup	5	2	0	1	1	1	1	2	1
Orange-flavored breakfast drink (prepared from mix)	1 cup	133	34	0	34	14	19	16	45	23
Orange drink	1 cup	122	31	0	31	13	17	15	41	21
Orange/apricot juice drink	1 cup	128	32	0	33	14	18	16	43	22
Orange/strawberry/banana juice	1 cup	108	29	0	28	11	15	13	37	18
Orange juice drink	1 cup	134	33	0	35	14	19	16	46	23
■ Grapefruit Juice										
Unsweetened grapefruit juice	1 cup	94	22	0	24	10	13	11	32	16
Sweetened grapefruit juice	1 cup	115	28	0	30	12	16	14	39	20
Grapefruit juice (prepared from frozen concentrate)	1 cup	101	24	0	26	11	14	12	34	17
Fresh pink grapefruit juice	1 cup	96	23	0	25	10	14	12	33	16
■ Tangerine Juice										
Fresh tangerine juice	1 cup	106	25	0	27	11	15	13	36	18
Sweetened tangerine juice	1 cup	124	30	1	32	13	18	15	42	21
Sweetened tangerine juice (prepared from frozen concentrate)	1 cup	111	27	0	29	12	16	13	38	19
■ Tropical Juices										
Fresh purple passion fruit juice	1 cup	126	34	0	32	13	18	15	43	21
Fresh yellow passion fruit juice	1 cup	148	36	0	38	16	21	18	50	25

FOOD	AMOUNT	CAL	CARBS	FAT	WALK	RUN	BIKE	SWIM	YOGA	DANCE
Unsweetened pineapple juice	1 cup	132	32	0	34	14	19	16	45	22
Unsweetened pineapple juice (prepared from frozen concentrate)	1 cup	130	32	0	34	14	18	16	44	22
Pineapple/grapefruit juice drink	1 cup	118	29	0	30	13	17	14	40	20
Pineapple/orange juice drink	1 cup	125	30	0	32	13	18	15	43	21
■ **Prune Juice**										
Prune juice	1 cup	182	45	0	47	19	26	22	62	31
■ **Nectars**										
Canned apricot nectar	1 cup	141	36	0	36	15	20	17	48	24
Papaya nectar	1 cup	142	36	0	37	15	20	17	48	24
Peach nectar	1 cup	134	35	0	35	14	19	16	46	23
Pear nectar	1 cup	150	39	0	39	16	21	18	51	26
Vegetable Juice										
Tomato juice	1 cup	41	10	0	11	4	6	5	14	7
Vegetable juice cocktail	1 cup	46	11	0	12	5	7	6	16	8
Carrot juice	1 cup	94	22	35	24	10	13	11	32	16
Mixed fruit and vegetable juice	1 cup	72	18	0	19	8	10	9	24	12
Clam and tomato juice	1 can (5.5 oz)	80	18	0	21	9	11	10	27	14
Campbell's Tomato Juice	1 cup	50	10	0	13	5	7	6	17	9
RW Knudsen Very Veggie Juice	1 cup	50	10	1	13	5	7	6	17	9
V8 Vegetable Juice	1 cup	50	10	0	13	5	7	6	17	9
Fruit Punch										
Fruit punch drink (prepared from frozen concentrate)	1 cup	114	29	0	29	12	16	14	39	19
Fruit punch flavored drink (prepared from mix)	1 cup	97	25	0	25	10	14	12	33	17
Fruit punch juice drink (prepared from frozen concentrate)	1 cup	124	30	1	32	13	18	15	42	21
Kool Aid Tropical Punch Bursts Soft Drink	6.7 oz	100	24	0	26	11	14	12	34	17
Snapple Drinks										
■ **Juice**										
Snapricot Orange, Snapple Apple	1 bottle (16 oz)	240	60	0	62	26	34	29	82	41
Fruit Punch, Mango Madness	1 bottle (16 oz)	220	58	0	57	23	31	27	75	37

FOOD	AMOUNT	CAL	CARBS	FAT	WALK	RUN	BIKE	SWIM	YOGA	DANCE
Grapeade, Cranberry-Raspberry, Orangeade, Raspberry-Peach	1 bottle (16 oz)	240	58	0	62	26	34	29	82	41
Kiwi-Strawberry	1 bottle (16 oz)	220	56	0	57	23	31	27	75	37
What-a-Melon	1 bottle (16 oz)	180	50	0	46	19	26	22	61	31
Diet Cranberry-Raspberry	1 bottle (16 oz)	20	4	0	5	2	3	2	7	3
Diet Kiwi-Strawberry	1 bottle (16 oz)	40	10	0	10	4	6	5	14	7
Diet Snapple Apple	1 bottle (16 oz)	30	8	0	8	3	4	4	10	5
■ **Lemonade**										
Lemonade and Pink Lemonade	1 bottle (16 oz)	220	56	0	57	23	31	27	75	37
Super Sour Lemonade	1 bottle (16 oz)	260	66	0	67	28	37	32	88	44
Diet Pink Lemonade	1 bottle (16 oz)	20	4	0	5	2	3	2	7	3
Brand Name Juices										
Apple & Eve Cranberry Apple Juice	1 cup	120	30	0	31	13	17	15	41	20
Apple & Eve Cranberry Grape Juice	1 cup	140	34	0	36	15	20	17	48	24
Apple & Eve Cranberry Raspberry Juice	1 cup	120	30	0	31	13	17	15	41	20
Apple & Eve Elmo's Punch	1 cup	120	29	0	31	13	17	15	41	20
Apple & Eve Organic Apple Juice	1 cup	110	26	0	28	12	16	13	37	19
Apple & Eve Organic Cranberry Blueberry Juice	1 cup	130	31	0	34	14	18	16	44	22
Apple & Eve Organic Peach Mango Juice	1 cup	130	31	0	34	14	18	16	44	22
Apple & Eve Organic Vintage Concord Grape Juice	1 cup	160	40	0	41	17	23	19	54	27
Ceres Guava Juice	1 cup	120	29	0	31	13	17	15	41	20
Ceres Mango Juice	1 cup	120	30	0	31	13	17	15	41	20
Ceres Papaya Juice	1 cup	120	30	0	31	13	17	15	41	20
Dole Pineapple Juice	1 cup	130	30	0	34	14	18	16	44	22
Mott's Apple Grape Juice	1 cup	130	32	0	34	14	18	16	44	22

FOOD	AMOUNT	CAL	CARBS	FAT	WALK	RUN	BIKE	SWIM	YOGA	DANCE
Mott's Apple Juice	1 cup	120	29	0	31	13	17	15	41	20
Mott's Apple Punch Juice	1 cup	120	30	0	31	13	17	15	41	20
Mott's Light Apple Juice	1 cup	60	15	0	15	6	9	7	20	10
Mott's Natural Apple Juice	1 cup	110	27	0	28	12	16	13	37	19
Ocean Spray Cran-apple Juice Cocktail	1 cup	130	33	0	34	14	18	16	44	22
Ocean Spray Cranberry Juice Cocktail	1 cup	140	34	0	36	15	20	17	48	24
Ocean Spray Cran-Raspberry Juice Cocktail	1 cup	140	34	0	36	15	20	17	48	24
Ocean Spray Pink Grapefruit Juice	1 cup	110	28	0	28	12	16	13	37	19
Ocean Spray Reduced Calorie Cranberry Juice Cocktail	1 cup	50	13	0	13	5	7	6	17	9
Ocean Spray White Grapefruit Juice	1 cup	100	24	0	26	11	14	12	34	17
POM Wonderful 100% Pomegranate Juice	1 cup	160	40	0	41	17	23	19	54	27
POM Wonderful Pomegranate & Blueberry Juice	1 cup	160	39	0	41	17	23	19	54	27
Red Jacket Apple Cider	1 cup	120	30	0	31	13	17	15	41	20
Red Jacket Cranberry Apple Cider	1 cup	120	30	0	31	13	17	15	41	20
Red Jacket Fuji Apple Cider	1 cup	120	30	0	31	13	17	15	41	20
Red Jacket Purple Apple Juice	1 cup	120	30	0	31	13	17	15	41	20
Red Jacket Raspberry Apple Juice	1 cup	120	30	0	31	13	17	15	41	20
Sambazon Acai Energy with Mango Banana Smoothie	1 cup	200	38	5	52	21	28	24	68	34
Sambazon Acai Energy with Soymilk Smoothie	1 cup	210	25	6	54	22	30	26	71	36
Sambazon Acai Energy with Strawberry Banana Smoothie	1 cup	185	33	4	48	20	26	23	63	32
Tropicana Berry Punch	1 cup	130	32	0	34	14	18	16	44	22
Tropicana Cranberry Cocktail	14 fl oz	240	59	0	62	26	34	29	82	41
Tropicana Cranberry Juice	1 cup	140	34	0	36	15	20	17	48	24
Tropicana Essentials with Fiber	1 cup	120	29	0	31	13	17	15	41	20
Tropicana Fruit Punch	1 cup	130	32	0	34	14	18	16	44	22
Tropicana Golden Grapefruit Juice	1 cup	90	22	0	23	10	13	11	31	15

FOOD	AMOUNT	CAL	CARBS	FAT	WALK	RUN	BIKE	SWIM	YOGA	DANCE
Tropicana Grape Juice	14 fl oz	270	67	0	70	29	38	33	92	46
Tropicana Healthy Heart Orange Juice	1 cup	110	26	0	28	12	16	13	37	19
Tropicana Healthy Kids Orange Juice	1 cup	110	26	0	28	12	16	13	37	19
Tropicana Homestyle Lemonade	14 fl oz	190	49	0	49	20	27	23	65	32
Tropicana Immunity Defense Orange Juice	1 cup	110	26	0	28	12	16	13	37	19
Tropicana Light 'n Healthy Orange Juice	1 cup	50	13	0	13	5	7	6	17	9
Tropicana Low Acid Orange Juice	1 cup	110	26	0	28	12	16	13	37	19
Tropicana Orangeade	1 cup	130	33	0	34	14	18	16	44	22
Tropicana Orchard Berry	1 cup	110	27	0	28	12	16	13	37	19
Tropicana Orchard Style Apple	14 fl oz	200	50	0	52	21	28	24	68	34
Tropicana Orchard Style Lemonade	1 cup	120	31	0	31	13	17	15	41	20
Tropicana Pure Premium Grovestand Orange Juice	1 cup	110	26	0	28	12	16	13	37	19
Tropicana Pure Premium Grovestand Orange Juice with Calcium and Vitamin D	1 cup	110	26	0	28	12	16	13	37	19
Tropicana Pure Premium Homestyle Orange Juice	1 cup	110	26	0	28	12	16	13	37	19
Tropicana Pure Premium Orange Juice	1 cup	110	26	0	28	12	16	13	37	19
Tropicana Pure Premium Orange Juice with Calcium and Vitamin D	1 cup	110	26	0	28	12	16	13	37	19
Tropicana Pure Premium Orange Pineapple Juice with Calcium	1 cup	130	31	0	34	14	18	16	44	22
Tropicana Pure Premium Orange Strawberry Banana Juice with Calcium and Vitamin D	1 cup	130	30	0	34	14	18	16	44	22
Tropicana Pure Premium Orange Tangerine Juice with Calcium	1 cup	110	25	0	28	12	16	13	37	19
Tropicana Pure Tropics Orange Kiwi Passion Juice	1 cup	100	26	0	26	11	14	12	34	17

FOOD	AMOUNT	CAL	CARBS	FAT	WALK	RUN	BIKE	SWIM	YOGA	DANCE
Tropicana Pure Tropics Orange Mango Peach Juice	1 cup	110	27	0	28	12	16	13	37	19
Tropicana Pure Tropics Orange Pineapple Juice	1 cup	120	29	0	31	13	17	15	41	20
Tropicana Pure Tropics Orange Strawberry Banana Juice	1 cup	110	27	0	28	12	16	13	37	19
Tropicana Ruby Red Grapefruit Juice	1 cup	90	22	0	23	10	13	11	31	15
Tropicana Sweet Grapefruit Juice	1 cup	130	31	0	34	14	18	16	44	22
Juice Boxes/Pouches										
Capri-Sun Fruit Punch Juice Drink	1 pouch (6.75 oz)	100	26	0	26	11	14	12	34	17
Capri-Sun Red Berry Juice Drink	1 pouch (6.75 oz)	100	25	0	26	11	14	12	34	17
Capri-Sun Wild Cherry Juice Drink	1 pouch (6.75 oz)	110	30	0	28	12	16	13	37	19
Capri-Sun Strawberry Cooler Juice Drink	1 pouch (6.75 oz)	90	25	0	23	10	13	11	31	15
Apple & Eve Apple Juice Box	1 box (8.45 oz)	110	26	0	28	12	16	13	37	19
Apple & Eve Elmo Punch Juice Box	1 box (4.23 oz)	60	15	0	15	6	9	7	20	10
V8 cans	1 can (5.5 oz)	35	7	0	9	4	5	4	12	6

FOOD	AMOUNT	CAL	CARBS	ALC. (G)	WALK	RUN	BIKE	SWIM	YOGA	DANCE

Alcoholic Beverages

Beer										
Regular beer	12 fl oz	153	13	14	39	16	22	19	52	26
Light beer	12 fl oz	103	6	11	27	11	15	13	35	18
Budweiser	12 fl oz	145	11	14	37	15	21	18	49	25
Bud Light	12 fl oz	110	7	12	28	12	16	13	37	19
Busch	12 fl oz	133	10	13	34	14	19	16	45	23
Busch Light	12 fl oz	95	3	12	24	10	13	12	32	16
Coors	12 fl oz	142	11	14	37	15	20	17	48	24
Coors Light	12 fl oz	102	5	12	26	11	14	12	35	17
Michelob Ultra Light	12 fl oz	95	3	12	24	10	13	12	32	16
Miller Genuine Draft	12 fl oz	143	13	14	37	15	20	17	49	24
Miller Lite	12 fl oz	96	3	13	25	10	14	12	33	16
Sierra Nevada Pale Ale	12 fl oz	200	12	16	52	21	28	24	68	34
Sierra Nevada Porter	12 fl oz	195	16	16	50	21	28	24	66	33
Sierra Nevada Wheat	12 fl oz	160	0	12	41	17	23	19	54	27
Mixed Drinks										
Daiquiri	8 fl oz	449	17	56	116	48	64	55	153	76
Martini	4 fl oz	274	2	38	71	29	39	33	93	47
Piña colada (also has 5 grams of fat)	8 fl oz	437	57	25	113	47	62	53	149	74
Whiskey sour	4 fl oz	193	19	17	50	21	27	23	66	33
Screwdriver	5.5 fl oz	160	14	14	41	17	23	19	54	27
Bloody Mary	8 fl oz	95	16	10	24	10	13	12	32	16
Jose Cuervo Margarita Mixer	4 fl oz	100	24	0	26	11	14	12	34	17
Margaritaville Margarita Mixer	4 fl oz	110	27	0	28	12	16	13	37	19
Bacardi Piña Colada Mixer	2.7 fl oz	140	38	0	36	15	20	17	48	24
Bacardi Strawberry Daiquiri Mixer	2.7 fl oz	140	40	0	36	15	20	17	48	24
Bacardi Margarita Mixer (10% frozen juice concentrate)	8 fl oz	90	25	0	23	10	13	11	31	15
Whiskey Sour mix	2 fl oz	57	14	0	15	6	8	7	19	10
Bloody Mary mix	8 fl oz	56	12	0	14	6	8	7	19	9

FOOD	AMOUNT	CAL	CARBS	ALC. (G)	WALK	RUN	BIKE	SWIM	YOGA	DANCE
Frozen nonalcoholic cocktail mix	2 oz	207	52	0	53	22	29	25	70	35
Lager										
Samuel Adams Lager	12 fl oz	180	19	13	46	19	26	22	61	31
Liquor										
Crème de Menthe	1.5 fl oz	187	21	15	48	20	27	23	64	32
Gin (90 proof)	1.5 fl oz	110	0	16	28	12	16	13	37	19
Rum (80 proof)	1.5 fl oz	97	0	14	25	10	14	12	33	17
Vodka (80 proof)	1.5 fl oz	97	0	14	25	10	14	12	33	17
Whiskey (86 proof)	1.5 fl oz	105	0	15	27	11	15	13	36	18
Coffee liqueur (53 proof)	1.5 fl oz	135	9	17	35	14	19	16	46	23
Cognac	1.5 fl oz	105	3	17	27	11	15	13	36	18
Kahlua	1.5 fl oz	135	9	17	35	14	19	16	46	23
Wine										
■ Cooking Wine										
Cooking wine	1 fl oz	14	2	1	4	1	2	2	5	2
Cooking sherry	1 fl oz	40	4	2	10	4	6	5	14	7
■ Dessert Wine										
Dry dessert wine	4 fl oz	179	14	18	46	19	25	22	61	30
Sweet dessert wine	4 fl oz	189	16	18	49	20	27	23	64	32
■ Table Wine										
Table wine	4 fl oz	99	3	12	26	11	14	12	34	17
Light wine	4 fl oz	59	1	8	15	6	8	7	20	10
■ Red Wine										
Red wine	4 fl oz	100	3	13	26	11	14	12	34	17
Barbera	4 fl oz	101	328	13	26	11	14	12	34	17
Burgundy	4 fl oz	103	4	12	27	11	15	13	35	18
Cabernet Franc	4 fl oz	99	3	12	26	11	14	12	34	17
Cabernet Sauvignon	4 fl oz	97	3	12	25	10	14	12	33	17
Carignane	4 fl oz	89	3	11	23	9	13	11	30	15
Claret	4 fl oz	99	4	12	26	11	14	12	34	17
Gamay	4 fl oz	93	3	12	24	10	13	11	32	16
Lemberger	4 fl oz	96	3	12	25	10	14	12	33	16
Merlot	4 fl oz	99	3	13	26	11	14	12	34	17
Mourvèdre	4 fl oz	105	3	13	27	11	15	13	36	18
Petite Syrah	4 fl oz	101	3	13	26	11	14	12	34	17

FOOD	AMOUNT	CAL	CARBS	ALC. (G)	WALK	RUN	BIKE	SWIM	YOGA	DANCE
Pinot Noir	4 fl oz	98	3	12	25	10	14	12	33	17
Sangiovese	4 fl oz	102	3	13	26	11	14	12	35	17
Syrah	4 fl oz	99	3	12	26	11	14	12	34	17
Red Zinfandel	4 fl oz	105	3	13	27	11	15	13	36	18
■ **White Wine**										
White wine	4 fl oz	98	3	12	25	10	14	12	33	17
Chenin Blanc	4 fl oz	96	4	11	25	10	14	12	33	16
Fume Blanc	4 fl oz	87	3	12	22	9	12	11	30	15
Gewurztraminer	4 fl oz	97	3	12	25	10	14	12	33	17
Muller Thurgau	4 fl oz	91	4	11	23	10	13	11	31	16
Muscat	4 fl oz	100	6	11	26	11	14	12	34	17
Pinot Blanc	4 fl oz	96	2	12	25	10	14	12	33	16
Pinot Grigio	4 fl oz	98	2	13	25	10	14	12	33	17
Riesling	4 fl oz	96	4	11	25	10	14	12	33	16
Sauvignon Blanc	4 fl oz	96	2	12	25	10	14	12	33	16
Semillon	4 fl oz	98	4	12	25	10	14	12	33	17
Other Beverages										
Malt beverage	1 cup	88	19	1	23	9	12	11	30	15
Nonalcoholic wine	8 fl oz	14	3	0	4	1	2	2	5	2
Sake	4 fl oz	125	5	15	32	13	18	15	43	21

References

Walk 231 calories burned per hour / 3.85 calories per minute
3.0 mph, level, moderate pace, firm surface / 3.3 METS

Run 564 calories burned per hour / 9.4 calories per minute
5.0 mph (12 min/mile) / 8 METS

Bike 423 calories burned per hour / 7.05 calories per minute
Bicycling, 10–11.9 mph, leisurely, slow, light effort / 6 METS

Swim 490 calories burned per hour / 8.17 calories per minute
Swimming laps, freestyle, slow, moderate or light effort / 7 METS

Yoga 175 calories burned per hour / 2.92 calories per minute
Hatha yoga / 2.5 METS

Dance 352 calories burned per hour / 5.88 calories per minute
Dancing / 5 METS

Based on 155-pound person; the greater the weight of the individual the more calories burned per hour.

Ainsworth BE, Haskell WL, Leon AS, Jacobs DR Jr., Montoye HJ, Sallis JF, Paffenbarger RS Jr. Compendium of physical activities: Classification of energy costs of human physical activities. *Medicine and Science in Sports and Exercise*, 1993; 25:71–80.

Ainsworth BE, Haskell WL, Whitt MC, Irwin ML, Swartz AM, Strath SJ, O'Brien WL, Bassett DR Jr., Schmitz KH, Emplaincourt PO, Jacobs DR Jr., Leon AS. Compendium of physical activities: An update of activity codes and MET intensities. *Medicine and Science in Sports and Exercise*, 2000; 32 (Suppl):S498–S516.

Acknowledgments

This book has been a longtime passion and I have many people to thank for helping me finally bring it to fruition.

I would like to thank Shira Isenberg, R.D., for her dedication and her unyielding commitment to help get this book in working order. She is just amazing. Next, I would like to thank my literary agent, Farley Chase, for believing in the idea from the start and pushing to make this book a reality.

Nancy Hancock, who has been a passionate advocate in getting this book produced, a great editor, and a smart marketer.

Alan Barnett and Alicia Fox for helping to design information so that readers see what is meant to be seen.

About the Author

Charles Stuart Platkin JD, MPH, is one of the country's leading nutrition and public health advocates, whose syndicated nutrition and fitness column appears in more than 165 daily newspapers nationally, including *The Miami Herald, The Buffalo News, The Honolulu Advertiser, Rochester Democrat and Chronicle, The State, The Fort Worth Star Telegraph, Omaha World Herald,* and *Richmond Times-Dispatch.* He is the founder and director of The Institute for Nutrition & Behavioral Sciences, a non-profit organization that conducts obesity-related research and designs public health programs.

Platkin has been quoted as a weight loss/nutrition expert in numerous publications, including *USA Today,* the *Los Angeles Times,* the *Chicago Tribune, Time, Newsweek, Ladies Home Journal, Men's Health, Shape,* and *Fitness.* He has also appeared on NBC's *The Today Show,* CNN, CNBC, CBS's *The Early Show,* the BBC, and others. He is a member of the American Society for Nutritional Sciences, the American Obesity Association, the North American Association for the Study of Obesity, American Public Health Association, Society for Public Health Educators, and the American Council on Exercise. He received his undergraduate degree from Cornell University, a law degree from Fordham University, and a Masters in Public Health from Florida International University. He is also a certified personal trainer and is currently pursuing his PhD in public health (2007).

Platkin is also the founder of Integrated Wellness Solutions, which designs health interventions combining behavioral print marketing and a sophisticated online software program that integrates the latest scientific and behavioral nutrition research. The program is used by insurance companies, pharmaceutical companies, and other large corporations.